Interprofessional Evidence-Based Practice

A Workbook for Health Professionals

Interprofessional Evidence-Based Practice

A Workbook for Health Professionals

Penelope A. Moyers, EdD, OT/L, FAOTA
Professor
Dean of the Henrietta Schmoll School of Health
St. Catherine University
St. Paul, Minnesota

Patricia L. Finch-Guthrie, PhD, RN
Assistant Professor
Coordinator of Interprofessional Education, Research, and Practice
Henrietta Schmoll School of Health
St. Catherine University
St. Paul, Minnesota

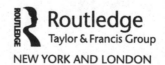

Routledge
Taylor & Francis Group

NEW YORK AND LONDON

First published 2016 by SLACK Incorporated

Published 2024 by Routledge
605 Third Avenue, New York, NY 10158

and by Routledge
4 Park Square, Milton Park, Abingdon, Oxon, OX14 4RN

Routledge is an imprint of the Taylor & Francis Group, an informa business.

Library of Congress Cataloging-in-Publication Data

Names: Moyers, Penelope, author. | Finch-Guthrie, Patricia L., - , author.
Title: Interprofessional evidence-based practice : a workbook for health
  professionals / Penelope A. Moyers, Patricia L. Finch-Guthrie.
Description: Thorofare, NJ : SLACK Incorporated, [2016] | Includes
  bibliographical references and index.
Identifiers: LCCN 2016005710 (print) | ISBN 9781630910983 (alk. paper)
Subjects: | MESH: Interprofessional Relations | Evidence-Based
  Practice--organization & administration | Planning Techniques | Health
  Personnel | Mentors | Program Development
Classification: LCC R834.5 (print) | NLM W 62 | DDC
  610.76--dc23
LC record available at http://lccn.loc.gov/2016005710

ISBN: 9781630910983 (pbk)
ISBN: 9781003524632 (ebk)

DOI: 10.4324/9781003524632

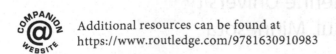 Additional resources can be found at
https://www.routledge.com/9781630910983

DEDICATION

We lovingly dedicate this book to our husbands; to Dock Franklin Cleveland for his thoughtfulness and generosity; and in memory of William Elmus Guthrie, who supports us every day in spirit.

DEDICATION

Contents

ACKNOWLEDGMENTS

We owe our gratitude to the faculty and students at St. Catherine University in the Henrietta Schmoll School of Health who gave their time to participate in the Interprofessional Evidence-Based Practice Program. Our Minnesota partners, Abbott Northwestern Hospital in Minneapolis and North Memorial Medical Center in Robbinsdale, were critical to the success of this project over the last three years. The nursing staff members from both of these health care organizations who participated as mentors and clinical scholars were incredible. We want to pay particular recognition to Janet Benz and Sue Sendelbach for their thoughtful work to ensure the success of the Abbott Evidence-Based Practice Fellows Program and the way in which this program helped us further develop our ideas for this book. John Fleming, Leah Johnson, and Jennie Strickland were invaluable in contributing extra time to make this book come to fruition. We would also like to give special acknowledgment to Alice Swan, professor emeritus from St. Catherine University, who worked with us in the North Memorial Clinical Scholar Program.

ABOUT THE AUTHORS

Penelope A. Moyers, EdD, OT/L, FAOTA, more often called "Penny," is the Dean of the Henrietta Schmoll School of Health and the Graduate College at St. Catherine University in St. Paul, Minnesota, and is a Professor of Occupational Therapy. The School of Health has over 35 programs in a variety of health professions and has provided Dr. Moyers an opportunity to observe how different professions learn and work together. She was the Department Chair for Occupational Therapy at the University of Alabama at Birmingham and was a Dean of the School of Occupational Therapy at the University of Indianapolis in Indiana. Penny is a Fellow and a past president of the American Occupational Therapy Association (AOTA), received the association's Award of Merit, and is board certified by AOTA in Mental Health.

Penny received her BS degree in occupational therapy from the University of Missouri in Columbia and has over 30 years of experience in the field. She went on to the University of Louisville in Kentucky, where she received an MS degree in community development. Her EdD is from Ball State University, Muncie, Indiana, in adult education. Her clinical expertise is in the areas of mental health, substance use disorders, HIV/AIDS, and upper extremity rehabilitation. She has published extensively on the occupational therapy interventions for persons with substance use disorders and those with co-occurring disorders. She also has expertise in the continuing competence of health care professionals and has authored many articles and book chapters on this topic.

In her role as Dean at St. Catherine University, she co-founded the Interprofessional Clinical Scholar Program with North Memorial Medical Center in Robbinsdale, Minnesota and then was invited to work with Abbott Northwestern Hospital, Minneapolis, Minnesota in their existing Evidence-Based Practice Fellows Program. Her desire was to bring groups of faculty, students, and staff together from multiple disciplines to solve problems in practice in a manner that places the patient and family at the center while considering the talents, expertise, and knowledge of professionals from multiple health care professions.

Patricia L. Finch-Guthrie, PhD, RN is the Director of Interprofessional Education, Practice and Research in the Henrietta Schmoll School of Health and is Assistant Professor in the Department of Nutrition and Exercise Science at St. Catherine University. In her role, Patricia has developed and taught interprofessional courses for baccalaureate students from multiple disciplines on teamwork, team roles and responsibilities, health care teams and quality, and research and evidence-based practice. Patricia has practiced as a Clinical Nurse Specialist in Gerontology and served as the Director of Education and Nursing Research at North Memorial Medical Center in Robbinsdale, Minnesota, overseeing many interprofessional evidence-based practice initiatives. Patricia co-founded the Interprofessional Clinical Scholar Program at North Memorial Medical Center and is now working with Abbott Northwestern Hospital in Minneapolis, Minnesota as part of their Evidence-Based Practice Fellows Program, bringing an interprofessional focus to the program.

Patricia received her BSN from the University of Iowa in Iowa City, a MS degree in nursing from the University of Minnesota in Minneapolis as a Clinical Nurse Specialist, and a PhD in nursing with a minor in gerontology from the University of Minnesota. Patricia has practiced as a bedside nurse in acute care for 14 years and in nursing administration for 21 years, with clinical and practice expertise in cardiovascular nursing care, the acute care of older adults, and advanced nursing practice. Patricia has published about the care of older adults regarding assessment, care planning, prevention of delirium, and decreasing pressure ulcer rates in critical care, and has served as a dissertation chair for PhD nursing students and as an advisor for master's level nursing projects as an educator.

Contributing Authors

Janet Benz, DNP, RN (Chapter 4)
Assistant Professor
Interprofessional Education
Henrietta Schmoll School of Health
St. Catherine University
St. Paul, Minnesota

Mark Blegen, PhD, FACSM (Chapter 13)
Associate Dean, Henrietta Schmoll School of Health
Associate Professor and Chair, Department of Nutrition
    and Exercise Sciences
St. Catherine University
St. Paul, Minnesota

David D. Chapman, PhD, PT/L (Chapters 10, 11)
Associate Professor
Doctor of Physical Therapy Program
Henrietta Schmoll School of Health
St. Catherine University
St. Paul, Minnesota

Therese Whalen Dlugosch, MA, OTR/L (Chapter 5)
Occupational Therapist
Hennepin County Medical Center
Minneapolis, Minnesota

John D. Fleming, EdD, OTR/L (Chapters 7, 8)
Assistant Professor
Occupational Therapy and Occupational Science
    Department
Henrietta Schmoll School of Health
St. Catherine University
St. Paul, Minnesota

Susan M. Hageness, DNP, RN, AHN-BC, CNE (Chapter 15)
Associate Professor
Department of Nursing; Department of Holistic Health
    Studies
Henrietta Schmoll School of Health
St. Catherine University
St. Paul, Minnesota

Vicky J. Larson, PhD, RN, CNE (Chapters 10, 11)
Assistant Professor
Department of Nursing
Henrietta Schmoll School of Health
St. Catherine University
St. Paul, Minnesota

VaLinda I. Pearson, PhD, RN, CRRN (Chapter 9)
Professor
Department of Nursing
Henrietta Schmoll School of Health
St. Catherine University
St. Paul, Minnesota

*Sue E. Sendelbach, PhD, APRN CNS, FAHA, FAAN
    (Chapter 6)*
Director of Nursing Research
Abbott Northwestern Hospital
Minneapolis, Minnesota

FOREWORD

The pace of change in health care continues to intensify. The healthcare problems encountered are increasingly complex as are the patients cared for who have multiple co-morbidities and chronic conditions. Concomitantly, expectations by consumers and regulatory and payment organizations to deliver optimal care and achieve optimal outcomes have never been higher.

In order to meet these challenges and expectations, it is essential that all information and evidence available are used in order to maximize outcomes while simultaneously decreasing waste and inefficiencies. There is an exponentially increasing amount of evidence being published and disseminated; yet, there remain significant gaps in strong evidence available for the pertinent and immediate questions faced every day in caring for patients. With this surge in evidence comes additional questions: How are sound decisions made when the evidence is unclear, contradictory, or nonexistent? How does one health care discipline stay on top of all the information that is being published? How does one health care discipline know all areas of evidence that directly impact the care they give? How does one discipline know how the care they provide impacts other disciplines and patient issues?

It is imperative that health care providers from all disciplines understand evidence-based practice, know how to interpret evidence, and know when problems are multidisciplinary in nature and therefore need to be addressed by all impacted stakeholders. It is necessary to share a common EBP language and understanding, a common approach regarding EBP, and a shared commitment to care for patients using the best evidence.

This book is a resource to establishing that common understanding and shared commitment through an interprofessional EBP program—forming teams, discussion of roles and communication skills, understanding basic EBP principles and a common EBP language, implementation of the evidence, and, finally, disseminating the outcomes and learnings of EBP projects.

The act of simply providing care by any single discipline can be challenging in today's environment. Evaluating and implementing evidence by interprofessional teams can take more time. However, health care providers can no longer afford to continue to work in silos. Yes, there are needs and opportunities that are specific and related to the work of a single discipline, but increasingly it is through interprofessional collaboration and care improvements that solutions will be found and implemented to address today's thorny patient care issues and ongoing challenges. This book is a valuable resource in developing the foundation to promote that interprofessional evidence-based practice.

Mary Fran Tracy, PhD, RN, APRN, CNS, FAAN
Critical Care Clinical Nurse Specialist
University of Minnesota Medical Center
Minneapolis, Minnesota

INTRODUCTION

The purpose of this book is to share our experience and expertise in designing and implementing an interprofessional evidence-based practice (EBP) program that involves a strong partnership between a health care organization and a university. The premise of this book is that EBP is more effective when conducted in interprofessional teams whose members are charged to bring multiple perspectives to bear upon vexing practice problems. It is not the intent of this book to advocate that an interprofessional EBP program is the primary or only way to address EBP and knowledge translation within a health care organization. Instead, the program is an adjunct to the other approaches in knowledge translation that simultaneously occurs within the health care organization and augments the other ways health professions educators teach evidence-based practice to their students.

Interprofessional EBP is challenging given that disciplines vary in the extent of their education in EBP and in the EBP models they use. These two factors contribute to the differences among disciplines in the ways EBP patient and population health questions are asked and in the ways evidence is defined, appraised, synthesized, and applied. Consequently, not all patient questions are amenable to an interprofessional EBP approach; however, given the shift to population-based health care, interprofessional EBP is becoming more the norm compared to EBP focused on a single discipline. Complex health questions are best addressed through an interprofessional EBP team in which a variety of perspectives examine the issue from a broader and more holistic perspective. Interprofessional EBP is defined as a dynamic team process that blends the patient's preferences and values, the expertise of practitioners from multiple disciplines, and multidisciplinary evidence to implement practice changes that challenge current disciplinary paradigms and biases to create an integrated approach to patient care, health care delivery, or population health. When deciding to engage in interprofessional EBP practice, this book helps describe the key decisions the team members must make as they go through the steps to address an important patient-centered or population health question. As universities add interprofessional education to their curricula, this book may be useful to courses that bring students from multiple disciplines together to engage in research and EBP.

The contributors to this book represent the disciplines of nursing, occupational and physical therapy, and exercise science from St. Catherine University in St. Paul, Minnesota, and the perspectives from two health care partners, North Memorial Medical Center in Robbinsdale, Minnesota, and Abbott Northwestern Hospital in Minneapolis, Minnesota. We demonstrate our excitement and belief in interprofessional collaboration and EBP as the interprofessional teams involved in this work have included other disciplines as well, such as physician assistants, respiratory care, holistic health, sonography, and library and information science. Physicians, pharmacists, social workers, and informaticists have provided consultations to the interprofessional teams along with many other university departmental and hospital leaders. The goal of the book is to encourage the development of effective interprofessional teams of evidence-based practitioners dedicated to improving the care and health of patients and the patient experience with the health care delivery system.

The bench strength of the team is enhanced as a result of partners combining resources to bring together staff from the health care organization and faculty and students from the university. Universities bring value to their health care partners when they engage in shared work that reduces the research-practice gap that currently exists. Health care organizations provide opportunities through a shared interprofessional EBP program for real-life learning experiences for students, as well as occasions for faculty and team scholarship. This book helps teams not only develop skills in interprofessional EBP, but also in implementation science so that a practice change will more likely occur.

Teamwork and communication are central to strong team performance in interprofessional EBP. Because teamwork is fundamental to an interprofessional EBP program, this book emphasizes team strategies and supports necessary strategies to sustain partnerships and for successful completion of each phase in the interprofessional EBP process. The interprofessional education and collaborative practice literature guides the understanding of how the teams should function in order to conduct a successful interprofessional EBP project from start to finish.

Why This Book?

The reader is assisted in making the determination of whether an interprofessional EBP program would be an advantage to a health care organization that has identified increasing EBP as a goal and whether partnering with a university would be advantageous in reaching such a goal. Take a moment to reflect on the importance of providing learning opportunities in interprofessional EBP as a way to prepare current and future practitioners. It is crucial to foster understanding of not only how to garner evidence leading to change, but also how to use implementation science to ensure a practice change is feasible, sustainable, and leads to improvements in patient outcomes. If you answer yes to any of the following questions, this book will guide you through the process of creating a successful interprofessional EBP program through organizational partnering.

Health Care Organizations

▶ Are you planning to start an interprofessional EBP program in your health care organization that prepares teams to conduct interprofessional EBP as part of their practice?

▶ Do your clinicians and practitioners need information about the steps in conducting interprofessional EBP?

▶ Do you have few EBP mentors or other key resources needed to run an interprofessional EBP program?

▶ Do you want to know how to partner with a university that has expertise in interprofessional EBP to augment your current organizational resources?

▶ Are you interested in expanding an existing EBP program to include more disciplines?

▶ Have you launched an interprofessional EBP program and found it difficult to achieve success in changing practice?

Universities

▶ Is your university interested in collaborating with interprofessional EBP teams in health care organizations?

▶ Do you want to explore with your existing clinical partners how to foster interprofessional EBP teams?

▶ Is your university looking for effective ways to provide interprofessional education to students that develops team competencies, preparing them for interprofessional practice?

▶ Are the faculty members of the university searching for opportunities for students to engage in practice change?

▶ Are the faculty members looking for opportunities to engage in scholarship with practitioners within an interprofessional team?

How Do Partners, Program Coordinators, and Teams Use the Book?

The book is divided into three major sections. Section I, Preparation for an Interprofessional Evidence-Based Practice Program, provides a basis for interprofessional EBP program development. Chapter 1 lays the foundation for an interprofessional EBP program through discussion of terminology, underlying theories, the roles of participants in the program, essential program elements, and key milestones for program completion. Chapter 2 focuses on how to develop a partnership between a health care organization and a university that facilitates the quality of team member efforts, as well as prepares the two organizations for engaging in interprofessional EBP. In Chapter 3, a theory of how program coordinators mentor interprofessional EBP mentors and how program coordinators and mentors work with teams is described. Mentoring is a key component of the interprofessional EBP program regardless of the skill levels of team members in EBP. Implementation of a practice change and enhancing its sustainability is a complicated process that fortunately can be facilitated with mentors who are experienced in EBP, implementation science, and interprofessional practice. Based on qualitative research of interprofessional EBP programs, this mentoring theory offers a new perspective on mentorship about mentor challenges and the mentor techniques and supports important for enhancing interprofessional EBP within a team context.

In describing well-known teamwork principles, Chapter 4 describes how to form an interprofessional EBP team and how to determine the roles of team members. Chapter 5 describes effective methods of communicating that lead to highly effective team performance. Poor communication is often the reason for ineffective teams and team conflict, as well as impacts practice change implementation and sustainability. Discussion of communication in teams sounds like commonsense principles; however, the fact remains that many teams do not implement needed communication strategies in a consistent, timely, and effective way. Communication is doubly important when adding teams with members used to operating within two different cultures, with each organization having its own language, hidden rules and standards, and traditions. Students on these teams may also perceive themselves as having a lower level of status and power, which actually may be the same experience that occurs among the disciplines. Power and status discrepancies affect communication and determine who might lead the team, rather than the team selecting leadership based upon who would be the most effective person to lead the team.

Chapters 6 through 9 in Section II (Immersion Into the Evidence) and Chapters 10 through 15 in Section III (Completion and Dissemination of the Interprofessional Evidence-Based Project) each focus on one phase of the interprofessional EBP or implementation process. The chapters are designed in a similar manner so that the learner understands the why, or the rationale for the phase; the what, or the essential focus of the interprofessional EBP practice phase; the how, or the steps and sequence of work in the phase; and the with what, or the resources and tools that can be used for the phase. Chapter 6 addresses the logistics of implementing an interprofessional EBP program and provides an effective approach to orient mentors and the interprofessional team to the program. Chapters 7 through 13 focus on the details of each interprofessional EBP phase. For those readers who may have knowledge of EBP, this book covers implications and crucial decisions for interprofessional EBP, which are quite different than carrying out EBP in a single discipline. In addition, the book provides helpful information about work tasks that are often more difficult to accomplish, such as conducting effectiveness research or a practice change pilot as part of implementing an EBP project, navigating the institutional review board process for safe and ethical conduct of research, writing a grant, and designing an evaluation of a practice change. In addition, each chapter discusses common issues and challenges teams and mentors may need to resolve during the interprofessional EBP phase.

Potential interprofessional EBP mentors have access to helpful techniques and supports to ensure the success of their teams as they engage in complicated but enjoyable work. The chapters include practical information borne out of experience combined with information from the literature that assists with anticipating and better preparing teams for doing the work of interprofessional EBP. Each chapter has accompanying resources offered on the website as a companion to this book, such as PowerPoint slides to support team education, forms and tools to guide the work of the team, and 1-minute updates to support the development of mentors. Appendix A lists these resources for each chapter that are housed on the book's accompanying website.

In the final two chapters (14 and 15) of the book in Section III, the EBP interprofessional team is guided through the strategies for disseminating the work to the organization, grant funders, and other professional audiences through reports, publications, and presentations. Chapter 14 takes a project management approach to help the team ensure completion of all the work of the team, the stakeholders are informed, and reports are delivered to program sponsors and grant funders. The purpose of Chapter 14 is to hold team members accountable for all the project completion and practice change sustainability tasks before the members are tempted to disperse. The need to recognize and celebrate the accomplishments of the team is highly critical in order for team members and partners in both organizations to end the experience with a high level of satisfaction. Ways in which to sustain over time the interprofessional EBP program is discussed as well. In Chapter 15, the team learns how to develop and implement a dissemination plan and to obtain resources needed for dissemination and knowledge translation. The chapter outlines the strategies for publication and presentation.

This work represents our efforts in designing and implementing interprofessional EBP programs over the last four years. We hope you will find our experience helpful in creating your own partnerships to design your own program. We believe you will benefit from challenges we have faced and have subsequently learned how to address. We wish you the best and encourage you to share your experience as we continue to modify and refine this work.

Penelope A. Moyers EdD, OT/L, FAOTA
Patricia L. Finch-Guthrie, PhD, RN

Section I

- **Preparation for an Interprofessional Evidence-Based Practice Program** — Section I

- **Immersion Into the Evidence** — Section II

- **Completion and Dissemination of the Interprofessional Evidence-Based Project** — Section III

Chapter 1	Getting Started	What is an interprofessional evidence-based practice program?
Chapter 2	Establishing Partnerships and Organizational Readiness	Who are the right partners to start an interprofessional evidence-based practice program?
Chapter 3	Developing Deliberative and Reflective Mentoring	How do you develop mentors for an interprofessional evidence-based practice program?
Chapter 4	Forming Interprofessional Teams and Clarifying Roles	How do you develop the interprofessional skills of evidence-based practice teams?
Chapter 5	Facilitating Effective Interprofessional Team Communication	How do you promote effective team communication for evidence-based practice?

1

Getting Started

Penelope A. Moyers, EdD, OT/L, FAOTA

CHAPTER TOPICS

- What is interprofessional evidence-based practice?
- Why is an interprofessional evidence-based practice team important?
- Why is interprofessional evidence-based practice challenging?
- What skills are needed for interprofessional evidence-based practice?
- How does an interprofessional evidence-based practice team use evidence to implement a practice change?
- What is an interprofessional evidence-based practice program?
- What are the theoretical underpinnings of an interprofessional evidence-based practice program?
- What are the essential elements of the interprofessional evidence-based practice program?
- How is an interprofessional evidence-based practice program evaluated?

PERFORMANCE OBJECTIVES

At the conclusion of this chapter, mentors and program coordinators will understand interprofessional evidence-based practice and be able to:

1. Use the overall process of interprofessional evidence-based practice to develop important patient change projects with deadlines for project milestones.

2. Determine the scope of the program and the resources needed to design the interprofessional evidence-based practice program.

3. Select outcome measurement tools to evaluate the interprofessional evidence-based practice program.

Moyers, P. A., & Finch-Guthrie, P. L.
*Interprofessional Evidence-Based Practice:
A Workbook for Health Professionals* (pp 3-22).
© 2016 Taylor and Francis Group.

This book describes an interprofessional evidence-based practice (EBP) program, sometimes referred to as a *clinical scholar program* or a *fellows program*. An interprofessional EBP program addresses important clinical questions arising from the work of staff from multiple disciplines in a health care organization. Such a program is designed to complement all of the other approaches the health care organization uses to address EBP and translate knowledge into practice. An interprofessional EBP program is not meant to function as a singular solution to maximizing EBP within a health care organization but is one of several important approaches. Unlike some EBP clinical scholar programs in which staff members each work on projects individually, the interprofessional EBP program's objective is to bring together persons from multiple professions to work in teams under the guidance of a mentor in order to focus on a clinical question of importance. The program promotes active learning of an interprofessional EBP process while answering a clinical question along with improvement in patient outcomes and experience, care process efficiency, effectiveness, and safety. Working in teams facilitates collaborative or interprofessional practice (IPP) to support patient-centered, holistic care.

Another distinctive aspect of this book is the discussion of how the program sponsors develop and foster collaboration between a university and a health care organization such that students and faculty participate on these interprofessional teams along with staff from the health care organization. Faculty and students bring a variety of skills and resources to the team; however, to equalize all roles, especially when teams have members from two separate organizations and have members with differing levels of perceived power, it is necessary to continually promote the motto for each team that everyone teaches, learns, and works to complete assigned tasks. This emphasis upon how all team members approach the interprofessional EBP project together is consistent with the definition of interprofessional education (IPE), which occurs when "two or more professions learn about, from, and with each other to enable effective collaboration and improve health outcomes" (World Health Organization [WHO], 2010, p. 13).

This book incorporates various points of view, including those who want to coordinate an interprofessional EBP program, who want to become an experienced mentor, or who want to be on an interprofessional EBP team. Therefore, not only does the design of this book acquaint an interprofessional team with the interprofessional EBP process, but it also addresses the communication and cross-organizational factors important for supporting the work of the team. For instance, this book clearly articulates common mentoring issues and challenges encountered in interprofessional EBP along with the iterative problem-solving approaches necessary to mitigate these temporary concerns. The book's website includes PowerPoint lectures and other resources to guide team learning about key interprofessional EBP topics, as well as to support the program coordinators and team mentors in their work with the interprofessional teams. The book includes a step-by-step process, thereby allowing teams to work in a systematic fashion according to plan.

WHAT IS INTERPROFESSIONAL EVIDENCE-BASED PRACTICE?

EBP is a broadening of the term *evidence-based medicine* (EBM). The Evidence-Based Medicine Working Group (1992) described EBM as a new paradigm involving a rational process for clinical decision making. The idea of EBM is for practitioners and clinicians to discern the best research findings and to incorporate these innovations into practice. Sackett, Rosenberg, Gray, Haynes, and Richardson (1996) added that the preferences of the patient are a necessary aspect of clinical decision making in addition to using research evidence and clinical expertise.

All health care disciplines have a body of theory and research; however, some fields, such as medicine, have a longer and deeper history of conducting randomized controlled trials (RCTs) to determine the efficacy of interventions. In some disciplines, RCTs are not always the best method for investigating the more applied aspects of the practice; and researchers may as a result use a broader array of research methodologies including qualitative research. Nursing, social work, and occupational and physical therapy are examples of disciplines with a rich body of qualitative research. Research in a field occurs at varying levels of design rigor and quality; but regardless, research forms an important foundation for EBP.

A field with an extensive body of research may have an advantage in engaging in EBP compared to disciplines with less research. Some fields have fewer researchers and have less government and foundation funding directed to answering practice questions relevant to the discipline. These disciplines may be more reliant on other types of evidence, such as organizational quality improvement and expert opinion. It is consequently important for all practitioners and clinicians to access research from a wide variety of relevant disciplines where there may be applicable research evidence for a particular patient or population health question. The practitioner or clinician can then combine this related research with other types of evidence within specific disciplines.

Regardless of an exponentially growing body of health care and population health research, the developers of EBM were concerned that a physician's experience or the seeking of expert opinion often overly influenced the selection of interventions. Prior to the advent of EBM, research utilization was a common topic in many professions, but seemed the most developed in nursing (Stetler, 2010). Research utilization, however, did not describe how to include patient

TABLE 1-1		
DEVELOPMENT OF EVIDENCE-BASED PRACTICE		
EVIDENCE-BASED MEDICINE	**EVIDENCE-BASED NURSING**	**EVIDENCE-BASED THERAPY**
• **1992:** Evidence-Based Medicine Working Group. (1992). Evidence-based medicine: A new approach in teaching the practice of medicine. *Journal of the American Medical Association, 268*, 2420-2425. • **1996:** Sackett, D. L., Rosenberg, W. M., Gray, J. A., Haynes, R. B., & Richardson, W. S. (1996). Evidence based medicine: What it is and what it isn't. *British Medical Journal, 312*, 71-72.	• **1998:** Flemming, K. (1998). Asking answerable questions. *Evidence Based Nursing 1*, 36-37. • **1999:** French, P. (1999). The development of EBN. *Journal of Advanced Nursing 29*, 72-78.	• **1997:** Occupational Therapy: Taylor, M. C. (1997). What is evidence-based practice? *British Journal of Occupational Therapy, 60*, 470-473. • **1998:** Physical Therapy: Clemence, M. L. (1998). Evidence-based physiotherapy: Seeking the unattainable? *British Journal of Therapy Rehabilitation 5*, 257-260

preference and clinical judgment in combination with the research findings. In addition, research utilization is really a subset of EBP because it only includes research as evidence and does not include evidence drawn from quality improvement and expert consensus panels.

As can be seen in Table 1-1, EBP began developing simultaneously in multiple disciplines and has since rapidly evolved. Dijkers, Murphy, and Krellman (2012) provided an overview of the current approaches to EBP in rehabilitation and the way the American Occupational Therapy Association (AOTA) and the American Physical Therapy Association (APTA) have both instituted resources to assist practitioners. For example, AOTA is currently publishing systematic evidence reviews on key topics in occupational therapy in the *American Journal of Occupational Therapy*. The organization's website provides access to many EBP resources including a resource directory, critically appraised topics (synopsis of a group of articles on a specific topic), and practice guidelines (http://www.aota.org/Practice/Researchers.aspx). APTA has similar resources for physical therapists, including links for evidence and research tools, implementing EBP, and a physical therapy outcomes registry (http://www.apta.org/EvidenceResearch/). Nursing has developed journals specifically devoted to EBP, such as the *Worldviews on Evidence-Based Nursing* (http://onlinelibrary.wiley.com/journal/10.1111/%28ISSN%291741-6787).

It is clear that many professions are educating their clinicians and practitioners about EBP. However, this book examines the way in which interprofessional EBP is different from EBP that is focused in a single discipline. Interprofessional EBP is defined as a dynamic team process that blends the patient's preferences and values, the expertise of practitioners, and multidisciplinary evidence to implement practice changes that challenge current disciplinary paradigms and biases to create an integrated approach to patient care, health care delivery, or population health. The main difference that occurs with interprofessional EBP is the melding of the work of multiple disciplines that may consequently require that the team directly address any misunderstandings they may have of other professions, including misperceptions of a discipline's interest in particular patient problems, the type of evidence available in each discipline, and the methods of appraisal developed within a discipline. The work of the team is squarely centered on the patient and not on the discipline, other than how each discipline works with others to solve patient problems.

WHY IS AN INTERPROFESSIONAL EVIDENCE-BASED PRACTICE TEAM IMPORTANT?

Health care is undergoing significant changes in terms of health care organizations working to improve the triple aim involving quality and the care experience while simultaneously decreasing cost (Berwick, Nolan, & Whittington, 2008; http://www.ihi.org/Engage/Initiatives/TripleAim/pages/default.aspx). Health care organizations that undervalue collaborative practice or teamwork typically struggle with patient outcomes as the result of poorly managed care transitions among providers and delivery systems. Because of the lack of collaboration among health care professionals, patients can be negatively affected in terms of receiving duplicative services, experiencing lapses in services or failures to obtain needed services, receiving care guided through conflicting care plans, and obtaining additional care that might not have been necessary. To help practitioners and clinicians provide competent care, the Institute of Medicine (IOM) created in 2003 a set of core competencies for all health professionals. These competencies emphasized quality improvement, EBP, patient-centered care, informatics, and interprofessional teamwork. This book focuses on the development of four of these competencies for health professionals through an interprofessional EBP team. The text does not address the informatics competency, but this competency may become important for teams who design interprofessional EBP projects in which the team extracts data from the electronic health record or develops care processes for inclusion in the electronic record.

As collaboration among disciplines improves, it becomes clearer how complicated cross-disciplinary translation of evidence into collaborative practice is for interprofessional teams. Health care practitioners differ in their training, vocabulary, theories guiding practice, research methods, and EBP frameworks. Satterfield et al. (2009) compared and contrasted EBP frameworks among the disciplines of medicine, nursing, psychology, social work, and public health. Each of these disciplines have a slightly different focus in the way EBP questions are asked, how evidence is defined and appraised in terms of its strength and quality, and the influence of contextual factors on the application of evidence. Social workers, in their practice reasoning, for example, pay close attention to organizational, economic, political, and community environments when applying evidence. As another example of differences among professions, medicine has focused on RCTs, whereas nursing derives value from qualitative data, patient satisfaction, and quality improvement and cost effectiveness data (Satterfield et al., p. 374). Psychology has identified empirically supported treatments and has integrated these treatments into professional-level curricula. Social work and public health emphasize public policy as an application for EBP. This book guides interprofessional EBP teams to examine carefully the perspectives and evidence from pertinent disciplines to broaden solutions to practice questions that place the patient or the population at the center of problem solving. The assumption is that learning to use evidence across disciplines leads to sound health care outcomes as opposed to approaching care from a singular discipline's body of evidence or approach to EBP.

WHY IS INTERPROFESSIONAL EVIDENCE-BASED PRACTICE CHALLENGING?

Education about EBP most often occurs within discipline-specific course work, which may result in addressing patient or public policy questions in a more narrow way that does not sufficiently acknowledge complex patient or population health needs. According to Newhouse and Spring (2010), fostering interprofessional EBP requires a paradigm shift in the way EBP is taught and supported. Current EBP models (Rycroft-Malone & Bucknall, 2010) need to change the emphasis on disciplinary-focused practice to one that addresses patient problems and population health needs with a team approach (Zwarenstein & Reeves, 2006).

Another challenge for an interprofessional EBP team is the variability across disciplines in the previous education each member has received about EBP. For some disciplines, EBP education occurs during advanced graduate degree programs rather than during basic entry to practice programs (Proctor, 2007), where creating awareness of EBP is more the norm. Some clinicians and practitioners graduated prior to EBP being part of the curriculum for their discipline (Melnyk, Fineout-Overholt, Gallagher-Ford, & Kaplan, 2012), or EBP was taught in a manner incongruent with the realities of actual practice (Forsyth, Melton, & Mann, 2005; Manns, Norton, & Darrah, 2015).

Many disciplines in their entry-level programs thoroughly cover how to form the EBP question, conduct a literature search and select literature, appraise the literature, and synthesize findings from the literature to answer the EBP question. However, because of the separation of didactic work from the practice experience in the way prelicensure curricula are often designed, these programs may not offer their students the opportunity to apply in practice the EBP recommendations they have synthesized from the research literature (Caldwell, Coleman, Copp, Bell, & Ghazi, 2007). Too often, EBP stops at making recommendations based on the research rather than going further to actually change practice through implementation of the recommended interventions or processes. The gap between knowledge of the need to change and making the actual change remains too large and often takes years (Westfall, Mold, & Fagnan, 2007).

Despite multiple challenges facing health care professionals when implementing EBP, fortunately this book guides the work of the interprofessional EBP team. The book helps program coordinators design an interprofessional EBP program that implements carefully chosen strategies and supports to prevent or strategically address challenges that typically occur within the interprofessional EBP process. For instance, the program develops and supports mentors in their role as facilitators of team performance. This support is needed to guide the work of the team through systematic processes. The book and its website provide mentors and team members with supporting tools and resources.

What Skills Are Needed for Interprofessional Evidence-Based Practice?

Gebbie et al. (2007) described interdisciplinary research competencies that inspired developing competencies to address the focus on the skills needed for interprofessional EBP. These competencies need verification over time as interprofessional EBP continues to develop. This book emphasizes how professionals from multiple disciplines develop these interprofessional EBP competencies, regardless of the professional's expertise in EBP used within his or her discipline. Competencies are helpful in developing assessment tools and educational programming to foster interprofessional EBP. The interprofessional EBP competencies include all team members being able to do the following:

- Advocate for an interprofessional EBP approach when addressing patient problems, even though it may first appear as a discipline-specific problem.

- Actively seek the perspectives of other disciplines when solving patient problems even when primarily using a disciplinary-focused EBP approach.

- Develop the habit of reading journals outside of one's discipline.

- Communicate regularly with EBP experts from multiple disciplines.

- Attend scholarly presentations of multiple disciplines.

- Employ EBP and implementation science frameworks and methods from multiple disciplines.

- Plan practice change EBP projects through the synthesis of interdisciplinary research.

- Share research from one's discipline with the interprofessional team using clear and easily understood language, avoiding discipline-specific jargon.

- Attend EBP and implementation science educational programs with professionals from other disciplines.

- Collaborate in interprofessional EBP and implementation science respectfully and equitably with professionals from other disciplines.

- Draft interprofessional EBP and implementation science funding proposals in partnership with professionals from other disciplines.

- Integrate concepts and methods from multiple disciplines in designing IPP change pilot protocols.

- Disseminate interprofessional EBP and practice change pilot results both within and outside one's discipline.

How Does an Interprofessional Evidence-Based Practice Team Use Evidence to Implement a Practice Change?

Practitioners and clinicians whether singly or in collaboration have difficulty changing practice in a system despite awareness of the evidence supporting a different intervention or delivery process and even desire to make the change (Melnyk et al., 2012). Systems often inadvertently prevent a health care practitioner or team of practitioners from changing to another more promising intervention or strategy due to cost, lack of equipment, inadequate training, or no support for the change from other professions and administrators (Salls, Dolhi, Silverman, & Hansen, 2009). Additionally, some changes may not be a priority for an institution given that competing change projects might deliver a greater value proposition for the patient population in terms of improving outcomes and decreasing costs. Even when these particular barriers do not exist and the organization is willing to implement change, there are other issues and challenges that arise throughout the implementation process. These challenges might derail the change or lead to ineffective implementation such that outcomes do not occur in the way the organization expected.

Practitioners and interprofessional EBP team members can learn strategies to address these various barriers to practice change through reading the growing body of knowledge referred to as *translation science* (Green, 2012). This science arose from the need to reduce the gap between the time when discoveries in research occur and when they are available for widespread use with patients. The term *implementation science* is a form of translation science (Green) and is particularly useful as an aspect of interprofessional EBP. Implementation science develops effective and efficient methods to overcome the human and financial resource constraints inherent in an organization or system. The most significant barrier to practice change relates to organizational inertia where change is a lower priority compared to addressing daily operational issues and challenges. This book has purposely included principles from implementation science as a strategic approach for systematically implementing practice changes supported through synthesis of the evidence.

TABLE 1-2

ROLES FOR AN INTERPROFESSIONAL EVIDENCE-BASED PRACTICE PROGRAM

ROLE	DESCRIPTION	WRITE THE NAMES OF PEOPLE IN THE ORGANIZATIONS WHO ARE OR WHO WILL BE IN THESE ROLES
Program sponsors	Leaders within the partnering organizations who widely communicate about the program, both internally and externally, invest resources into the program and help remove organizational barriers that might negatively impact the program success.	
Program developers and coordinators	The program sponsors appoint at least one person from each organization to develop and conduct the program. Developers and Coordinators may be a single role or two separate roles. The number of needed coordinators depends on the number of teams in a single program cycle.	
EBP team mentors	Staff members from the health care organization who lead the team through the steps of an evidence-based project in a manner that results in on-time completion within budget.	
Clinical scholars or evidence-based fellows	This is a staff member(s) from the health care organization who has the original idea for a project and desires mentoring and assistance from a team in order to learn EBP.	
Faculty and student team members	These are team members from multiple disciplines who are interested in the EBP topic of the clinical scholar and who are willing to become a part of a team as a learning and scholarship opportunity.	

WHAT IS AN INTERPROFESSIONAL EVIDENCE-BASED PRACTICE PROGRAM?

An interprofessional EBP program typically lasts 12 to 18 months. The program design promotes the development and implementation of a practice change in a health care organization because of completing a systematic interprofessional evidence-based process inclusive of implementation science. The program includes collaborative partnerships, such as between a health care organization and a university, or involves multiple health care organizations and universities. Typically, the goals of a program include the following:

- For the health care organization: Bring about sustainable and effective practice change supportive of the quality improvement goals of the health care organization in a way that develops staff in all disciplines about interprofessional EBP.

- For the university: Provide student and faculty learning about and experience in the process and scholarship of interprofessional EBP inclusive of practice change.

- For both organizations: To foster capacity to build highly functioning interprofessional teams dedicated to interprofessional EBP and to implementation science as an aspect of patient-centered care.

Another aspect of an interprofessional EBP program is the specific roles needed to conduct a successful program. These roles include the program coordinators, mentors, clinical scholars or EBP fellows, and faculty and student team members (Table 1-2). The roles are not prescribed to any specific discipline because the goal is to create teams composed of members from several disciplines. The program coordinators and mentors may want to use Table 1-2 to educate each team member about his or her role on the team.

What Are the Theoretical Underpinnings of an Interprofessional Evidence-Based Practice Program?

When starting an interprofessional EBP program as a joint collaborative between a health care organization and a university, the program developers, who are often the program coordinators, should use specific theoretical principles to ensure that the results and products of the teams actually change care and improve patient outcomes. Program developers will want to consider the theoretical underpinnings derived from the literature in six areas (Figure 1-1). Theoretical principles from these six areas include EBP models, clinical scholar programs, implementation science, interprofessional competencies, highly functioning teams, and mentoring (Table 1-3). These theoretical principles support the key team roles and interprofessional EBP program elements. Program developers should use these references to guide the development of their programs and to support the program coordinators, program mentors, and interprofessional teams throughout the program.

Evidence-Based Practice Models

It was important for the interprofessional EBP program to select a particular organizational model for EBP. No one particular model is better than another, so university/health care organizational partners may decide whether a different model would be more effective depending on the practice setting, disciplines involved, and patient populations. A review of the literature resulted in finding only a couple of interprofessional EBP models (Goode, Fink, Krugman, Oman, & Traditi, 2011; Satterfield et al., 2009), while most were discipline specific for occupational therapy (Caldwell, Whitehead, Fleming, & Moes, 2008), physical therapy (Stevens et al., 2015), and nursing (Stetler, 2010; Titler et al., 2001). One model developed in occupational therapy (Plastow, 2006) was designed for a system's organizational change process, which has similarities to the organizational focus of the nursing models (Stetler; Titler et al.).

This book is based on the experiences of St. Catherine University in St. Paul, Minnesota, collaboratively running an interprofessional EBP program for 1 year at North Memorial Medical Center in Robbinsdale, Minnesota, and for 2 years at Abbott Northwestern Hospital in Minneapolis. The Iowa model of EBP to promote quality care (referred to throughout the book as the *Iowa model*) (Titler et al., 2001) guided the interprofessional EBP program not only because of the model's organizational emphasis, but also due to both aforementioned health care organizations' use of the model to direct their EBP and research efforts (Figure 1-2).

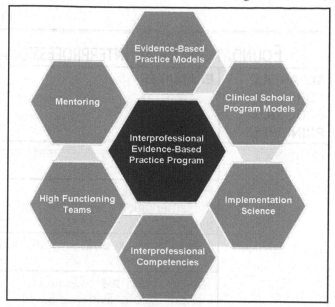

Figure 1-1. Theoretical foundation for interprofessional EBP program.

In following the Iowa model as described in Chapter 6, the design of the interprofessional EBP project began with potential clinical scholars submitting practice issues arising from knowledge-focused or problem-focused triggers. A committee of the health care organization decides whether the issue is a priority for the organization, and then if it is a priority, an interprofessional team is formed to address the issue through the formulation of a specific EBP question. The interprofessional team gathers, appraises, and synthesizes the appropriate evidence in order to decide whether there is enough research or other relevant evidence for a practice change. If not enough evidence, the interprofessional EBP project takes more of a research focus in terms of the team deciding to conduct an effectiveness study or some other type of descriptive study to gather more information about the issue. If there is enough evidence, the interprofessional team designs a practice change implementation plan, implements the plan, monitors and evaluates the results of the change, and then decides whether the change should be widely implemented. If the change is widely implemented and sustained, the organization then monitors and assesses the overall change outcomes and disseminates the results. A decision not to implement the practice change once the change pilot is completed may lead to further revision of the practice change and another implementation pilot. Another possibility is for the organization to continue to monitor developments in the research literature, thereby waiting for a knowledge trigger in order to continue further with the particular issue.

Clinical Scholar Program Models

This book primarily derived its interprofessional EBP program concepts from the nursing literature about clinical

TABLE 1-3

FOUNDATION FOR AN INTERPROFESSIONAL EVIDENCE-BASED PRACTICE PROGRAM

SIX AREAS FOR PROGRAM PRINCIPLES	EXAMPLES	SOURCE	WHAT RESOURCES/MODELS WILL WE USE FOR OUR PROGRAM?
EBP models	Iowa Model of Evidence-Based Practice to Promote Quality Care	Titler et al., 2001	
	Promoting Action on Research Implementation in Health Services (PARIHS)	Kitson, Harvey, & McCormack, 1998; Rycroft-Malone & Bucknall, 2010	
	The Johns Hopkins Nursing EBP Model	Newhouse, Dearholt, Poe, Pugh, & White, 2007	
	The Colorado Patient-Centered Interprofessional Evidence-Based Practice Model	Goode et al., 2011	
	Advancing Research and Clinical Practice Through Close Collaboration (ARCC)	Ciliska et al., 2011	
	Stetler Model	Stetler, 2010	
Clinical scholar program models	EBP program at the Unit Level for oncology nurses	Cooke et al., 2004	
	EBP program for nurses in a pediatric academic hospital	Steurer, 2010	
	EBP program for nurses and allied health professionals in a children's hospital	Hockenberry, Brown, Walden, & Barrera, 2009	
	Advanced EBP program for nurses in leadership roles responsible for guiding teams and mentoring	Cullen, Titler, & Rempel, 2010	
	Describes the program outcomes of an interprofessional clinical scholar program that forms the basis of this book	Moyers, Finch Guthrie, Swan, & Sathe, 2014	
Interprofessional competencies	Core competencies for interprofessional collaborative practice	Interprofessional Education Collaborative Expert Panel, 2011	
	Identifies the mechanisms that shape successful collaborative teamwork	World Health Organization (WHO), 2010	
	Toronto model for IPE and practice: Competencies progress from exposure, immersion, and competence for entry into practice	Nelson, Tassone, & Hodges, 2014	

(continued)

| TABLE 1-3 (CONTINUED) |||| |

FOUNDATION FOR AN INTERPROFESSIONAL EVIDENCE-BASED PRACTICE PROGRAM				
SIX AREAS FOR PROGRAM PRINCIPLES	**EXAMPLES**	**SOURCE**	**WHAT RESOURCES/MODELS WILL WE USE FOR OUR PROGRAM?**
Implementation science	Provides a framework and strategies for EBP project implementation	van Achterberg, Schoonhoven, & Grol, 2008	
	Review of implementation science frameworks. Provides phases and steps for implementation	Meyers, Durlak, & Wandersman, 2012; Meyers et al., 2012	
	Synthesizes implementation research literature	Fixsen et al., 2005	
	Use of translation science as a context for nursing practice	Titler, 2010	
	Describes the theory of diffusion of innovation into practice through identification and description of phases	Rogers, 2010	
High functioning teams	Discusses the types of health care teams, roles, and evaluating, and improving team effectiveness	Mosser & Begun, 2014	
	Study to identify predictors of team success	Pentland, 2012	
	Describes methods for promoting collaboration among team members	Gratton & Erickson, 2007	
	Team Strategies and Tools to Enhance Performance and Patient Safety (TeamSTEPPS) developed by the Agency for Healthcare Research and Quality (AHRQ) and the U.S. Department of Defense (DoD)	Agency for Health Research Quality, 2006	
Mentoring	EBP mentoring program for nurses working on a Neonatal Intensive Care Unit	Mariano et al., 2009	
	Evidence on the outcomes of mentoring	Melnyk, 2007	
	Model for mentoring nursing students	Andrews & Chilton, 2000	

scholar programs. No other disciplines have written about these types of programs, although the discipline of occupational therapy reported some similar approaches (Crist, Munoz, Witchger Hansen, Benson, & Provident, 2005). In reviewing the nursing literature, it is clear that clinical scholar programs are implemented in health care organizations to increase the amount of EBP projects that nursing staff conduct in order to improve the quality of patient care (Cooke et al., 2004). They were not originally designed to have an interprofessional focus. Clinical scholar programs typically require the selected nursing staff scholar to work with a mentor, often an advanced practice nurse

who has a background in EBP (Mariano et al., 2009). Along with time spent developing the project with a mentor, the scholar usually attends an EBP course (Soukup & McCleish, 2008). Often these EBP projects end with proposed recommendations for practice change submitted to the nursing leadership for implementation (Everett, 2011). These same components are included in the interprofessional clinical scholar program described in this book; however, we have added both the interprofessional focus and the implementation of the practice change as a part of the interprofessional EBP process.

Figure 1-2. The Iowa Model of Evidence-Based Practice to Promote Quality Care. (Used/ Reprinted with permission from the University of Iowa Hospitals and Clinics and Marita G. Titler, PhD, RN, FAAN. Copyright 1998. For permission to use or reproduce the model, please contact the University of Iowa Hospitals and Clinics.)

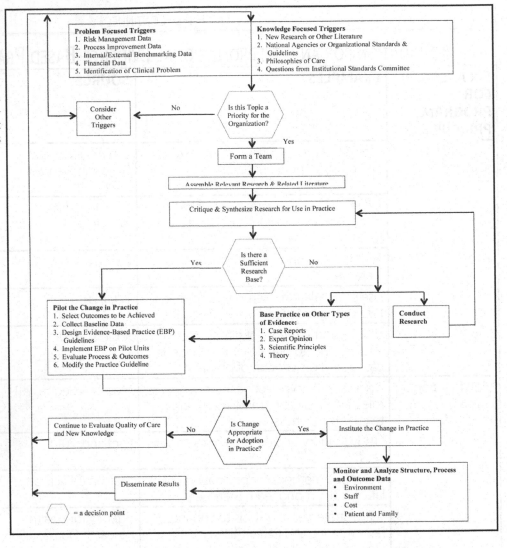

Crist et al. (2005) and Crist (2010) described and evaluated a practitioner-scholar program in which the goal was to develop occupational therapy services in community agencies that did not normally provide these services. This goal is quite different than the goals of clinical scholar programs reported in the nursing literature; however, similar to nursing clinical scholar programs, there was a focus on developing and implementing practices supported by the evidence and on disseminating scholarly work related to the new practice. Crist et al. articulated the importance of the university partnering with a community agency and involving students and faculty. Partnerships and the involvement of faculty and students are central to the interprofessional EBP program.

Glegg, Livingstone, and Montgomery (2015) developed an ongoing EBP process for occupational therapists and other clinicians and practitioners with many similarities to clinical scholar programs described in nursing. These authors constructed a Web-based toolkit designed to assist implementation of EBP within a pediatric rehabilitation setting. The toolkit contained resources and templates to streamline, quantify, and document outcomes throughout the EBP process, including the implementation of an EBP change. With this book, we have included a toolkit housed on a companion website after developing such resources for the interprofessional EBP teams.

Implementation Science

Thomas and Law (2014) analyzed data from a cross-sectional survey of 368 members of the Canadian Association of Occupational Therapists indicating that practitioners, although viewing the importance of EBP positively, had yet to integrate EBP fully into clinical practice. These data substantiated the need for additional supports for EBP and research utilization if evidence is going to be moved more quickly into practice. Manns et al. (2015) similarly noted inconsistency between the emphases on EBP for physical therapy at the university versus at the workplace, where support for EBP often occurs inconsistently. In addition, most of the clinical scholar programs described in the nursing literature indicate that few of the recommendations from the evidence-based projects were actually implemented by the health care organization (Fineout-Overholt & Johnston, 2006). Consequently, it is important for an interprofessional EBP program to include strategies for implementation of a practice change.

The implementation science literature (Fixsen, Naoom, Blasé, Friedman, & Wallace, 2005) was incorporated into the interprofessional EBP program as part of the program phases (see Chapter 12) in which implementation plans are devised to test the synthesized practice change before recommending widespread implementation in the health care organization (see Figure 1-2). Burke and Gitlin (2012) in occupational therapy regard the nursing literature in implementation science as helpful in translating research into practice in a way that is sensitive to the practitioner and specific to the site and patient population. In nursing, van Achterberg et al. (2008) discussed a useful framework for implementation that starts with the description of operational change objectives and a thorough analysis of current practice, the target group, and the context in which change should take place. Based on this foundation for implementation, an implementation plan is developed using strategies best addressing the needs of the target group and the context. The implementation plan is operationalized through the determination of who does what and when it is done. Additionally, implementation includes assessment of both the processes and outcomes of the plan and the sustainability of the implementation.

Chapter 12 discusses how the interprofessional EBP program teaches team members to develop a sound implementation plan that includes implementation strategies selected to address the implementation facilitator or barrier. These barriers or facilitators include knowledge, attitudes, self-efficacy, social norms, organization, and financing (van Achterberg, Schoonhoven, and Grol, 2008). Knowledge implementation strategies include active learning and advanced organizers, while strategies for promoting supportive attitudes include shifting perspectives and anticipating regret related to giving up current practice methods. Modeling is an example of a self-efficacy strategy and a method of establishing social norms. Priority setting is an important implementation strategy for the organization, as is offering financial incentives to partially finance the change.

Interprofessional Competencies

The interprofessional EBP program should include competencies regarding team roles and responsibilities, value and ethics, communication, teamwork, and team-based practice throughout the interprofessional EBP learning modules (Interprofessional Education Collaborative Expert Panel, 2011). Although these competencies guide interprofessional behavior in general, this book focuses on their

application to interprofessional EBP. Chapter 4 addresses teams and teamwork and Chapter 5 focuses on team communication for the interprofessional EBP program. Values and ethics for teamwork and for project accountability are clearly articulated in each team's charter (see Chapter 4 and the book's website), which is meant to be a living document that the team can use when changes need to be made in team functioning or when problems occur that require renewal of the original agreements made among team members. In addition, values and ethics related to EBP, informed consent and protection of human subjects, stewardship of project funds and meeting expectations of grant funders, and honoring inclusion in decision making of key stakeholders throughout the project are emphasized in the appropriate interprofessional EBP phase.

In addition to the interprofessional competencies, several current IPE models were helpful in designing the interprofessional EBP program. These models include the Toronto Model for Interprofessional Education and Practice (Nelson et al., 2014), the team-based learning for health professions education (Michaelsen, Parmelee, McMahon, & Levine, 2008), the Promoting Interprofessional Education Model (PIPE) (Howkins & Bray, 2008), and the Effective Interprofessional Education for Effective Practice Model (Freeth, Hammick, Reeves, Koppel, & Barr, 2005). Each of these models offers a unique contribution to the development of an interprofessional EBP program. The Toronto model has a different set of IPE competencies when compared to the competencies described in the work of the Interprofessional Education Collaborative Expert Panel (2011). The Toronto model takes a developmental approach to IPE competencies involving exposure, immersion, and competence for entry into practice. Building IPE educational experiences developmentally helps mentors and program coordinators structure learning from the basic to the more advanced levels depending on the skills of the interprofessional EBP team. All of the IPE educational models focus on ways for facilitators and educators to enable interprofessional learning and practice in terms of professional development, curriculum design, and teaching methods.

Although the use of these models is not yet widespread in higher education, key organizations are working to expand IPE. The Josiah Macey Foundation (http://macyfoundation.org/about) provides grant funding in support of education and training of health professionals to which they have directed substantial resources in support of IPE. The National Center for Interprofessional Practice and Education at the University of Minnesota is focusing on leading, coordinating, and studying the advancement of IPE (https://nexusipe.org/about). The Institute of Medicine (IOM, 2013, 2015) along with the other organizations, provides valuable information, resources, and tools that assist in developing the team education and teamwork aspects of an interprofessional EBP program.

Highly Functioning Teams

The term *interprofessional professionality* is important for understanding how teams in health care should evolve into highly functioning teams. Stern (2006) defined interprofessional professionality as "consistent demonstration of core values evidenced by professionals working together, aspiring to and wisely applying principles of altruism and caring, excellence, ethics, respect, communication, accountability to achieve optimal health and wellness in individuals and communities" (p. 19). To improve the patient's quality experience, IPP places the emphasis upon members of the health service delivery team participating in the team's activities in order to rely on one another to accomplish common goals and improve health care delivery (Australasian Interprofessional Practice and Education Network [AIPEN], http://www.aippen.net/what-is-ipe-ipl-ipp).

Models for IPP are still evolving and tend to focus on one type of patient care service (e.g., rehabilitation, mental health, hospice, or geriatric-based care) or are ad hoc in nature in that disciplines come together to address specific quality improvement needs (Mosser & Begun, 2014). However, newer team models for primary care are developing in response to the need to switch to preventive health care, proactive management of chronic illnesses, and improved team functioning (Goldberg, Beeson, Kuzel, Love, & Carver, 2013; Zawora, O'Leary, & Bonat, 2015). Key components from the literature for developing effective team-based care include the following (Doherty & Crowley, 2013; Goldberg et al., 2013; Mosser & Begun; Zawora, O'Leary, & Bonat):

- An organizational culture for team-based care
- A leader or champion for interprofessional team-based care
- A focus on the specific needs of the population served, creating a patient-centered approach
- Education about the purpose and benefits of team-based care
- Assignment of responsibilities to team members given their expertise, experience, and talent in order to fit the specific needs of patients
- Willingness within the team to take on added responsibilities to facilitate receipt of needed services and to identify shared team responsibilities
- Respect for diversity in the perspectives and training of team members
- Management of team workflow processes and responsibilities
- Clear team communication processes
- Evaluation of team function and outcomes with a focus on improving quality

The interprofessional EBP program, through its support and training of mentors as well as through the way the team process is operationalized, has incorporated these main principles of highly functioning teams. Chapter 4 describes how the interprofessional EBP program uses TeamSTEPPS (team strategies and tools to enhance performance and patient safety) developed by the Agency for Healthcare Research and Quality (AHRQ) and the U.S. Department of Defense (DoD) (AHRQ, 2006). The TeamSTEPPS curriculum focuses on five core competencies of teamwork: team structure, leadership, situational monitoring, mutual support, and communication. The tools from this curriculum are useful in helping teams structure their work processes and communication strategies.

Mentoring

The availability of mentors for staff ensures that EBP occurs within a health care organization (Melnyk, Fineout-Overholt, Giggleman, & Cruz, 2010). Mentorship is partially needed because of variation in EBP education, attitudes, experience, and confidence of clinicians and practitioners within and across disciplines in conducting EBP (Thomas & Law, 2014; Zidarov, Thomas, & Poissant, 2013; Ziviani, Wilkinson, Hinchliffe, & Feeney, 2015). In addition, mentorship is needed because of the evolving nature of EBP in terms of the changes in approaches and methods for forming questions, for conducting appraisal and synthesis, as well as in terms of the increasing complexity of implementing a sustainable practice change. In addition, interprofessional EBP is in its infancy in terms of how to address the differences in EBP approaches across disciplines.

While mentorship is primarily positive, researchers evaluating the effectiveness of these mentorship programs concluded that mentoring may promote or limit an EBP culture, beliefs about EBP, and the implementation of practice change projects grounded in evidence (Wallen et al., 2010). Haas (2008) noted that mentors who lack training in EBP are likely to promote negative attitudes toward it. Carefully preparing mentors to provide the leadership necessary to facilitate an EBP process is critical (Zwarenstein & Reeves, 2006). Because of the variation in results from mentoring, mentors need development (Ramani, Gruppen, & Kachur, 2006) to establish cultures that advance EBP (Melnyk, Fineout-Overholt, Giggleman, & Cruz, 2010).

In examining the literature on mentoring, several categories emerge, including mentoring in the workplace, developing students and young people, and advancing new academicians. No matter the particular foci, mentoring typically occurs to enable an individual's personal and professional development. Complex mentoring involves mentors working with several individuals from multiple disciplines, as well as mentees receiving mentoring from multiple individuals at the same time depending on the needs of the mentee or the organization (Eby, Allen, Evans,

Ng, & DuBois, 2008). Regardless of the complexity of mentoring relationships, there is consensus about teaching/learning as a critical component of the mentoring process (Andrews & Chilton, 2000; Eby et al.; Melnyk, 2007).

Mentoring theory for the interprofessional EBP program was developed in a grounded-theory qualitative study of the initial offering of the program occurring as a partnership between St. Catherine University and North Memorial Medical Center. This interprofessional EBP program mentoring theory is described in Chapter 3 and was based on the work of Andrews and Chilton (2000) and the nursing mentoring research of Darling (1984), who is widely cited, including in occupational therapy (Scheerer, 2007). Darling describes attraction (mutual between mentor and mentee), action (time and energy), and affect (mutual respect) as absolute requirements of mentoring. Mentors have three basic mentoring roles (inspirer, investor, and supporter) and nine action roles. Andrews and Chilton increased the action roles to 14 when combining the three main roles with the action roles and adding new ones discovered in their survey research. Program developers and mentors should examine these roles in order to strategize how they will enact them throughout the program (Figure 1-3).

Our work with the interprofessional EBP program has shown the importance of mentoring regardless of the skill level of team members in EBP and in interprofessional teamwork. Likewise, Morgan (2012) described positive changes in the experiences of nurses to EBP barriers prior to and after participation in an EBP mentoring intervention. In general, few studies assess the influence of mentoring on EBP and knowledge translation. Abdullah et al. (2014) completed a systematic review to examine the effectiveness of mentoring in knowledge translation and found only 10 studies over a period from 1988 to 2012. These studies showed mixed results of mentoring, as some aspects of practitioner behavior were not changed; however, there were studies that showed that mentoring led to improvement in knowledge, changes in beliefs about evidence, and successful change throughout the organization.

WHAT ARE THE ESSENTIAL ELEMENTS OF THE INTERPROFESSIONAL EVIDENCE-BASED PRACTICE PROGRAM?

Now that the theoretical principles guiding an interprofessional EBP program have been articulated and described, the reasoning behind the creation of the essential elements of the program becomes clearer. Based on the supporting literature, there are integral components that ensure the success of an interprofessional EBP program. Table 1-4 includes the key elements of an interprofessional EBP

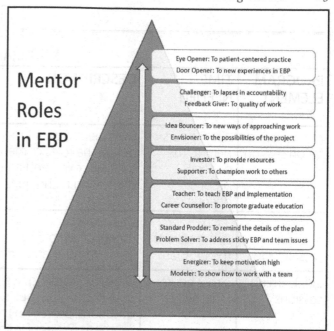

Figure 1-3. Mentor roles for interprofessional teams.

program as a helpful resource for program coordinators to indicate how they will incorporate these elements in their program. Although program developers may create other elements for the interprofessional EBP program that fit the needs of the partnering organizations, we have found after three iterations that these main components are effective in creating successful program outcomes. Chapter 6 provides greater detail about these major program elements.

A mentor orientation ensures that mentors firmly grasp their roles and demands upon their time; understand how the program operates; buy into the program's outcome expectations for each team; are familiar with the interprofessional EBP methods and tools; are aware of interprofessional team competencies; and learn about mentoring roles, techniques, and mentor supports (see Chapter 3). Mentors should also plan to meet regularly with program coordinators throughout the program to solve team issues and obtain clarity on each phase of the interprofessional EBP program. Program coordinators meet regularly to keep the program moving forward and to make changes in the program and its resources and materials as needed.

Teams should also come together for a program orientation that provides an opportunity for participants to become acquainted with each team member and decide through generation of a team charter how each team will operate. The orientation is designed to provide an overview of interprofessional EBP and the program's goals and objectives, a calendar of the program's activities, and some time to practice with communication tools if needed (e.g., wikis, learning platforms, Google docs and chats, and virtual meeting software), and to complete pre-program evaluation survey instruments about EBP and IPP. Typically, it is

TABLE 1-4

PROGRAM SCOPE

PROGRAM ELEMENT	TIME NEEDED	DESCRIPTION	PROGRAM SCOPE (DATES AND PERSONS RESPONSIBLE)
Mentor orientation session	2 to 3 hours prior to the general program orientation	Designed to orient mentors to the program, fully define the roles of mentors, and acquaint the mentors with expected mentoring challenges and mentoring techniques	
Program orientation session	3 to 6 hours at the start of the program	Designed to orient all team members to the elements of the program, EBP, roles on the team, and key communication methods and technologies	
EBP learning sessions	1 to 2 hours bimonthly	Designed to bring in experts to educate and discuss 8 to 10 EBP topics, such as EBP overview, PICO questions, Searching the Literature, Appraisal & Synthesis, Project Design, Project Implementation, Evaluation and Analysis, and Project Dissemination. Some topics require more than one session.	
Team and scholar work time and consultation sessions with experts and organizational leaders	6 to 8 hours bimonthly	Designed to give the team work time within their work/school day to complete EBP tasks as a team and as individual team members while having access to help to answer questions or to give guidance. Health care organizations will need to consider whether this time is paid work time for staff. Universities have to coordinate faculty and student schedules (or use communication technologies). Universities will need to address faculty load assigned to the project (e.g., 1 to 3 course loads).	
Mentor meetings with program coordinators	1 hour bimonthly	Designed to identify mentoring issues related to team progress and performance and to proactively develop strategies to support the team's work	
Mentoring workshops	Two to four times over the 18 months; either half or full days	Designed to offer in depth training for mentors on mentor-identified topics where the mentors want better preparation to work with their teams	
Program coordinator meetings	1 hour weekly	Designed to assist program coordinators to proactively address program issues as they develop	

best if prior to volunteering, all team members understand when the interprofessional EBP and implementation science education sessions occur, when teams will meet either face-to-face or virtually, when work should be completed, and when consultation with stakeholders and experts should happen. The mentors and team members learn through the program calendar that there are nine phases in the interprofessional EBP process and implementation of a practice change. Chapters 6 through 15 describe in detail these nine phases. In Table 1-5, these phases are briefly described and serve as the milestones for interprofessional project completion.

	TABLE 1-5			
	INTERPROFESSIONAL TEAM MILESTONES			
CHAPTER	STAGES OR MILESTONE	DESCRIPTION	DATE FOR EXPECTED MILESTONE ACHIEVEMENT	DATE ACHIEVED
6	Orienting	An overview of the interprofessional EBP and implementation processes, problem identification, identifying team roles, meeting times, minute taking, team communication methods, and decision-making strategies		
7	Figuring it out	Conducting a background literature search to further explore the practice trigger and developing the EBP question. Determining the extent of the problem in the organization		
8	Settling in	Conducting the foreground literature search to answer the EBP question, documenting the search process, and selecting the literature for appraisal		
9	Transitioning	Appraising the selected literature and synthesizing the results into a practice recommendation		
10 and 11	Designing	Designing the practice change incorporating stakeholder involvement, selecting measures to document the change outcomes, seeking institutional review board approval, and obtaining funding for personnel and equipment		
12	Implementing	Consenting patients/staff, following the intervention design protocol, ensuring fidelity, troubleshooting, managing data, and meeting deadlines. Designing and implementing practice change sustainability		
13	Analyzing	Cleaning and analyzing data and drawing conclusions		
14	Wrapping up	Finalizing the practice recommendation, celebrating hard work, recognizing team members, finishing up loose ends, ensuring sustainability of projects and program		
15	Disseminating	Preparing abstracts, posters, and papers for presentation or publication. Planning other mechanisms of external and internal dissemination		

HOW IS AN INTERPROFESSIONAL EVIDENCE-BASED PRACTICE PROGRAM EVALUATED?

It is important to the sponsors of the interprofessional EBP program from both organizations to have data indicating positive results of the program. Tools and surveys are available to measure changes in the knowledge of and beliefs in EBP and attitudes toward interprofessional teams and IPE (Table 1-6). There is a variety of outcome measures available given the priorities of the interprofessional EBP program. It is therefore important for program coordinators to review the assessment literature on EBP learning outcomes and the literature on

TABLE 1-6

PROGRAM MEASUREMENT INSTRUMENTS

OUTCOME	INSTRUMENT	DESCRIPTION	REFERENCE	WHAT MEASUREMENT TOOLS WILL WE USE FOR THE EBP PROGRAM OUTCOME MEASURES?
Knowledge of EBP	Terminology subscale from the *Evidence-Based Practice Profile*	Participants rank their understanding of EBP concepts on a 5-point Likert scale, with 1 indicating having never before heard the term *EBP* and 5 indicating ability to explain the concept to others. The terminology subscale has acceptable internal consistency (Cronbach's α = .94) and test–retest reliability (intraclass correlations ranging from .67 to .86).	McEvoy, Williams, & Olds, 2010	
EBP attitudes and beliefs	*The Evidence-Based Practice Belief Scale*	Participants rate on a scale ranging from *strongly disagree* to *strongly agree* their level of agreement with 16 items indicating confidence in ability to engage in EBP. Evidence-Based Practice Belief Scale achieved internal consistency with a Cronbach's α of .90.	Melnyk et al., 2008	
Interprofessional teamwork attitudes and beliefs	*The Attitudes Toward Interprofessional Teamwork and Education Scale*, faculty and student versions. Two subscales: Attitudes Toward Interprofessional Health Care Teams and The Attitudes Toward Interprofessional Education	The Attitudes Toward Interprofessional Health Care Teams scale includes 14 items rated on a 5-point Likert scale ranging from *strongly disagree* to *strongly agree*. It has a Cronbach's α of .8 for internal consistency. The Attitudes Toward Interprofessional Education subscale was given only to students, mentors, and clinical scholars. It contains 14 items rated on a 5-point Likert scale and has a Cronbach's α of .91.	Curran, Sharpe, & Forristall, 2007 Curran, Sharpe, Forristall, & Flynn, 2008	

(continued)

		TABLE 1-6 (CONTINUED)		
		PROGRAM MEASUREMENT INSTRUMENTS		
OUTCOME	INSTRUMENT	DESCRIPTION	REFERENCE	WHAT MEASUREMENT TOOLS WILL WE USE FOR THE EBP PROGRAM OUTCOME MEASURES?
Productivity of EBP teams	Frequencies	Grants submitted and awarded Poster presentations Juried presentations Publications Products developed	Moyers et al., 2014	

interprofessional team performance in order to select the most important outcome measurement tools. The National Center for Interprofessional Practice and Education at the University of Minnesota provides information about assessment instruments for IPE and practice (https://nexusipe.org/about).

In addition to the quantitative tools, mentors and program coordinators may want to keep journals to note key learnings, issues, and experiences of the teams and team members. Interviews of team members and mentors may also provide qualitative data to describe the experience within the interprofessional EBP program. Course feedback after each interprofessional EBP learning session is important for course revision as is the maintenance of careful attendance records of all participants. Program coordinators need to document the outcomes of each team in terms of grants obtained, EBP products developed, and presentations and publications submitted and accepted.

SUMMARY

The interprofessional EBP and implementation processes are not easy because there will be challenges ahead of the interprofessional team. The advantage of having a team is that team members have a variety of skills and abilities and can share the workload. No matter how experienced, each person not only brings a set of strengths but also has learning needs. Using each other's strengths while honoring the learning goals of each team member will create an environment of respect and mutual support and reciprocity. A team should expect some conflict, as having disagreements actually strengthens a project when the team considers a variety of perspectives. An effective team knows how to dialogue within a specified time period and then agrees to make a decision in order to move on to the next steps and phases.

Members have to learn how to give and receive feedback and how to hold each other accountable for work task completion and work quality. The mentor's job is to facilitate each team's progression through the interprofessional EBP experience. The opportunities for learning how to improve care are tremendous. Practitioners and clinicians will find that, upon engaging in interprofessional EBP, they will feel reinvigorated about their practice and will have a renewed spirit that comes from knowing the work made a difference to the lives of patients and their families.

REFLECTION QUESTIONS

1. Think about the potential challenges (e.g., team members with different education and experience in EBP) to interprofessional EBP and determine how you would resolve at least three of them as a mentor or team member.

2. Whether you are a mentor or team member, decide which mentoring roles might be the most difficult and determine how you would develop yourself in this role.

REFERENCES

Abdullah, G., Rossy, D., Ploeg, J., Davies, B., Higuchi, K., Sikora, L., & Stacey, D. (2014). Measuring the effectiveness of mentoring as a knowledge translation intervention for implementing empirical evidence: A systematic review. *Worldviews on Evidence-Based Nursing, 11,* 284-300. doi:10.1111/wvn.12060

Andrews, M., & Chilton, F. (2000). Student and mentor perceptions of mentoring effectiveness. *Nurse Education Today, 20,* 555-562. doi:10.1054/nedt.2000.0464.

Agency for Healthcare Research and Quality. (2006). *TeamSTEPPS instructor's guide: Team strategies and tools to enhance performance and patient safety.* Rockville, MD: author.

Berwick, D. M., Nolan, T. W., & Whittington, J. (2008). The Triple Aim: Care, health, and cost. *Health Affairs, 27,* 759-769. doi:10.1377/hlthaff.27.3.759

Burke, J. P., & Gitlin, L. N. (2012). The issue is—How do we change practice when we have the evidence? *American Journal of Occupational Therapy, 66,* e85-e88. doi:10.5014/ajot.2012.004432

Caldwell, K., Coleman, K., Copp, G., Bell, L., & Ghazi, F. (2007). Preparing for professional practice: How well does professional training equip health and social care practitioners to engage in evidence-based practice. *Nursing Education Today, 27,* 518-528. doi:10.1016/j.nedt.2006.08.014

Caldwell, E., Whitehead, M., Fleming, J., & Moes, L. (2008). Evidence-based practice in everyday clinical practice: Strategies for change in a tertiary occupational therapy department. *Australian Occupational Therapy Journal, 55,* 79-84. doi:10.1111/j.1440-1630.2007.00669.x

Ciliska, D., DiCenso, A., Melynk, B. M., Fineout-Overholt, E., Stettler, C. B., Cullent, L.,...Dang, D. (2011). Models to guide implementation of evidence-based practice. In B. M. Melynk, E. Fineout-Overholt, E. (Eds.), *Evidence-Based Practice in Nursing and Healthcare: A Guide to Best Practice,* pp. 241-275. Philadelphia, PA: Wolters Kluwer.

Clemence, M. L. (1998). Evidence-based physiotherapy: Seeking the unattainable? *British Journal of Therapy Rehabilitation, 5,* 257-260.

Cooke, L., Smith-Idell, C., Dean, G., Gemmill, R., Steingass, S., Sun, V., ...Borneman, T. (2004). "Research to practice": A practical program to enhance the use of evidence-based practice at the unit level. *Oncology Nursing Forum, 31*(4), 825. doi:10.1188/04.onf.825-832

Crist, P. (2010). Adapting research instruction to support the scholarship of practice: Practice scholar partnerships. *Occupational Therapy in Health Care, 24,* 39-55. doi:10.3109/07380570903477000

Crist, P., Munoz, J. P., Witchger Hansen, A. M., Benson, J., & Provident, I. (2005). The practice scholar program: An academic-practice partnership to promote the scholarship of best practices. *Occupational Therapy in Health Care, 19* (1/2), 71-93. doi:10.1080/j003v19n01_06

Cullen, L., Titler, M. G., & Rempel, G. (2010). An advanced educational program promoting evidence-based practice. *Western Journal of Nursing Research, 33,* 345-364. doi:10.1177/0193945910379218

Curran, V. R., Sharpe, D., & Forristall, J. (2007). Attitudes of health science faculty towards interprofessional teamwork and education. *Medical Education, 41,* 892-896. doi:10.1111/j.1365-2923.2007.02823.x.

Curran, V. R., Sharpe, D., Forristall, J., & Flynn, K. (2008). Attitudes of health science students toward interprofessional teamwork and education. *Learning in Health and Social Care, 7,* 146-156. doi:10.1111/j 1473-6861.2008.00184.x

Darling, L. A. (1984). What do nurses want in a mentor? *The Journal of Nursing Administration, 14,* 42-44. doi:10.1097/00006223-198501000-00012

Dijkers, M. P., Murphy, S. L., & Krellman, J. (2012). Evidence-based practice for rehabilitation professionals: Concepts and controversies. *Archives of Physical Medicine Rehabilitation, 93,* Supplement 2, S164-S176. doi:10.1016/j.apmr.2011.12.014

Doherty, R. B., & Crowley, R. A. (2013). Principles supporting dynamic clinical care teams: An American College of Physicians Position Paper. *Annals of Internal Medicine, 159,* 620-626. doi:10.7326/0003-4819-159-9-201311050-00710

Eby, L. T., Allen, T. D., Evans, S. C., Ng, T., & DuBois, D. L. (2008). Does mentoring matter? A multidisciplinary meta-analysis comparing mentored and non-mentored individuals. *Journal of Vocational Behavior, 72,* 254-267. doi:10.1016/j.jvb.2007.04.005

Everett, L. (2011). Transformational leadership required to design and sustain evidence based practice: A system exemplar. *Western Journal of Nursing Research, 33*(3), 398. doi:10.1177/0193945910383056

Evidence-Based Medicine Working Group. (1992). Evidence-based medicine: A new approach in teaching the practice of medicine. *Journal of the American Medical Association, 268,* 2420-2425. doi:10.1001/jama.268.17.2420

Fineout-Overholt, E., & Johnston, L. (2006). Teaching EBP: Implementation of evidence: Moving from evidence to action. *Worldviews on Evidence-Based Nursing, 3*(4), 194. doi:10.1111/j.1741-6787.2006.00070.x

Fixsen, D.L., Naoom, S. F., Blasé, K. A., Friedman, R. M., & Wallace, F. (2005). *Implementation research: A synthesis of the literature.* Tampa, FL: University of South Florida, Louis de la Parte Florida Mental Health Institution, The National Implementation Research Network (FMHI Publication #231).

Flemming, K. (1998). Asking answerable questions. *Evidence Based Nursing, 1,* 36-37.

Forsyth, K., Melton, J., & Mann, L. S. (2005). Achieving evidence-based practice: A process of continuing education through practitioner-academic partnership. *Occupational Therapy in Health Care, 19*(1/2), 211-227. doi:10.1080/j003v19n01_15

Freeth, D. S., Hammick, M., Reeves, S., Koppel, I., & Barr, H. (2005). *Effective interprofessional education: Development, delivery, and evaluation.* Hoboken, NJ: Wiley-Blackwell.

French, P. (1999). The development of EBN. *Journal of Advanced Nursing, 29,* 72-78.

Gebbie, K. M., Meier, B. M., Bakken, S., Carrasquillo, O., Formicola, A., Aboelela, S. W., ... Larson, E. (2007). Training for interdisciplinary health research. Defining the required competencies. *Journal of Allied Health, 37,* 65-70.

Glegg, S. M. N., Livingstone, R., & Montgomery, I. (2015). Facilitating interprofessional evidence-based practice in paediatric rehabilitation: Development, implementation and evaluation of an online toolkit for health professionals. *Disability Rehabilitation, Early Online,* 1-9. doi:10.3109/09638288.2015.1041616

Goldberg, D. G., Beeson, T., Kuzel, A. J., Love, L. E., & Carver, M. C. (2013). Team-based care: A critical element of primary care practice transformation. *Population Health Management, 16* (3), 150-156. doi:10.1089/pop.2012.0059

Goode, C. J., Fink, R. M., Krugman, M., Oman, K. S., & Traditi, L. K. (2011). The Colorado Patient-Centered Interprofessional Evidence-Based Practice Model: A framework for transformation. *Worldviews on Evidence-Based Nursing, 8,* 96-105. doi:10.1111/j.1741-6787.2010.00208.x

Gratton, L., & Erickson, T. (2007). 8 ways to build collaborative teams. *Harvard Business Review, 85,* 100-109.

Green, J. (2012). Editorial: Science, implementation, and implementation science. *Journal of Child Psychology and Psychiatry, 53,* 333-336. doi:10.1111/j.1489-7610.2012.00531.x

Haas, S. (2008). Resourcing evidence-based practice in ambulatory care nursing. *Nursing Economics, 26,* 319-322.

Hockenberry, M., Brown, T., Walden, M., & Barrera, P. (2009). Teaching evidence-based practice skills in a hospital. *The Journal of Continuing Education in Nursing, 40*(1), 28. doi:10.3928/00220124-20090101-08

Howkins, E., & Bray, J. (2008). *Preparing for interprofessional teaching: Theory and practice.* New York, NY: Radcliffe.

Institute of Medicine. (2003). *Health professions education: A bridge to quality.* Washington, DC: National Academies Press.

Institute of Medicine. (2013). *Interprofessional education for collaboration: Learning how to improve health from interprofessional models across the continuum of education to practice: Workshop summary.* Washington, DC: The National Academies Press.

Institute of Medicine. (2015). *Measuring the impact of interprofessional education on collaborative practice and patient outcomes.* Washington, DC: The National Academies Press.

Interprofessional Education Collaborative Expert Panel. (2011). *Core competencies for interprofessional collaborative practice: Report of an expert panel.* Washington, DC: Interprofessional Education Collaborative.

Kitson, A., Harvey, G., & McCormack, B. (1998). Enabling the implementation of evidence based practice: A conceptual framework. *Quality and Safety in Health Care, 7,* 149-158. doi:10.1136/qshc.7.3.149.

Manns, P. J., Norton, A. V., & Darrah, J. (2015). Cross-sectional study to examine evidence-based practice skills and behaviors of physical therapy. *Physical Therapy, 95*(4), 568-578. doi:10.2522/ptj.20130450

Mariano, K. D., Caley, L. M., Eschberger, L., Woloszyn, A., Volker, P., Leonard, M. S., & Tung, Y. (2009). Building evidence-based practice with staff nurses through mentoring. *Journal of Neonatal Nursing, 15*(3), 81. doi:10.1016/j.jnn.2009.01.005

McEvoy, M. P., Williams, M. T., & Olds, T. S. (2010). Development and psychometric testing of a trans-professional evidence-based practice profile questionnaire. *Medical Teacher, 32,* e373-e380. doi:10.3109/0142159X.2010.494741.

Melnyk, B. M. (2007). The latest evidence on the outcomes of mentoring. *Worldviews on Evidence-Based Nursing, 4,* 170-173. doi:10.1111/j.1741-6787.2007.00099.x

Melnyk, B. M., Fineout-Overholt, E., Giggleman, M., & Cruz, R. (2010). Correlates among cognitive beliefs, EBP implementation, organizational culture, cohesion, and job satisfaction in evidence-based mentors from a community hospital system. *Nursing Outlook, 58,* 301-308. doi:10.1016/j.outlook.2010.06.002

Melnyk, B. M., Fineout-Overholt, E., Gallagher-Ford, L., & Kaplan, L. (2012). The state of evidence-based practice in US nurses. Critical implications for nurse leaders and educators. *Journal of Nursing Administration, 42,* 410-417.doi:10.1097/nna.0b013e3182664e0a

Melnyk, B. M., Fineout-Overholt, E., & Mays, M. Z. (2008). The evidence-based practice beliefs and implementation scales: Psychometric properties of two new instruments. *Worldviews on Evidence-Based Nursing, 5,* 208-216.

Meyers, D. C., Durlak, J. A., & Wandersman, A. (2012). The quality implementation framework: A synthesis of critical steps in the implementation process. *American Journal of Community Psychology, 50,* 462-480. doi:10.1007/s10464-012-9522-x

Meyers, D. C., Katz, J., Chien, V., Wandersman, A., Scaccia, J. P., & Wright, A. (2012). Practical implementation science: Developing and piloting the quality implementation tool. *American Journal of Community Psychology, 50,* 481-496. doi:10.1007/s10464-012-9521-y

Michaelsen, L. K., Parmelee, D. X., McMahon, K. K., & Levine, R. E., (2008). *Team-based Learning for Health Professions Education.* Sterling, VA: Stylus.

Morgan, L. A. (2012). A mentoring model for evidence-based practice in a community hospital. *Journal for Nurses in Staff Development, 28,* 233-237. doi:10.1097/NND.0b013e318269feof

Mosser, G., & Begun, J. (2014). *Understanding teamwork in health care.* Columbus, OH: McGraw Hill Education.

Moyers, P. A., Finch Guthrie, P. L, Swan, A. R., & Sathe, L. A. (2014). Interprofessional evidence-based clinical scholar program: Learning to work together. *American Journal of Occupational Therapy, 68,* S23-S31. doi:10.5014/ajot.2014.012609

Nelson, S., Tassone, M., & Hodges, B. D. (2014). *Creating the health care team of the future: The Toronto Model for Interprofessional Education and Practice.* Ithaca, NY: Cornell University Press.

Newhouse R., Dearholt, S. L., Poe, S. S., Pugh, L. C., & White, M. (2007). *Johns Hopkins nursing evidence-based practice: Model and guidelines.* Indianapolis, IN: Sigma Theta Tau International.

Newhouse, R. P., & Spring, B. (2010). Interdisciplinary evidence-based practice: Moving from silos to synergy. *Nursing Outlook, 58*(6), 309-317. doi:10.1016/j.outlook.2010.09.001

Pentland, A. (2012). The new science of building great teams. *Harvard Business Review, 90,* 60-70.

Plastow, N. A. (2006). Implementing evidence-based practice: A model for change. *International Journal of Therapy and Rehabilitation, 13,* 464-469. doi:10.12968/ijtr.2006.13.10.22194

Proctor, E. (2007). Implementing evidence-based practice in social work education: Principles, strategies, and partnerships. Research on Social Work Practice, Online publication http://rsw.sagepub.com/content/early/2007/05/31/1049731507301523.

Ramani, S., Gruppen, L., & Kachur, E. K. (2006). Twelve tips for developing effective mentors. *Medical Teacher, 28,* 404-408. doi:10.1080/01421590600825326

Rogers, E. M. (2010). *Diffusion of innovations* (4th ed.). New York, NY: The Free Press.

Rycroft-Malone J., & Bucknall T. (2010). *Models and frameworks for implementing evidence-based practice: Linking evidence to action.* West Sussex, UK: Wiley-Blackwell.

Sackett, D. L., Rosenberg, W. M., Gray, J. A., Haynes, R. B., & Richardson, W. S. (1996). Evidence based medicine: What it is and what it isn't. *British Medical Journal, 312,* 71-72. doi:10.1136/bmj.312.7023.71

Salls, J., Dolhi, C., Silverman, L., & Hansen, M. (2009). The use of evidence-based practice by occupational therapists. *Occupational Therapy in Health Care, 23,* 134-145. doi:10.1080/07380570902773305.

Satterfield, J. M., Spring, B., Brownson, R. C., Mullen, E. J., Newhouse, R. P., Walker, B. B., & Whitlock, E. P. (2009). Toward a transdisciplinary model of evidence-based practice. *Milbank Quarterly, 87*(2), 368-390. doi:10.1111/j.1468-0009.2009.00561.x

Scheerer, C. R. (2007). Mentoring in occupational therapy: One state's status. *Occupational Therapy in Health Care, 21,* 17-33. doi:10.1300/j003v21n03_02

Soukup, S. ,& McCleish, J. (2008). Advancing evidence-based practice: A program series. *The Journal of Continuing Education in Nursing, 39*(9), 402-406.

Stern, D. T. (2006). *Measuring medical professionalism.* New York, NY: Oxford University Press.

Stetler, C. B. (2010). Stetler model. In J. Rycroft-Malone & T. Bucknall (Eds.), *Models and frameworks for implementing evidence-based practice: Linking evidence to action* (pp. 51-88). West Sussex, UK: Wiley-Blackwell.

Steurer, L. (2010). An evidence-based practice scholars program: One institution's journey toward excellence. *The Journal of Continuing Education in Nursing, 41*(3), 139-143. doi:10.3928/00220124-20100224-04

Stevens, J. M., Bise, C. G., McGee, J. C., Miller, D. L., Rockar, P. Jr., & De litto, A. (2015). Evidence-based practice implementation: Case report of the evolution of a quality improvement program in a multicenter physical therapy organization. *Physical Therapy, 95,* 588-599. doi:10.2522/ptj.201 30541

Taylor, M. C. (1997). What is evidence-based practice? *British Journal of Occupational Therapy, 60,* 470-473.

Thomas, A., & Law, M. C. (2014). Evidence-based practice supports among Canadian occupational therapists. *Canadian Journal of Occupational Therapy, 81*(2) 79-92. doi:10.1177/0008417414526972

Titler, M. G. (2010). Translation science and context. *Research and Theory for Nursing Practice, 24* (1), 35-55.

Titler, M. G., Kleiber, C., Steelman, V. J., Rakel, B. A., Budreau, G., Everett, L. Q., & Goode, C. J. (2001). The Iowa model of evidence-based practice to promote quality care. *Critical Care Nursing Clinics of North America, 13*(4), 497-509.

Van Achterberg, T., Schoonhoven, L., & Grol, R. (2008). Nursing implementation science: How evidence-based nursing requires evidence-based implementation. *Journal of Nursing Scholarship, 40*(4), 302-310. doi:10.1111/j.1547-5069.2008.00243.x

Wallen, G. R., Mitchell, S. A., Melnyk, B., Fineout-Overholt, E., Miller-Davis, C., Yates, J., & Hastings, C. (2010). Implementing evidence-based practice: Effectiveness of a structured multifaceted mentorship programme. *Journal of Advanced Nursing, 66,* 2761-2771.

Westfall, J., Mold, J., & Fagnan, L. (2007). Practice-based research: Blue highways on the NIH roadmap. *JAMA: The Journal of the American Medical Association, 297*(4), 403-406. doi:10.1001/jama.297.4.403

World Health Organization (WHO). (2010). *Framework for action on interprofessional education and collaborative practice.* Geneva: author.

Zawora, M. Q., O'Leary, C. M., & Bonat, J. (2015). Turning team-based care into a winning proposition. *The Journal of Family Practice, 64*(3), 159-164.

Zidarov, D., Thomas, A., & Poissant, L. (2013). Knowledge translation in physical therapy: from theory to practice. *Disability and Rehabilitation, 35* (18), 1571-1577. doi:10.3109/09638288.2012.748841

Ziviani, J., Wilkinson, S. A., Hinchliffe, F., & Feeney, R. (2015). Mapping allied health evidence-based practice: Providing a basis for organizational realignment. *Australian Health Review.* doi:10.1071/AH14161.

Zwarenstein, M., & Reeves, S. (2006). Knowledge translation and interprofessional collaboration: Where the rubber of evidence-based care hits the road of teamwork. *Journal of Continuing Education in the Health Professions, 26,* 46-54. doi:10.1002/chp

---

Supplemental materials for this chapter are available online.
Please refer to the sticker in the front of the book and enter the access code provided.

Establishing Partnerships and Organizational Readiness

Patricia L. Finch-Guthrie, PhD, RN

CHAPTER TOPICS

- Value of a partnership between a health care organization and a university
- What is a partnership?
- Types of partnerships
- Choosing a university or a health care organization for partnering
- Organizational readiness for interprofessional evidence-based practice
- Interprofessional evidence-based practice teamwork
- Mentor challenges
- Mentor techniques and mentor supports

PERFORMANCE OBJECTIVES

After reading this chapter, those developing an interprofessional evidence-based practice program will be able to do the following:

1. Identify the type of partnership between a health care organization and a university needed to develop a successful interprofessional evidence-based practice program.

2. Select a partner for an interprofessional evidence-based practice program that matches articulated expectations.

3. Use successful strategies for ensuring and maintaining the quality of a partnership for an interprofessional evidence-based practice program.

4. Select an interprofessional evidence-based practice framework or model that will drive the interprofessional evidence-based practice program.

5. Assess the readiness of the organization for interprofessional evidence-based practice.

Moyers, P. A., & Finch-Guthrie, P. L.
*Interprofessional Evidence-Based Practice:
A Workbook for Health Professionals* (pp 23-39).
© 2016 Taylor and Francis Group.

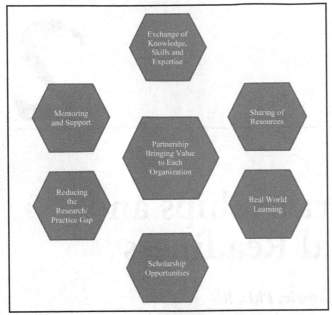

Figure 2-1. Mutually beneficial partnerships.

Interprofessional practice (IPP) and education (IPE) involve developing a variety of partnerships among disciplines within a health care organization, across several health care organizations, and within universities. Chapter 1 described a basic framework for an interprofessional evidence-based practice (EBP) program. This chapter focuses specifically on creating partnerships between health care organizations and a university in the process of developing an interprofessional EBP program. Creating a *strong education-practice interface* is essential for developing clinicians and practitioners in interprofessional EBP. According to the Toronto model for IPE and IPP (Nelson, Tassone, & Hodges, 2014, p. 81), the education–practice interface is about a reciprocal relationship between two organizations in which value for both occurs through new learning opportunities for clinicians and practitioners and through opportunities for students and faculty to be part of a health care team.

Unfortunately, universities have generally added IPE to the curricula without seeking input from the employers of health professionals and from patients and their families (Josiah Macy Jr. Foundation, 2013). IPE created solely within a university results in limited alignment with the priorities of health care organizations. IPE has a benefit for students who require preparation in team-based practice, faculty who need to role-model relevant team skills to students, and clinicians and practitioners who need development and strengthening of their interprofessional team skills.

Collaboration varies among disciplines and depends upon the setting of practice, such as long-term care, assistive living, home care, and clinics. Lack of collaboration lengthens the time it takes for the translation of evidence into practice regardless of the practice setting (Westfall, Mold, & Fagnan, 2007). Conducting interprofessional EBP through partnerships between a university and a health care organization is one method for creating a synergistic approach that benefits both organizations. Universities are often unable to provide opportunities for students that go beyond making recommendations from the literature to implementing and evaluating EBP solutions that address significant practice questions. Typically, the EBP curriculum housed within a university does not consider the time constraints practitioners experience in practice, address the varying skill needs of practicing clinicians, or include the full EBP process that ends with practice change and sustainability. Thus, clinicians often find it difficult to incorporate EBP into their daily practice in a meaningful way.

According to Lindbloom, Ewigman, and Hickner (2004), there is often a gap between the "possible" and the "practical" in delivering high-quality health care. Research networks or partnerships between health care organizations and universities assist with identifying important issues and outcomes that otherwise might go unexplored (pp. III-45). There is a need for practice to inform research and EBP questions, as well as for research to guide practice. Multiple disciplines recommend the use of partnerships between health care organizations and universities as an effective approach to advance EBP and to address the variation in the EBP and implementation knowledge and skills of practitioners and clinicians (Austin, Richter, & Frese, 2009; Bledsoe-Monsori et al., 2013; Crist, Munoz, Hansen, Benson, & Provident, 2005; Fineout-Overholt, Melnyk, & Schultz, 2005; Forsyth, Melton, & Mann, 2005; Proctor, 2007; Salls, Dolhi, Silverman, & Hansen, 2009; Thomas & Law, 2013).

VALUE OF A PARTNERSHIP BETWEEN A HEALTH CARE ORGANIZATION AND A UNIVERSITY

The elements of a mutually beneficial partnership include the following: (1) exchanging knowledge, skills, and experience; (2) sharing resources; (3) situating learning in real-world contexts; (4) providing scholarship opportunities; (5) reducing the research/practice gap; and (6) mentoring and supporting the EBP project (Figure 2-1). Partnerships create an exchange of knowledge, skills, and expertise between staff from the health care organization and the faculty and students from the university. Practitioners tend to have greater experience in practice, and faculty have more advanced EBP and research skills and experience with these processes. Practitioners understand the culture of a particular unit or department of the health care organization as embedded within the entire organizational culture. They are experts in understanding how this culture influences the workflow and practice patterns critical for interprofessional EBP implementation.

In terms of situating learning, faculty gain additional understanding of EBP as it is applied to daily practice, access to practice sites to further their scholarship, and real-world learning venues for students. Each organization contributes resources that have potential to strengthen the overall program and to reduce the research-to-practice gap, with faculty bringing their knowledge of EBP and research. Universities often have continuing education and research infrastructures that are beneficial for running an interprofessional EBP program, while the health care organization provides practice access to faculty and students, as well as financial support for practitioners to participate in the program.

Partnerships, while beneficial, require an understanding of the roles that each organization plays, the resources that each partner provides, the responsibilities unique to each, and the outcomes that are jointly expected. Each partner needs to ensure a return on investment considering the time, effort, commitment, and resources devoted to the interprofessional EBP program and its initiatives. Effective partnerships require mutual trust, openness, and equal opportunities for each organization in order to create a collaborative, interprofessional EBP learning experience. Before embarking on a university–health care organization partnership for an interprofessional EBP program, it is important to do the following: (1) define the word *partnership*, (2) identify the type of possible partnerships, (3) develop criteria for selecting a partner, (4) examine the assumptions guiding an effective partnership, and (5) determine criteria for success.

What Is a Partnership?

In business, a partnership is a legal entity formalized in contractual agreements that describe co-ownership of a business. Outside of a business context, the word *partnership* is used more loosely to mean a group that works together. The term *partnering* is often used to mean the same thing as the word *collaborating*. For the purpose of this chapter, a partnership is a relationship in which entities agree to work together to advance common interests through collaboration in order to achieve specific results. The important words in this definition are *relationship*, *agree*, *common interests*, and *results*. Positive relationships built on respect are the cornerstone of a partnership. Partners seek agreements prior to launching the interprofessional EBP program regarding the program elements, roles and responsibilities, and resources. Identifying common interests for the partnership serves to create a foundation for articulating expected results that become the goals for the interprofessional EBP program.

Types of Partnerships

An organization that is seeking a partner for an interprofessional EBP program should start with identifying the type of relationship or partnership wanted for their interprofessional EBP program. Two basic types of partnerships are *limited* or *full*. Limited partnership includes two types: participatory or consultative, which is based on the level of involvement and accountability of each entity. For example, a limited partnership may involve one partner who participates but who is not making decisions about the program itself and who instead provides more consultative support. Full partnerships do not necessarily have to be equal in terms of decision making, but generally both partners are involved in developing the program. Table 2-1 identifies the basic partnership types and their characteristic relationships among the entities involved.

No one type of partnership is better than another, but it is important to understand the differences between them. The type of partnership may depend on whether the health care organization or university seeks to develop a new program or expand an existing clinical scholar program into an interprofessional EBP program. If an EBP scholar program already exists within a health care organization, the university might receive an invitation to assist with expanding the program. The health care organization may have clear ideas and needs they want the university to develop and address. Health care organizations often view universities as a valuable resource, as long as the university partnership addresses issues, proposes solutions relevant to the patient/client populations, and most importantly is a university partner known for its history of sustaining partnerships (Checkoway, 2001). Universities may initiate a partnership with a health care organization for developing a stronger connection between research and practice and as such need to select a partner with similar goals. Thus, determining the type of partnership for the interprofessional EBP program and defining the boundaries of the partnership are important steps for identifying the best fit to meet the needs for both the health care organization and the university.

Choosing a University or a Health Care Organization for Partnering

It is important to get to know potential partners prior to launching a joint interprofessional EBP program. Partners who want to establish long-term relationships are more likely to continuously improve their level of collaboration and to remain committed to the relationship. Checklists in Table 2-2 and Table 2-3 are designed to help a health care organization or university select an appropriate partner.

TABLE 2-1	
TYPES OF PARTNERSHIPS	
TYPE OF PARTNERSHIP	**DESCRIPTION OF THE RELATIONSHIP**
Limited partnerships	1. *Participatory:* One partner participates fully in the work at the EBP team level, but is not involved in the overall program development or decisions regarding the overall program. 2. *Consultative:* One partner may serve in a consultative role, providing advice and recommendations for the program, but is not responsible for decisions about the program.
Full partnerships	1. *Unequal:* Both partners collaborate on the development and design of the program; however, one partner may have more decision-making power than the other partner. Accountability and responsibility may be less for the partner that has limited decision-making authority. 2. *Equal:* Both partners fully collaborate on the development and design of the program in which the decisions, accountability, and responsibilities for the program are shared.

TABLE 2-2
HEALTH CARE ORGANIZATION CHECKLIST FOR CHOOSING A UNIVERSITY PARTNER
√
Leadership: Strong, stable leadership, ability to deliver on agreements and represent the organization, sufficient power for decision making
Mission/vision: Compatible and complementary organizational mission and vision
Accountability: Doctoral prepared faculty, with a history of leadership, to serve as co-program coordinators with the health care organization
Capacity: Faculty experienced in clinical practice, IPE and IPP, EBP, research, grantsmanship, and dissemination
Commitment: Robust and resilient, sees projects through, history of delivering more than promised, capable of shared ownership
Diversity: Wide range of interprofessional health care degree programs and students
Culture: Track record of collaboration, cooperation, and willingness to understand the historical and social context of the health care organization
Innovation: History of developing innovative learning approaches
Resources: Ability to provide additional resources, such as learning technology platforms, learning modules, library access, continuing education accreditation, project management support, grant management
Finances: Financially stable organization
Reputation: High quality graduates, well known in the community, region, and nationally
* Grey shading denotes similar elements in both organizations

Both checklists have the same evaluation categories, specifically leadership, mission and vision, accountability, capacity, commitment, diversity, culture, innovation, resources, finances, and reputation. Some of the elements within the categories on the checklists are the same for both organizations, such as under the leadership category. Other elements described within the categories are unique to the type of setting. For example, under the category of diversity, a health care organization should have practitioners from a wide range of disciplines willing to serve as interprofessional EBP scholars. Interprofessional EBP is more likely to flourish with transformational leaders in health care organizations and in universities that encourage participatory decision making and a sense of inquiry that result in organizational learning.

TABLE 2-3		
UNIVERSITY CHECKLIST FOR CHOOSING A HEALTH CARE ORGANIZATION PARTNER		
√		
	Leadership: Strong, stable leadership, ability to deliver on agreements and represent the organization, sufficient power for decision making	
	Mission/vision: Compatible and complementary organizational mission and vision	
	Accountability: Doctoral or masters prepared clinician(s), with a history of leadership, to serve as co-coordinator with the university	
	Capacity: Health care clinicians with EBP education to serve as mentors	
	Commitment: Robust and resilient, sees projects through, history of delivering more than promised, capable of shared ownership	
	Diversity: Wide range of interprofessional health care clinicians willing to participate as scholars	
	Culture: Track record of collaboration, cooperation, and support for clinical research, demonstrates readiness for EBP (see section on organizational readiness for EBP).	
	Innovation: History of developing and implementing innovation in practice	
	Resources: Ability to provide resources, such as release time for scholars and mentors to participate, meeting space, clinical, quality improvement, and leadership experts	
	Finances: Financially stable organization	
	Reputation: High quality care and services, well known in the community	

* Grey shading denotes similar elements in both organizations

Bledsoe-Mansori et al. (2013) identified that universities with doctoral programs, those with older health care programs, and those more highly ranked were more likely to engage in a school-wide partnership effort around EBP with a health care organization. These authors also recommended that universities place a high priority on faculty participation in community partnerships in order to sustain a partnership long term. Preliminary meetings between potential partners are important in order for both organizations to explore whether there is a fit for working together to create and implement an interprofessional EBP program. Once partners determine they are willing to work together, the next step is to explore the assumptions that each partner has about the necessary relationship needed to ensure a successful program.

Assumptions for a Successful Partnership

Assumptions are beliefs that partners have about the proposed relationship; however, these assumptions are often not clearly articulated and can become the source of problematic relationships. In order to ensure a successful partnership for an interprofessional EBP, both organizations should articulate and operationalize the following assumptions:

- Partnering is a valuable endeavor based on a spirit of inclusivity.
- True participation within a partnership occurs with shared work and commitment.
- Follow-through is necessary to keep the partnership functioning.
- Open and frequent communication is central to maintaining a lasting partnership.
- Interdependency between partners, in which reciprocity (Green, Daniel, & Novick, 2001) exists with fair distribution of costs and benefits, is necessary.
- Emphasis on ongoing learning is a shared interest for all partners.
- Coordinators or leaders of the interprofessional EBP program pursue the highest degree of productivity, credibility, impact, and accountability (Jones & Wells, 2007).

Once assumptions or beliefs are articulated, the partners should formalize agreements in a memorandum of understanding or a similar type of formalized agreement to clarify provision of resources and to clarify the ownership of materials for the program (Jones & Wells, 2007). Memoranda of understanding are not as formal as a contract and are generally not as complex. However, in comparison to verbal agreements, memoranda of understanding are more formal and are more effective in making agreements transparent.

An effective memorandum of understanding addresses the purpose of the partnership, outlines the guiding principles behind the partnership, describes the responsibilities of the partners, and includes an overall statement of agreement. Leaders in both organization should work together to create the agreement, and those with the authority to deploy the resources must sign the agreement. If the partnership for the interprofessional EBP program continues, the memorandum of understanding needs annual review and updating. Table 2-4 offers an example of a memorandum of understanding that includes all of the important elements for outlining an effective agreement.

Criteria for a Successful Partnership

Themes in the literature regarding successful partnerships are shared goals and outcomes, strong relationships, information sharing, transparent decision making, ongoing assessment and evaluation, dissemination of results, sharing costs and products, and methods to ensure sustainability (Aikins et al., 2012; Crist et al., 2005; Rodgers et al., 2014; Szilagyi et al., 2014). The American College of Nursing (http://www.aacn.nche.edu/leading-initiatives/academic-practice-partnerships/tool-kit) and others (Christopher, Watts, McCormick, & Young, 2008; Meyer, Armstong-Cohen, & Batista, 2005) have identified important guiding principles for partnering between academic and health care organizations. Table 2-5 provides a list of strategies that partners should discuss and incorporate into their routines for delivering the interprofessional EBP program.

ORGANIZATIONAL READINESS FOR INTERPROFESSIONAL EVIDENCE-BASED PRACTICE

Prior to engaging in program development, it is important for both the university and the health care organization to conduct an organizational assessment for readiness for interprofessional EBP. To assess institutional readiness, a model that focuses on the organizational support systems necessary for EBP is helpful in enabling the partners to proactively identify and address potential barriers for the program. While different disciplines have created EBP models to guide the EBP process (see Chapter 1), many of these models focus on the process and assist in teaching the EBP steps to incorporate research and other forms of evidence into practice (Darrah, Loomis, Manns, Norton, & May, 2006; Schaffer, Sandau, & Diedrick, 2012). Some models are practice models that support using EBP in daily practice (Caldwell, Whitehead, Fleming, & Moes, 2008).

However, an extensive literature review did not identify an interprofessional organizational-level framework for EBP or an organizational EBP framework that was not discipline specific.

The advancing research and clinical practice through close collaboration (ARCC; Cliska et al., 2011) and the promoting action on research in health services (PARIHS; Rycroft-Malone, 2004) frameworks are two well-known organizational nursing models. These models were primarily developed for health care organizations when implementing EBP nursing practice; however, other disciplines and universities benefit when examining the framework in terms of the barriers that all disciplines face when implementing EBP and in terms of the way in which faculty prepare students to work in health care organizations. This chapter uses the PARIHS framework, which includes as core components evidence, context or quality of the organization or practice environment, and facilitation. Facilitation refers to strategies individuals and organizations use to make implementation of a practice change occur more smoothly.

Evidence

The evidence domain of the PARIHS framework concerns the value that individuals place on the use of research and other types of evidence in guiding practice. In universities, faculty members encourage students throughout the curricula to use evidence to support selection of assessment instruments and patient interventions. In health care organizations, clinicians and practitioners use evidence to develop standards of practice. While important evidence comes from studies that practitioners and clinicians review and deem relevant, research is only part of the evidence necessary for changing practice. The evidence domain also includes data and information stemming from practice and the patient/client experience, as well as from organizational quality improvement efforts.

A health care organization should explore how practitioners and clinicians use evidence and should identify the type of evidence they value. If practitioners and clinicians use research infrequently, then implementing an interprofessional EBP program is potentially more difficult. For example, Profetto-McGrath, Negrin, Hugo, and Smith (2010) found that nurses primarily valued knowledge stemming from practice and patient preferences. When using research, nurses often prefer qualitative approaches because of the focus on the patient experience. Manns, Norton, and Darrah (2015) found in a cross-sectional study that physical therapists primarily thought of evidence as research and saw patient experience and values as mutually exclusive from evidence. Some practicing physical therapists participating in the study stated that they did not like EBP because they perceived it as excluding patients from making decisions about their own care. Some faculty may value research over practice evidence and thus may prefer

TABLE 2-4

ELEMENTS OF A MEMORANDUM OF UNDERSTANDING

ELEMENT	FOCUS	EXAMPLE CONTENT
Statement of purpose	Reason for the partnership	This Memorandum of Understanding is entered into by the parties to identify the role of "put name of university" in supporting "put name of health care organization" in conducting its Interprofessional EBP in "year."
Guiding principles	Discussion about ownership of products and materials developed for the program, as well as sharing of evaluation data and costs	Both parties agree to co-own the learning modules created for the interprofessional EBP, allowing both parties to use the modules in other learning activities provided jointly or separately by the two institutions. Neither party will charge for use, except concerning normal use in the curriculum of the university, or will allow use of the modules by any third party without notification and mutual agreement of the two institutions. Both parties agree to share costs related to the educational aspects of the interprofessional EBP program (e.g., books, materials, etc.) with "name of health care organization" assuming responsibility for the clinical scholars and mentors; and "name of university" assuming responsibility for the students and faculty.
Responsibilities of the parties	Discussion of in-kind support for each partner	A university may provide the following type of resources and support: 1. A program coordinator for the EBP program who assumes responsibility for program management with the health care organization 2. Access to electronic learning platforms for learning modules and communication 3. Support for copyright clearance and access to university library resources 4. Support for conducting program evaluation 5. Support for technology to create learning modules 6. Provision of faculty experts in EBP and research 7. Education for EBP mentors for their development in EBP 8. Continuing Education credits A health care organization may provide the following resources and support: 1. Coordinator from the health care organization to work with the coordinator from the university 2. Time and financial support for EBP mentors and clinical scholars to participate 3. Provide access to students to participate, including agency orientation 4. Meeting space 5. Access to organization's learning platform for EBP modules 6. Parking for participants 7. Financial support for obtaining continuing education credits for different disciplines

(continued)

TABLE 2-4 (CONTINUED)

ELEMENTS OF A MEMORANDUM OF UNDERSTANDING

ELEMENT	FOCUS	EXAMPLE CONTENT
Statement of agreement and signature lines	At the end of the document, a statement should indicate that both partners agree to the elements identified in the agreement.	Both parties agree to principles and in-kind support outlined in the Memorandum of agreement. Date and year Places for each decision leader of the institutions to sign

TABLE 2-5

SUPPORTS AND STRATEGIES FOR SUCCESSFUL PARTNERSHIPS

1. Mutually established goals and objectives for the program and for the individual projects: goals and outcomes set for the program as a whole and for each phase of the program, objectives developed for the EBP learning modules

2. Development of strong relationships built on trust and accountability: criteria determined for selecting program coordinators, interprofessional team members, and participants, identification of responsibilities for co-coordinators from the university and health care organization, roles and responsibilities clarified for mentors of the interprofessional teams

3. Specific methods for communicating that include planned meetings (virtual and face-to-face) throughout the program for co-coordination of the EBP program: planning sessions for developing the program, routine meetings focusing on solving problems and issues that occur with program implementation, formative program evaluation meetings at critical points of the program

4. Routine information sharing: occurs as part of basic operations, progress in meeting goals and objectives of the program, updates on progress of the work from the interprofessional EBP teams, reporting of incurred costs

5. Transparency in decision making: needed decisions are clearly described, who makes the decision is identified, impact of decisions are explored prior to making final decisions, the right expertise is sought when needed to make informed decisions

6. Ongoing assessment and evaluation of the partnership: proactive problem solving, timely resolution of issues between partners, creating a safe environment for honest discussions, co-created summative evaluation processes, methods to assist with continuous improvement of the EBP program and supports shared learning between partners.

7. Follow through: shared plans for dissemination within and between organizations, locally, regionally, nationally, and internationally for the work of the EBP teams, as well as the outcomes of the partnership

8. Sharing of products, technology, and costs: Use of memorandums of understanding to outline costs and in-kind support prior to implementing an EBP program, discussion of costs and products not identified prior to the program as developed or incurred, sharing technology for virtual meetings, learning, document management, managing and analyzing data

9. Plans for sustainability and building on the partnership: public recognition and marketing of the partnership internally and externally, development of reports on program outcomes, planned celebration

quantitative methods, especially randomized controlled trials. Faculty may need to learn to listen to the practice experience of practitioners and clinicians from various disciplines and develop openness to other research traditions and perspectives.

In independent EBP surveys, physical therapists, occupational therapists, social workers, and allied health workers identified that while they support EBP, it was difficult to implement because it requires additional searching, appraisal, and literature synthesis skills (Graham, Robertson, & Anderson, 2013; Jette et al., 2003; Lyons, Brown, Tseng, Casey, & McDonald, 2011; Parrish & Oxhandler, 2015; Thomas & Law, 2013; Ziviani, Wilkinson, Hinchliffe, & Feeney, 2015). As documented in various studies from a variety of disciplines, skill issues for EBP are not unique to any one discipline (Hadley, Hassan, & Khan, 2008; Melnyk et al., 2004; Rezazadeh, Hachesu, Rezapoor, & Alireza, 2014). Faculty members who have not learned EBP as a part of their initial professional and graduate education may also need more learning opportunities (Blanco, Capello, Dorsch, Perry, & Zanetti, 2014; Bledsoe-Mansori et al., 2013). Faculty members might not have experience working for health care organizations that valued EBP prior to entering academia.

To address the skill issues regarding the use of research, the partnering organizations might offer interprofessional EBP learning modules and sessions to all staff and faculty rather than only to participants in the interprofessional EBP program. Additionally, putting the EBP learning modules online makes the program offerings available to staff, faculty, and students who cannot physically attend. In addition, the interprofessional EBP team may need to design educational sessions for staff throughout the implementation phases of a practice change the team is launching.

Practitioners from multiple disciplines have consistently reported time restrictions for using EBP since discipline-focused surveys were first conducted about EBP (Fairhurst & Huby, 1998; Graham et al, 2013; Jette et al., 2003; Kajermo, Nordstrom, Krusebrant, & Bjorvell, 1998; Lyons et al., 2011; Manns et al., 2015; McColl, Smith, White, & Field, 1998; Nilsagard & Lohse, 2010; Turner & Whitfield, 1997). In addition, time is also a barrier cited most frequently for health care organization and university research and EBP partnerships (Bledsoe-Mansori et al., 2013). The commonality of time as an issue for implementing EBP and maintaining a partnership indicates that those developing an interprofessional EBP program must strategically address time as a factor; otherwise, time creates barriers for program success.

Strategies for addressing time management include thoughtful discussions about team composition, team roles, and preparation for assuming team roles. Interprofessional EBP teams should include enough members to enable dividing the work in order to lessen the time that any one discipline spends on each EBP step. Effective learning modules that improve team skills decrease the wasted time that can occur when searching and appraising evidence. Including experts such as librarians and library science students as members of the interprofessional EBP teams facilitate the searching skills of all team members. In addition, faculty should find ways that students' team experience and work can become part of their course work (e.g., research papers, graduate student projects, practicums, and capstone projects).

Health care organizations and universities need to provide time for the coordinators of the program, clinical scholars, mentors, and faculty to participate in the interprofessional EBP program as part of their roles within their institutions. For example, the university could include the role of the interprofessional EBP program coordinator as part of the course load of the individual faculty member who takes on this very important role rather than adding responsibilities onto an already full annual assignment. To incorporate the work as a team member into the faculty member's course load, universities should examine sources of funding to cover release time or ways to incorporate the interprofessional EBP program into courses the faculty members are already teaching, such as practicum, fieldwork, or leadership experiences. Increased external funding opportunities for supporting the collaboration is one of the most important facilitators of health care organization and university partnerships for EBP (Bledsoe-Mansori et al., 2013). Funding includes not only national sources, but also those from regional and local institutions.

Focusing the interprofessional EBP program on an area of practice that the health care organization has identified as a priority for improvement may make it easier for mentors and practitioners to have project time. The focus on health care organizational initiatives means that the interprofessional EBP team has the potential to affect the organization's overall improvement strategy with their project. The interprofessional EBP program could select a theme, such as pain management, fall prevention, pressure ulcers, or delirium prevention. Each team identifies a unique project that addresses the overall theme of the organization's quality improvement goals.

Faculty and students may have trouble initially viewing the focus of the health care organization as pertinent to their disciplines. Consequently, they may push the interprofessional EBP team to change the clinical scholar's original topic, or they may not volunteer to participate in the first place. In these situations, the program coordinator from the university side of the partnership will need to facilitate a broader understanding of a patient-centered focus rather than approaching the EBP project from only a disciplinary perspective. In fact, the EBP team members may be surprised how a variety of disciplines can address the topic.

Context of the Interprofessional Evidence-Based Practice Program

The context domain of the PARIHS framework includes having a receptive environment for EBP, which comprises not only adequate physical space, presence of computers, and access to EBP databases, but also encompasses supportive professional and social networks within the health care organizational or university systems that facilitate teamwork and team-based care. Context for interprofessional EBP is also dependent on each practitioner's understanding and support of EBP and, in the case of the university, the faculty member's knowledge of EBP. Several researchers (Graham et al., 2013; Hadley et al., 2008; Melnyk, Fineout-Overholt, Giggleman, & Cruz, 2010) have determined that the beliefs of individuals about EBP influence their ability to implement EBP. While EBP skills are necessary, positive beliefs play a major role in facilitating implementation of EBP. Thus, assessing the EBP beliefs of staff, faculty, and students may assist in determining EBP readiness for both the health care organization and the university. Based on the assessment, interprofessional EBP learning modules and classes can include strategies that create a belief that EBP is doable, essential for patient care, and part of the roles of all practitioners and clinicians, faculty, and students.

Other essential elements of context include organizational and university culture, type of leadership practiced, and use of feedback mechanisms normally used to make change happen. Learning organizations routinely evaluate their processes and outcomes, building effective feedback systems for individuals, teams, and the system. Organizations with strong hierarchical structures and authoritarian approaches for problem solving may find it difficult to support interprofessional EBP. The organizational and university culture, including the institution's beliefs and values, significantly affects either positively or negatively the clinical practice in health care organizations and the educational practice in universities (Bledsoe-Mansori et al., 2013; Crist et al., 2005; Estrada, 2009).

Interprofessional EBP is more likely to flourish with transformational leaders in health care organizations and in universities that encourage participatory decision making and a sense of inquiry that results in organizational learning. Caldwell et al. (2008) and Wilkinson, Nutley, and Davies (2011) argue that the attitudes and actions of leaders significantly affect EBP implementation independent of the overall organizational culture. Thus, the support for EBP of frontline leaders in the health care organization and the support of deans in schools of nursing, medicine, health professions, or public health are essential for an effective interprofessional EBP program. Prior to starting an interprofessional EBP program, leaders in the health care organization and the university may need education about the leadership role for EBP so that they can support staff members and faculty and students participating in the program. Ongoing meetings between the manager of a unit or department within the health care organization and the interprofessional EBP team should be geared toward sharing evidence and obtaining input. These consistent communications between the EBP team and the manager of the unit or department within the health care organization lead to stronger support for the practice change.

Facilitation of Evidence-Based Practice

Facilitation, as described in the PARIHS framework, is critical for EBP and occurs when mentors or advisors assist staff, faculty, and students in implementing EBP and when systems within the health care organization and the university exist that support health professionals using EBP in daily practice (Melnyk, Fineout-Overholt, Gallagher-Ford, & Kaplan, 2012; Melnyk, Fineout-Overholt, Gallagher-Ford, & Stillwell, 2011; Nilsagard & Lohse, 2010). Mentors need clear roles for working with clinical scholars and the interprofessional team on EBP initiatives, as well as skills and expertise for mentoring, interprofessional teaming, and EBP (see Chapter 3). When a health care organization has few mentors or universities have few faculty with the skills needed, several strategies and supports exist that are helpful. The interprofessional EBP partners can design and offer education programs just for mentors focused on EBP, interprofessional teamwork, and mentoring (Forsyth et al., 2005). Scheduling and planning problem-solving meetings for the mentors are essential for creating a successful experience (see Chapter 3).

Other EBP facilitators and supports that assist with EBP implementation include systems in the health care organization that link EBP guidelines, library databases, and other evidence sources to the electronic health record. Making EBP resources easily available and embedding them in the workflow processes of the practitioner makes the use of evidence more likely and facilitates interprofessional EBP as the standard approach for providing care. An interprofessional EBP program should incorporate the health care organization's evidence sources that are routinely accessible as a strategy to re-enforce their routine use. University faculty and students may not know about specific national guidelines that are in use and may benefit from accessing the health care organization's EBP resources with their assigned interprofessional EBP team. When EBP facilitation systems are not available in the health care organization, the interprofessional EBP program coordinators may need to brainstorm about methods for introducing EBP sources to the practice areas, such as posting evidence on the unit's bulletin boards, conducting journal clubs on the topic, creating email evidence updates, and attending the clinical area practice meetings to present new information.

Another important strategy (Dearholt & Dang, 2012; Tilter et al., 2001) for preparing an effective interprofessional EBP program is for the program planning team to select a specific EBP model or framework as identified in

Chapter 1 (e.g., the Iowa model of evidence-based practice to promote quality care [Titler et al., 2001] or the Johns Hopkins nursing EBP model [Dearholt & Dang, 2012]). A specified interprofessional EBP model assists the program coordinators in developing education, structuring the program and the EBP process, and devising communications about the program to partnering organizations and staff, faculty, and students. A visual representation of the selected EBP framework helps to create shared mental models for the work of the interprofessional EBP team (see Chapter 4). It is important to understand, however, that differences in EBP occur among staff with different health care roles. For example, EBP for social workers and public health practitioners includes more of a focus on the community. It is beneficial for the creators of the interprofessional EBP program to consider adopting the transdisciplinary model of EBP (Satterfield et al., 2009) that includes universal EBP concepts.

In summary, the primary principle of the PARIHS framework is that successful implementation of EBP within an organization is a function of the three domains and their interrelationships. Thus, the planning team for an interprofessional EBP program should consider the potential effect of evidence, context, and facilitation on the success of the program and based on that assessment develop strategies to address any gaps. A variety of assessment instruments exist that may assist with determining readiness (Table 2-6).

INTERPROFESSIONAL EVIDENCE-BASED PRACTICE TEAMWORK

Interprofessional teamwork is essential for the success of the interprofessional EBP program (see Chapter 1). Frequently, practitioners in a variety of health care disciplines believe they are collaborating and do not recognize the need to improve teamwork abilities and skills. Common conflicts among disciplines result from misunderstandings and assumptions about the roles of each professional; poor communication; and differences in perspectives, values, beliefs, culture, and language (Hall, 2005). In addition, health care organizations often have not structured the practice areas, or the university has not created departments to promote interprofessional EBP collaboration. For example, health care organizations may not have meeting rooms in the care areas, department leaders may not build the time for meetings into care routines, and job descriptions may not include interprofessional EBP collaboration. Universities may not have space for bringing the faculty and students together from multiple programs, or program schedules might be out of sync with the class schedules of other programs. Caseloads and reimbursement that focus on the number of patients/clients seen sometimes preclude interprofessional EBP teamwork in health care organizations.

In general, best practices for IPE and team-based practice overall are still not well-defined (Abu-Rish et al., 2012). Thus, it is important for the planners of an interprofessional EBP program to assess the skills, knowledge, and attitudes that disciplines have about interprofessional EBP education and practice within both organizations (see Chapter 1). Based on these organizational assessments of collaboration, the interprofessional EBP planning committee may need to incorporate team learning and evaluation of teamwork into the program.

MENTOR CHALLENGES

Mentors of the interprofessional EBP teams may face issues and challenges regarding the interprofessional EBP partnership because of the cultural differences between the academic and health care organizations. Because many clinical staff are hourly paid employees, the health care organization needs to ensure that practitioners in the program are managing their time and not working overtime because of the interprofessional EBP program. This focus on hourly paid time might seem foreign to academic team members. Faculty and students may not understand the importance of the focus, especially when faculty classify their involvement on the team as university service. In addition, the health care organization may not realize that faculty and student time is based on an academic calendar. Consequently, students may graduate prior to completing the project, and faculty may have 9-month contracts and be off contract during summer months. When time commitments are not discussed proactively, staff of the health care organization may feel unsupported during some of the phases of the project. Team members may need to change mid-project. Consequently, the mentors and program coordinators need to anticipate and plan for transitions in team membership.

Team members from the health care organization and the university may have different ways they approach decision making based on their organizational culture. In the health care organization, patient care decisions are often immediate, whereas academic team members may prefer a decision-making style that includes more dialogue and debate. Practitioners may perceive an extended dialogue as wasting time and may see debate as interprofessional conflict rather than a scholarly exchange. Practitioners may view faculty as having an "ivory tower" perspective that is impractical or unrealistic, whereas faculty may believe the team is ignoring research evidence in developing a project plan. In addition, because faculty are used to guiding students, they may inadvertently treat clinical scholars as students, forgetting that clinicians are their colleagues. As a result, the clinical scholar may believe that faculty team members are taking over the project because of their advanced research and interprofessional EBP knowledge.

Table 2-6

Assessment Instruments for Determining Interprofessional EBP Readiness

INSTRUMENTS	SOURCES	DESCRIPTION
Evidence-Based Practice Assessment of Clinicians		
Knowledge of Research Evidence Competencies (K-REC)	Lewis, Williams, & Olds, (2011). Development and psychometric testing of an instrument to evaluate cognitive skills of evidence based practice in student health professionals. *BMC Medical Education, 11*, 77.	Assessment of cognitive skills of EBP in entry-level student health professionals
Evidence-Based Practice Beliefs and Implementation Scales	Melnyk, Fineout-Overholt, & Mays, (2008). The evidence-based practice beliefs and implementation scales: Psychometric properties of two new instruments. *Worldviews on Evidence-Based Nursing, 5(4)*, 208-216.	Measurement of an individual's beliefs about the importance of EBP and the capacity to implement
Evidence-Based Practice Attitude Scale (EBPAS)	Melas, Zampetakis, Dimopoulou, & Moustakis, (2012). Evaluating the properties of the evidence-based attitude scale (EBPAS) in health care. *Psychological Assessment, 24(4)*, 867-876.	Measures the attitudes toward the adoption of innovation and EBP in mental health service settings
Evidence-Based Practice Questionnaire	Upton & Upton, (2005). Nurses' attitudes to evidence-based practice: Impact of a national policy. *British Journal of Nursing, 14*, 284-288.	Assessment of knowledge, skills, and attitudes of EBP, as well as barriers to EBP
Self-Efficacy in Evidence-Based Practice (SE-EBP) and Outcome Expectancy for Evidence-Based Practice (OE-EBP)	Chang & Crowe, (2011). Validation of scales measuring self-efficacy and outcome expectancy in evidence-based practice. *Worldviews on Evidence-Based Nursing, 8 (2)*, 106-115.	Measures health professionals' confidence in the EBP process and the outcomes for a practice based on evidence
Evidence-Based Practice Confidence Scale	Salbach, Jaglal, & Williams, (2013). Reliability and validity of the evidence-based practice. confidence (EPIC) scale. *Journal of Continuing Education in the Health Care Professions, 33 (1)*, 33-40.	Measures self-efficacy and belief regarding EBP for physical therapists
Evidence-Based Practice Survey	Dopp, Stultjen, & Radel (2012). A survey of evidence-based practice among Dutch occupational Therapists. *Occupational Therapy International, 19*, 17-27.	Measures occupational therapists perceptions of EBP and the barriers for implementing EBP
Trans-professional Evidence-Based Practice Profile Questionnaire	McEvoy, Williams, & Olds, (2010). Development and psychometric testing of a trans-professional evidence-based practice profile questionnaire. *Medical Teacher, 32*, e366-373.	Designed for use across health professions and includes items that will change with education
Assessment of Evidence-Based Practice Environment		
Evidence-Based Practice Nursing Leadership and Work Environment Scales	Pryse, McDaniel, & Schafer, (2014). Psychometric analysis of two new scales: The evidence-based practice nursing leadership and work environment scales. *Worldviews on Evidence-Based Nursing, 11 (4)*, 240-247.	Designed to examine the practice environment and nursing leadership in which staff nurses practice. The aim is to measure elements that facilitate or serve as a barrier to evidence-based practice.

(continued)

TABLE 2-6 (CONTINUED)		
ASSESSMENT INSTRUMENTS FOR DETERMINING INTERPROFESSIONAL EBP READINESS		
INSTRUMENTS	**SOURCES**	**DESCRIPTION**
Assessment of Evidence-Based Practice Environment (continued)		
Organizational Readiness to Change Assessment (ORCA)	Helfrich, Li, Sharp, & Sales, (2009). Organizational readiness to change assessment (ORCA): Development of an instrument based on the Promoting Action on Research in Health Services (PARISH). *Implementation Science, 4*, 38.	Measures the quality of the evidence used in an organization's quality improvement program, organizational context for improvement, and the ability to facilitate change in practice
Context Assessment Index	McCormack, McCarthy, Wright, Slater, & Coffey, (2009). Development and testing of the context assessment index (CAI). *Worldviews on Evidence-Based Nursing. 6* (1), 27-35.	Used to assess the work context for EBP.
Questions to assess environmental readiness for using EBP to change practice	Smith, & Donze, (2010). Assessing environmental readiness: First steps in developing an evidence-based practice implementation culture. *Journal of Perinatal& Neonatal Nursing, 24* (1), 61-71.	Provides an extensive list of questions that an organization and interprofessional teams should ask prior to embarking on EBP that address organization structure, interdisciplinary teams, considerations for each discipline on the team, and patients/families
Assessment of Interprofessional Teams		
Attitudes Toward Interprofessional Teamwork and Education Scale	Curran, Sharpe, & Forristall, (2007). Attitudes of health science faculty towards interprofessional teamwork and education. *Medical Education, 1*, 892-896. Curran, Sharper, Forristall, & Flynn, (2008). Attitudes of health science students toward interprofessional teamwork and education. *Learning in Health and Social Care, 7* (3).	Assessment of attitudes regarding working on interprofessional health teams and the value of IPE
The Readiness for Interprofessional Learning Scale	McFadyen, Webster, Strachan, Figgins, Brown, & McKenchnie, (2005). The readiness for interprofessional learning scale: A possible more stable sub-scale model for the original version of RIPLS. *Journal of Interprofessional Care, 19* (6), 595-603.	Used to measure the attitudes of health students and professionals towards interprofessional learning
Assessment of Interprofessional Team Collaboration Scale (AITCS)	Orchard, King, Khalili, & Bezzina, M.B, (2012). Assessment of Interprofessional Team Collaboration Scale (AITCS): Development and testing of the instrument. *Journal of Continuing Education in The Health Professions, 32* (1), 58-67.	Measures elements of collaboration (i.e., partnership, cooperation, coordination, and shared decision making).

Differences in governance structures in health care organizations and universities may also lead to confusion regarding the team's decision-making process. Implementation of an interprofessional EBP project may require approval from multiple leaders or committees within the health care organization, which may delay implementation of the project. Universities may provide leadership in obtaining grants for the interprofessional EBP team's project, with the academic setting managing the project funds. The university's grant management systems may create an imbalance in power for the team because of the partner who controls the funds.

Health care organizations, on the other hand, control clinical access to some EBP team members. Health care organizational policies and procedures may limit faculty and student involvement in the project unless they go through the required on-boarding or credentialing processes. In addition, student involvement and level of work may require approval from other faculty and the chair of the respective academic department, who may not be part of the interprofessional EBP team. Thus, the team may have trouble delegating work to students on the team. While problems do occur between partners at the EBP interprofessional team level, mentor techniques and mentor supports help mentors and teams address problems proactively with the partnership.

MENTOR TECHNIQUES AND MENTOR SUPPORTS

The mentor assists the team in recognizing partnership issues, identifying resources that support the partnership, solving problems related to partnership issues, and ensuring implementation of improvement strategies. Some key mentoring techniques and mentor supports from the program coordinators that manage the partnership include the following:

- Creating a team environment that is transparent and safe for discussing issues among team members

- Anticipating differences in organizational culture that may affect team performance

- Supporting the team in creating a decision-making process that fits both organizational cultures

- Facilitating discussions about differences in organizational governance structures

- Maintaining awareness of situations that can destabilize the partner relationships

- Addressing behaviors of difficult team members

- Obtaining support from program sponsors when assistance is needed regarding potential clashes in culture

- Ensuring equal work load from team members from the different institutions

- Using the expertise and skills that each team member from the different organizations brings to the partnership

SUMMARY

Partnerships between a university and a health care organization for conducting an interprofessional EBP program provide mutual benefits for both organizations. Each partner brings skills and expertise, resources, and opportunities needed to decrease the research-to-practice gap

that currently exists. Understanding the type of partnership needed (i.e., limited or full), using selection criteria to examine organizational fit and capability, and addressing the strategies, techniques, and supports for successful partnerships help mitigate partnership issues. Prior to engaging in a partnership, it is important to assess each organization's readiness to engage in interprofessional EBP, as well determine the ability of employees from each organization to work in teams. Based on these assessments, the organizations may need to do some pre-work to prepare for participating in an interprofessional EBP program, such as educating mentors to understand the potential partnership issues and the mentor techniques that support the development and continuation of a strong partnership between the health care organization and the university.

REFLECTION QUESTIONS

1. Discuss the culture of your organization using the PARIHS framework and determine readiness issues that may exist for starting an interprofessional EBP program.

2. How developed is your organization concerning disciplines working together as an interprofessional team? Think about the disciplines that work well together, as well as those that may not routinely work in a team-based approach and the learning they may need.

REFERENCES

Abu-Rish, E., Kim, S., Choe, L., Varpio, L., Malik, E., White, A. A., ... Zieler, B. (2012). Current trends in interprofessional education of health sciences students: A literature review. *Journal of Interprofessional Care, 26*, 444-451. doi:10.3109/13561820.2012.715604

Aikins, A. D., Arhinful, D., Pitchforth, E., Ogedegbe, G., Allotey, P., & Agyemang, C. (2012). Establishing and sustaining research partnerships in Africa: A case study of the UK-Africa Academic Partnership on Chronic Disease. *Globalization and Health, 8*, (29). doi:10.1186/1744-8603-8-29

Austin, T. M., Richter, R. R., & Frese, T. (2009). Using a partnership between academic faculty and a physical therapist liaison to develop a framework for an evidence-based journal club: A discussion. *Physiotherapy Research International, 14*(4), 213-223. doi: 10.1002/pri.444

Blanco, M. A., Capello, C. F., Dorsch, J. L., Perry, G., & Zanetti, M. L. (2014). A survey study of evidence-based medicine training in US and Canadian medical schools. *Journal of Medical Library Association, 102*(3), 160-168. doi:10.3163/1536-5050.102.3.005

Bledsoe-Mansori, S. E., Bellamy, J. L., Wike, T., Grady, M., Dinata, E., Killian-Farrell, C., & Rosenberg, K. (2013). Agency-university partnerships for evidence-based practice: A national survey of schools of social work. *Social Work Research, 37*(3), 179-193. doi:10.1093/swr/svt015

Caldwell, E., Whitehead, M., Fleming, J., & Moes, L. (2008). Evidence-based practice in everyday clinical practice: Strategies for change in a tertiary occupational therapy department. *Australian Occupational Therapy Journal, 55,* 79-84.doi:10.1111/j.1440-1630.2007.00669.x

Chang, A. M. & Crowe, L. (2011). Validation of scales measuring self-efficacy and outcome expectancy in evidence-based practice. *Worldviews on Evidence-Based Nursing, 8*(2), 106-115. doi:10.1111/j.1741-6787.2011.00215.x

Checkoway, B. (2001). Renewing the civic mission of the American Research University. *Journal of Higher Education, 72*(2), 125-147. doi:10.2307/2649319

Christopher, S., Watts, V., McCormick, A., & Young, S. (2008). Building and maintaining trust in a community-based participatory research partnership. *American Journal of Public Health, 98*(8), 1398-1406. doi:10.2105/ajph.2007.125757

Cliska, D., DiCenso, A., Melynk, B. M., Fineout-Overholt, E., Stettler, C. B., Cullent, L.,...Dang, D. (2011). Models to guide implementation of evidence-based practice. In B. M. Melynk & E. Fineout-Overholt (Eds.) *Evidence-Based Practice in Nursing and Healthcare: A Guide to Best Practice* (pp. 241-275). Philadelphia, PA: Wolters Kluwer.

Crist, P., Munoz, J. P., Hansen, A. M. W., Benson, J., & Provident, I. (2005). The practice scholar program: An academic-practice partnership to promote the scholarship of best practices. *Occupational Therapy in Health Care, 19*(1/2), 71-93. doi:10.1300/j003v19n01_06

Curran, V. R., Sharpe, D., & Forristall, J. (2007). Attitudes of health science faculty towards interprofessional teamwork and education. *Medical Education, 1,* 892-896. doi:10.1111/j.1365-2923.2007.02823.x

Curran, V. R., Sharpe, D., Forristall, J., & Flynn, K. (2008). Attitudes of health science students toward interprofessional teamwork and education. *Learning in Health and Social Care, 7*(3), 146-156. doi:10.1111/j.1473-6861.2008.00184.x

Darrah, J., Loomis, J., Manns, P., Norton, B., & May, L. (2006). Role of conceptual models in a physical therapy curriculum: Application of an integrated model of theory, research, and clinical practice. *Physiotherapy Theory and Practice, 22* (5) 239-250. doi:10.1080/09593980600927765

Dearholt, S. L., & Dang, D. (2012). Johns Hopkins nursing evidence-based practice: Models and Guidelines (2nd ed.) Indianapolis: Sigma Theta Tau International Honor Society of Nursing. doi:10.1016/j.nedt.2012.07.001

Dopp, C. M., Steultjens, E. M., & Radel, J. (2012). A survey of evidence-based practice among Dutch occupational therapists. *Occupational Therapy International, 19,* 17-27. doi:10.1002/oti.324

Estrada, N. (2009). Exploring perceptions of a learning organization by RNs and relationship to EBP beliefs and implementation in the acute care setting. *Worldviews on Evidence-Based Nursing, 6* (4), 2000-2009.

Fairhurst, K., & Huby, G. (1998). From trial data to practical knowledge: Qualitative study of how general practitioners have accessed and used evidence about statin drugs in their management of hypercholesterolemia. *British Medical Journal, 317,* 1130-1134. doi:10.1136/bmj.317.7166.1130

Fineout-Overholt, E., Melnyk, B. M., & Schultz, A. (2005). Transforming health care from the inside out: Advancing evidence-based practice in the 21st century. *Journal of Professional Nursing, 21*(6), 335-344.

Forsyth, K., Melton, J., & Mann, L. S. (2005). Achieving evidence-based practice: A process of continuing education through practitioner-academic partnership. *Occupational Therapy in Health Care, 19* (1/2), 211-227.

Graham, F., Robertson, L., & Anderson, J. (2013). New Zealand occupational therapists' views on evidence-based practice: A replicated survey of attitudes, confidence and behaviors. *Australian Occupational Therapy Journal, 60,* 120-128. doi:10.1111/1440-1630.12000

Green, L., Daniel, M., & Novick, L. (2001). Partnerships and coalitions for community based research. *Public Health Reports, 116* (Supplement 1), 20-31.

Hadley, J., Hassan, I., & Khan, K. S. (2008). Knowledge and beliefs concerning evidence-based practice amongst complementary and alternative medicine health care practitioners and allied health care professionals: A questionnaire survey. *BMC Complementary Alternative Medicine, 8,* 45. doi:10.1186/1472-6882-8-45

Hall, P. (2005). Interprofessional teamwork: Professional cultures as barriers. *Journal of Interprofessional Care, Supplement 1,* 188-196. doi:10.1080/13561820500081745

Helfrich, C. D., Li, Y., Sharp, N. D., & Sales, A. E. (2009). Organizational readiness to change assessment (ORCA): Development of an instrument based on the Promoting Action on Research in Health Services (PARISH). *Implementation Science, 4,* 38. doi:10.1186/1748-5908-4-38

Jette, D. U., Bacon, K., Batty, C., Carlson, M., Ferland, A., Hemingway, R. D., Hill, J. C., Ogilvie, L., & Volk, D. (2003). Evidence-based practice: Beliefs, attitudes, knowledge, and behaviors of physical therapists. *Physical Therapy, 83,* 786-805.

Jones, L., & Wells, K. (2007). Strategies for academic and clinician engagement in community-participatory partnered research. *Journal of the American Medical Association, 297*(4), 407-410. doi:10.1001/jama.297.4.407

Josiah Macy Jr. Foundation. (2013). Transforming patient care: Aligning interprofessional education with clinical practice redesign. Conference Recommendations, January 17-20, Atlanta, GA: www.macyfoundation.org.

Kajermo, K. N., Nordstrom, G., Krusebrant, A., & Bjorvell, H. (1998). Barriers to and facilitators of research utilization, as perceived by a group of registered nurses in Sweden. *Journal of Advanced Nursing, 27,* 798-807. doi:10.1046/j.1365-2648.1998.00614.x

Lewis, L. K., Williams, M. T., & Olds, T. S. (2011). Development and psychometric testing of an instrument to evaluate cognitive skills of evidence based practice in student health professionals. *BMC Medical Education, 11,* 77. doi:10.1186/1472-6920-11-77

Lindbloom, E. J., Ewigman, B. G., & Hickner, J. M. (2004). Practice-based research networks: The laboratories of primary care research. *Medical Care, 42,* Suppl, III-45-49. doi:10.1097/01.mlr.0000119397.65643.d4

Lyons, C., Brown, T., Tseng, M. H., Casey, J., & McDonald, R. (2011). Evidence-based practice and research utilization: Perceived research knowledge, attitudes, practices and barriers among Australian pediatric occupational therapists. *Australian Occupational Therapy Journal, 58*(3), 178-186. doi:10.1111/j.1440-1630.2010.00900.x

Manns, P. J., Norton, A. V., & Darrah, J. (2015). Cross-sectional study to examine evidence-based practice skills and behaviors of physical therapy. *Physical Therapy, 95*(4), 568-578.

McColl, A., Smith, H., White, P., & Field, J. (1998). General practitioners' perceptions of the route to evidence-based medicine: A questionnaire survey. *British Medical Journal, 316,* 361-365. doi:10.2522/ptj.20130450

McCormack, B., McCarthy, G., Wright, J., Slater, P., & Coffey, A. (2009). Development and testing of the context assessment index (CAI). *Worldviews on Evidence-Based Nursing. 6*(1), 27-35. doi:10.1111/j.1741-6787.2008.00130.x

McEvoy, M. P., Williams, M. T., & Olds, T. S. (2010). Development and psychometric testing of a trans-professional evidence-based practice profile questionnaire. *Medical Teacher, 32,* (9), e366-e380. doi:10.3109/0142159x.2010.494741

McFadyen, A. K., Webster, V., Strachan, K., Figgins, E., Brown, H., & Mckenchnie, J. (2005). The readiness for interprofessional learning scale: A possible more stable sub-scale model for the original version of RIPLS. *Journal of Interprofessional Care, 19*(6), 595-603. doi:10.1080/13561820500430157

Melas, C. D., Zampetakis, L. A., Dimopoulou, A., & Moustakis, V. (2012). Evaluating the properties of the evidence-based attitude scale (EBPAS) in health care. *Psychological Assessment, 24*(4), 867-876. doi:10.1037/a0027445

Melnyk, B. M., Fineout-Overholt, E., Feinstein, N., Li, H., Small, L., Wilcox, L., & Kraus, R. (2004). Nurses' perceived knowledge, beliefs, skills, and needs regarding evidence-based practice: Implications for accelerating the paradigm shift. *Worldviews of Evidence Based Nursing, 1*(3), 185-193. doi:10.1111/j.1524-475x.2004.04024.x

Melnyk, B.M., Fineout-Overholt, E., Gallagher-Ford, L., & Kaplan, L. (2012). The state of evidence-based practice in US nurses: Critical implications for nurse leaders and educators. *Journal of Nursing Administration, 42,* 9, 410-417. doi:10.1097/nna.0b013e3182664e0a

Melnyk, B. M., Fineout-Overholt, E., Gallagher-Ford, L., & Stillwell, S. B. (2011). Sustaining evidence-based practice through organizational policies and an innovative model. *American Journal of Nursing, 111*(9), 57-60. doi:10.1097/01.naj.0000405063.97774.0e

Melnyk, B. M., Fineout-Overholt, E., Giggleman, M., & Cruz, R. (2010). Correlates among cognitive beliefs, EBP implementation, organizational culture, cohesion and job satisfaction in evidence-based practice mentors from a community hospital system. *Nursing Outlook, 58*(6), 301-308. doi:10.1016/j.outlook.2010.06.002

Melnyk, B. M., Fineout-Overholt, E., & Mays, M. Z. (2008). The evidence-based practice beliefs and implementation scales: Psychometric properties of two new instruments. *Worldviews on Evidence-Based Nursing, 5*(4), 208-216. doi:10.1111/j.1741-6787.2008.00126.x

Meyer, D., Armstrong-Cohen, A., & Batista, M. (2005). How a community-based organization and an academic health center are creating an effective partnership for training and service. *Academic Medicine, 80*(4), 327-333. doi:10.1097/00001888-200504000-00004.

Nelson, S., Tassone, M., & Hodges, B. D. (2014). Creating the health care team of the future: The Toronto Model for Interprofessional Education and Practice. Ithaca, NY: Cornell University Press. doi:10.3163/1536-5050.103.2.014

Nilsagard, Y., & Lohse, G. (2010). Evidence-based physiotherapy: A survey of knowledge, behavior, attitudes and prerequisites. *Advances in Physiotherapy, 12,* 179-186. doi:10.3109/14038196.2010.503812

Orchard, C. A., King, G. A., Khalili, H., & Bezzina, M. B. (2012). Assessment of Interprofessional Team Collaboration Scale (AITCS): Development and testing of the instrument. *Journal of Continuing Education in The Health Professions, 32* (1), 58-67. doi:10.1002/chp.21123

Parrish, D. E., & Oxhandler, H. K. (2015). Social work field instructors' views and implementation of evidence-based practice. *Journal of Social Work Education, 51,* 270-286.

Proctor, E. (2007). Implementing evidence-based practice in social work education: Principles, strategies, and partnerships. Research on Social Work Practice, Online publication http://rsw.sagepub.com/content/early/2007/05/31/1049731507301523.

Profetto-McGrath, J., Negrin, K. A., Hugo, K., & Smith, K. B. (2010). Clinical nurse specialists' approaches in selecting and using evidence to improve practice. *Worldviews on Evidence-Based Nursing 7*(1), 36-50. doi:10.1111/j.1741-6787.2009.00164.x

Pryse, Y., McDaniel, A., & Schafer, J. (2014). Psychometric analysis of two new scales: The evidence-based practice nursing leadership and work environment scales. *Worldviews Evidence Based Nursing, 11*(4), 240-247. doi:10.1111/wvn.12045

Rezazadeh, E., Hachesu, P. R., Rezapoor, A., & Alireza, K. (2014). Evidence-based medicine: Going beyond improving care provider viewpoints, using and challenges upcoming. *Journal of Evidence Based Medicine, 7*(1), 26-31. doi:10.1111/jebm.12083

Rodgers, K. C., Akintobi, T., Thompson, W. W., Evans, D., Escoffery, C., & Kegler, M. C. (2014). A model for strengthening collaborative research capacity: Illustrations form the Atlanta Clinical Translational Science Institute. *Health Education & Behavior,* published online http://heb.sagepub.com/content/early/2013/12/04/1090198113511815.

Rycroft-Malone, J. (2004). The PARIHS framework: A framework for guiding the implementation of evidence-based practice. *Journal of Nursing Care Quality, 19*(4), 297-304. doi:10.1097/00001786-200410000-00002

Salbach, N. M., Jaglal, S. B., & Williams, J. I. (2013). Reliability and validity of the evidence-based practice confidence (EPIC) scale. *Journal of Continuing Education in the Health Professions, 33*(1), 33-40. doi:10.1002/chp.21164

Salls, J., Dolhi, C., Silverman, L., & Hansen, M. (2009). The use of evidence-based practice by occupational therapists. *Occupational Therapy in Health Care, 23*(2), 134-145. doi:10.1080/07380570902773305

Satterfield, J. M., Spring, B., Brownson, R. C., Mullen, E. J., Newhouse, R. P., Walker, B. B., & Whitlock, E. P. (2009). Toward a transdisciplinary model of evidence-based practice. *Milbank Quarterly, 87*(2), 368-390. doi:10.1111/j.1468-0009.2009.00561.x

Schaffer, M. A., Sandau, K. E., & Diedrick, L. (2012). Evidence-based practice models for organizational change: Overview and practical applications. *Journal of Advanced Nursing, 69*(5), 1197-1209. doi:10.1111/j.1365-2648.2012.06122.x

Smith, J. R. & Donze, A. (2010). Assessing environmental readiness: First steps in developing an evidence-based practice implementation culture. *Journal of Perinatal& Neonatal Nursing, 24*(1), 61-71. doi:10.1097/jpn.0b013e3181ce1357

Szilagyi, P. G., Shone, L. P., Dozier, A. M., Newton, G. L., Green, T., & Bennett, N. M. (2014). Evaluating community engagement in an academic medical center. *Academic Medicine, 89*(4), 585-595. doi:10.1097/acm.0000000000000190

Thomas, A., & Law, M. (2013). Research utilization and evidence-based practice in occupational therapy: A scoping study. *American Journal of Occupational Therapy, 67*, e55-e65. doi:10.5014/ajot.2013.006395

Titler, M. G., Kleiber, C., Steelman, V. J., Rakel, B. A., Budreau, G., Everett, C. L. Q., ... Goode, C. J. (2001). The Iowa model of evidence-based practice to promote quality care. *Critical Care Nursing Clinics of North America, 13*(4), 497-509.

Turner, P. A., & Whitfield, T. W. (1997). Journal readership amongst Australian physiotherapists: A cross-national replication. *Australian Journal of Physiotherapy, 43*, 197-202.

Upton, D. & Upton, P. (2005). Nurses' attitudes to evidence-based practice: Impact of a national policy. *British Journal of Nursing 14*(5), 284-288. doi:10.12968/bjon.2005.14.5.17666

Westfall, J. M., Mold, J., & Fagnan, L. (2007). Practice-based research—"Blue Highways" on the NIH roadmap, *Journal of American Medical Association, 297*(4), 403-406. doi:10.1001/jama.297.4.403.

Wilkinson, J. E., Nutley, S. M., & Davies, H. T. (2011). An exploration of the roles of nurse managers in evidence-based practice implementation. *Worldviews on Evidence-Based Nursing, 8*(4), 236-246. doi:10.1111/j.1741-6787.2011.00225.x

Ziviani, J., Wilkinson, S. A., Hinchliffe, F., & Feeney, R. (2015). Mapping allied health evidence-based practice: Providing a basis for organizational realignment. *Australian Health Review*. doi:10.1071/AH14161

Supplemental materials for this chapter are available online.
Please refer to the sticker in the front of the book and enter the access code provided.

3

Developing Deliberative and Reflective Mentoring

Penelope A. Moyers, EdD, OT/L, FAOTA and Patricia L. Finch-Guthrie, PhD, RN

CHAPTER TOPICS

- Overview of the mentor study
- Deliberative and reflective mentoring practice
- Putting it all together
- Future research

PERFORMANCE OBJECTIVES

With the completion of this chapter, the program coordinators and mentors will be able to do the following:

1. Design a program structure to support deliberative and reflective mentoring practice.

2. Assess the characteristics of team members as it might influence team productivity.

3. Identify potential macro-contextual barriers to team member work effort.

4. Assess the task demand of interprofessional EBP and implementation science tasks in order to modify these tasks to match team member capacity.

The previous two chapters provided an overview of an interprofessional evidence-based practice (EBP) program and strategies for developing a university and health care organization partnership. The guiding theories described in Chapter 1 for the interprofessional EBP program included literature regarding highly functioning teams. Chapter 2 continued the discussion regarding teams concerning organizational readiness for engaging in an interprofessional EBP program. This chapter furthers the team discussion and focuses on the team's mentor role as a facilitator of

optimal team performance for developing a highly functioning interprofessional EBP team. Often, health care organizations lack available mentors adequately trained in interprofessional EBP. The university might supplement the needs of the team with faculty mentors; however, this solution is not viable long term given that an important aspect of the mentoring role is knowledge of and comfort with the health care organization's workflow, priorities, and leadership.

Moyers, P. A., & Finch-Guthrie, P. L.
*Interprofessional Evidence-Based Practice:
A Workbook for Health Professionals* (pp 41-61).

Mentors are critical for continuing and accelerating the implementation of EBP within an organization (Melnyk et al., 2004; Melnyk & Fineout-Overholt, 2002; Melnyk, 2007; Novak & McIntyre, 2010; Wallen et al., 2010). Not only do clinical scholars and interprofessional EBP mentors need mentoring, but members of the entire team benefit from ongoing mentoring. In fact, support of mentoring is important for even the most experienced mentors given the demands on their time, the growing complexity of EBP and implementation science, and the rising expectations for EBP within the health care organization (Abdullah et al., 2014). In addition to knowledge and skills in interprofessional EBP, mentors must be adept at fostering the interprofessional competencies needed to support success of the interprofessional EBP project. These competencies include team values and ethics, roles and responsibilities for collaborative practice, communication, teamwork, and team-based care (Interprofessional Education Collaborative Expert Panel, 2011).

This chapter presents a mentoring theory for interprofessional EBP programs derived from our grounded theory study, which the Minnesota Nurses Foundation provided $10,000 in funding, conducted from January of 2012 through February of 2013. Two theoretical models informed the initial work in developing understanding of the mentoring process in interprofessional EBP programs. These two models were advancing research and clinical practice through close collaboration (ARCC) (Melnyk & Fineout-Overholt, 2012) and Darling's (1984) description of positive mentor roles and functions.

According to the ARCC model (Melnyk & Fineout-Overholt, 2012), clinicians who receive mentoring in interprofessional EBP have stronger beliefs associated with EBP and are more likely to implement evidence into practice (Wallen et al., 2010). Strengthening of the beliefs about EBP of clinicians and practitioners occurs as long as mentors have advanced knowledge and skills in EBP, mentorship, and practice change (Haas, 2008). While the ARCC model links mentoring with EBP implementation, the model does not clearly describe the mentoring process that leads to EBP implementation. Darling (1984) extrapolated three requirements for successful mentoring, which included attraction (between mentor and mentee), action (time and energy), and affect (mutual respect). Darling's work provided a conceptual place to start in understanding mentoring in terms of the roles mentors assume during the mentoring process. However, Darling's discussion of mentoring roles primarily focused on one-to-one mentoring and did not examine the mentoring roles specific to an interprofessional team and EBP. Thus, exploring the actual mentoring process that occurs within an interprofessional EBP program was necessary to determine whether these same mentoring concepts were relevant.

OVERVIEW OF THE MENTOR STUDY

As employees of St. Catherine University in St. Paul, Minnesota, and North Memorial Medical Center in Robbinsdale, Minnesota, respectively, when conducting the study, we collaboratively devised and implemented an interprofessional EBP program involving 37 participants distributed on five interprofessional teams. Each team's EBP project addressed the Medical Center's goal of improving pain management and enhancing patient comfort (Table 3-1).

Although clinicians from multiple disciplines may serve as mentors, the mentors in our study were advanced practice nurses or master's prepared nurse educators. When possible, the program coordinators should select mentors who have some knowledge of EBP; however, the ability to mentor others is the primary criteria as often these skills are the most difficult to develop in comparison to the more technical skills of EBP. It is crucial for the program coordinators to avoid the temptation to select mentors based primarily on organizational titles (e.g., director of rehabilitation) or disciplines with the greatest traditional sources of power, such as physicians. Physicians should provide mentorship if they have the requisite mentoring skills combined with knowledge in EBP. Most importantly, physicians and staff from other disciplines selected to mentor must have time for active involvement throughout the program.

In the mentoring study, because of limitations within the organization for implementing an interprofessional EBP program for the first time, the mentors had basic EBP knowledge and limited experience in mentoring an interprofessional team regarding EBP. The mentors graduated from master's degree programs before EBP was part of their respective curricula. Instead, their graduate programs focused on learning about the research process. The mentors had excellent interpersonal skills in interacting, leading, and serving on many different quality improvement and clinical teams, which made them good candidates for team mentors. However, most of the mentors had experience developing individual clinicians rather than an interprofessional team.

In these types of circumstances when few experienced mentors are available, the program coordinators need to implement plans to foster skill development so that mentors and the teams have a positive learning experience. Because of the mentor's lack of interprofessional EBP experience, three program coordinators mentored the mentors in the clinical scholar program; two of the coordinators are authors of this chapter. Although our first set of mentors did not quite have the requisite experience, we have since implemented another round of the interprofessional EBP program. Even though the second group of mentors was more experienced in EBP, the tenets of the mentoring theory and the components of the mentor supports as

TABLE 3-1

TEAM MEMBERS AND PROJECTS

PROJECT LENGTH	DISCIPLINES ON TEAMS	NUMBER OF TEAM MEMBERS	PROJECTS
1-year–long project	Occupational therapy; nursing; holistic health	2 students 3 faculty 2 mentors 2 scholars	Use of aromatherapy in managing pain for patients in the emergency department and on the trauma specialty care unit
6-month project	Occupational therapy; nursing; holistic health; physical therapy	2 students 2 faculty 1 mentor 1 scholar	Back pain post-angioplasty prior to sheath removal
1-year–long project	Occupational therapy; nursing; respiratory care	3 students 3 faculty 2 mentors 1 scholar	Assessing pain in the ventilated intensive care unit patient
1-year–long project	Occupational therapy; nursing; holistic health; physician assistant	3 students 3 faculty 1 mentor 1 scholar	Effectiveness of a clinical guideline and staff education to improve chronic pain management
1-year–long project	Exercise & sports science; nursing; holistic health	1 student 2 faculty 1 mentor 1 scholar	Use of aromatherapy prior to surgery for preventing nausea and vomiting in the post-anesthesia care unit

delineated in this mentoring study were helpful in ensuring that mentoring occurred for an interprofessional team in an efficient and effective manner.

The program coordinators designed and implemented the mentoring study, as well as triangulated data from multiple sources to derive the mentoring theory. The seven nursing mentors participated in an advanced interprofessional EBP course at St. Catherine University, attended three seminars on team mentoring, engaged in bimonthly mentor meetings that occurred throughout the program, and received monthly mentoring newsletters on such issues as improving communication, having crucial conversations, and maintaining motivation (see book website). It is important for program coordinators to assess the needs of mentors in terms of their knowledge and skills in EBP and implementation science, but also in leading and facilitating interprofessional teams. Frequently, the skill requiring the most development for mentors is EBP team leadership regardless of experience within a discipline, with a role within the health care organization, or with experience in EBP and implementation science.

Research Design and Methods

Because an initial theory of mentoring roles guided this study (Darling, 1984), grounded theory was selected to elaborate and further develop the theory as it might be used with interprofessional EBP teams. A grounded theory approach uses specific coding methods (Strauss, 1987; Strauss & Corbin, 1998). In open coding, where the concepts of the theory are discovered, constant comparison methods were used when triangulating data collected from participant observations, field notes, and interviews with mentors and team members. Axial coding verified the concepts and assisted with discovering relationships among concepts. Memos that explicated the details of the concept from the data and proposed relationships for further examination of the data were written during this phase of the study. Selective coding of the data linked the concepts together in a theoretical model around a central category of the mentoring phenomenon within an interprofessional EBP program. Table 3-2 provides a brief description of the grounded theory study methods, procedures, and analysis

TABLE 3-2

INTERPROFESSIONAL EVIDENCE-BASED PRACTICE PROGRAM MENTORING STUDY

STUDY DESIGN ELEMENTS	STUDY METHODS	DESCRIPTION OF METHODS
Data gathering	• Two mentor interviews of each mentor midpoint of program and at end of program; one interview with each team member about his or her experience on the team • Six group data gathering sessions involving mentors • Program coordinator and mentor participant observation of interprofessional EBP and mentor team meetings	*Mentor interview questions:* a) What has been your biggest challenge in mentoring? b) How did you use your mentoring strategies to address this challenge? c) What has been the relationship between your mentoring strategies and your team's development of interprofessional competencies? *Data gathering sessions:* card sorting, concept matching, and thematic verification
Procedures	• Audio recordings • Field notes • Transcription of audio recordings • Mentor and team member review of interview transcripts • Memos to triangulate data	Mentor and team member interviews Mentor data gathering sessions Mentor meetings Mentor workshops Interprofessional team meetings Project coordinator meetings EBP educational and team work sessions
Data analysis for triangulating data sources	• Open • Axial • Selective coding	*Open coding* involves constant comparison to elicit categories along with their properties and dimensions. *Axial coding* focuses on cause-and-effect relationships among categories. *Selective coding* involves integrating categories with the central theoretical concept that emerged.

strategies (Strauss, 1987; Strauss & Corbin, 1998). The study had institutional review board approval from both St. Catherine University and North Memorial Medical Center. All mentors and team members gave consent to participate in the study.

The research question for the study was: What is the process for mentoring an interprofessional EBP team in an interprofessional EBP program? There were two subquestions, as follows:

1. What is the process the program coordinators use to mentor the mentors and team members of interprofessional EBP teams?

2. What is the process the mentors use to mentor the interprofessional EBP team?

Grounded theory analysis of the data produced an understanding of two types of mentoring, from the program coordinators to the mentors and team members and from the mentors to their team members. Theory development also led to understanding the way in which the mentoring from program coordinators and mentors converged to facilitate the overall progress of the interprofessional EBP teams. The goal of this chapter is not to report the findings as one would in a research article, but instead to describe the theory that emerged from the study. Readers may contact the authors of this chapter to receive a more complete description of the study or refer to program results published elsewhere (Moyers, Finch Guthrie, Swan, & Sathe, 2014). In addition, this chapter lays out some suggestions for future research to continue studying the mentoring process used in an interprofessional EBP program.

REVIEW OF TENETS FROM THE MENTORING THEORY

To provide a background for an in-depth discussion throughout the chapter regarding the theory for mentoring an interprofessional EBP team, the basic mentoring tenets derived from the grounded theory study are summarized. All of the tenets and the description of these tenets were inductively derived from extensive data, including field notes, participant observations, and interviews of the mentors and team members conducted throughout the year-long interprofessional EBP program. Program coordinators and mentors should review this list of tenets because, in doing so, they will discover that mentoring is complex, the mentoring needs of the scholar and team change and become more difficult as the interprofessional EBP process is enacted, and the team itself and the environment affect mentoring. These tenets may lead the program coordinators to question whether they understand or know what mentor supports are needed throughout an interprofessional EBP program. Program coordinators should use this information when designing their interprofessional EBP program. Table 3-3 defines the concepts associated with these tenets and provides data or sample quotes from the interviews to support each proposition.

- Tenet 1: A successful interprofessional EBP program is carefully designed to create a supportive structure that fosters the reflective and deliberative mentoring practice of the mentors and the program coordinators.

- Tenet 2: Each of the nine phases of interprofessional EBP has its own characteristics involving mentor challenges, complexity of EBP and implementation science tasks, and team micro- and macro-contexts.

- Tenet 3: The characteristics of the phases interact to influence the work output and work quality of the teams on their EBP projects.

- Tenet 4: Mentor challenges indicate the team members' or the scholars' need for mentoring because of questions, barriers, disagreements, confusion, team relationship difficulties, and novel opportunities.

- Tenet 5: The complexity of the interprofessional EBP and implementation science tasks creates demands on team performance and may create mentor challenges.

- Tenet 6: The micro-context arises from the team dynamics because of individual team member and mentor personalities and the kinds of expertise and experience of team members and mentors.

- Tenet 7: The macro-context involves the external environment (e.g., the health care policy environment), the culture of the health care organization and its units or divisions, and the mixing of this culture with the culture of the university.

- Tenet 8: The interaction among mentor challenges, the interprofessional EBP and implementation science task demands, the phases of the work, and the micro- and macro-contexts prompts mentors to use specific techniques to mentor their teams and scholars.

- Tenet 9: Program coordinators use a variety of mentor supports to mentor the mentors and other team members.

- Tenet 10: The outcome of the work of the teams and the evolving micro- and macro-contexts and project phases lead to additional mentor challenges, task demands, and subsequent need for mentoring techniques and supports.

Deliberative and Reflective Mentoring Practice (Tenets 1 and 8)

From the results of the study of mentoring in an interprofessional EBP program, it became clear that the design of the interprofessional EBP program must include a structure to support a reflective and deliberative mentoring practice of the mentors and the program coordinators. Because deliberative mentoring occurs immediately when it is needed, it is a more conscious and active approach to assisting a team or, in the case of program coordinators, assisting the mentor and the team. Reflective mentoring occurs when thinking about what happened in the team, what mentoring strategies worked or did not work, and how the mentor or program coordinator might want to help the team move forward; or in the case of the program coordinator, devise ways to help the mentor to facilitate progress. When the program coordinators and mentors actually apply the strategies devised during reflective mentoring, deliberative mentoring occurs as an ongoing cycle of reflection to action. Writing field notes after every interprofessional team meeting, interprofessional EBP workday, mentor meetings, and a mentor workshop (see the book's website for the field note form) is an effective way for mentors and program coordinators to develop this reflective mentoring practice.

Programs can incorporate other methods of promoting reflection instead of or in addition to field notes, such as mentor meetings and program coordinator meetings. During the regular mentor meetings, the program coordinators should encourage the mentors to share their field notes generated from the interprofessional EBP team meetings with each other. The ensuing discussion of common issues occurring across the teams helps the mentors assume a problem-solving posture to devise mentor techniques. For example, a mentor may indicate that the team has not grasped the synthesis process of EBP.

TABLE 3-3

THEORETICAL TENETS AND SUPPORTING DATA

TENET	DEFINITIONS	SUPPORTING DATA
Tenet 1: A successful interprofessional EBP program is carefully designed to create a supportive structure that fosters the reflective and deliberative mentoring practice of the mentors and the program coordinators.	**Reflective mentoring practice:** Reflective mentoring occurs after a mentor or program coordinator has taken time to ponder an experience to consider the challenges, the task demands, and the capabilities of the team in order to devise potential strategies that will lead to a positive resolution of a mentor challenge. **Deliberative mentoring practice:** Deliberative mentoring of mentors and program coordinators occurs within an experience and includes offering strategies that will lead to an immediate positive resolution of a mentor challenge. Deliberative mentoring also occurs when enacting the selected mentor techniques or mentor supports arising from reflective mentoring. **Supportive structure:** Supportive structure includes mentor meetings, mentor workshops, program coordinator meetings, and newsletters to encourage reflective mentoring.	**Mentor and reflective mentoring:** "I learned the process is messy at times. I would talk to the program coordinator to vet my plan for the team and she would coach me. During the team meeting, I was then better prepared to mentor." **Program coordinator and deliberative mentoring:** "I could tell that the student on the team was getting frustrated. The team was not listening to the student and the mentor did not notice this problem. One team member in particular kept talking over the student. I asked the team to stop for a minute and check with the student about why she seemed frustrated. I helped the student dialogue about wanting to be listened to when she had something to offer. The team throughout the session listened carefully whenever the student talked and even started asking her for her opinion."
Tenet 2: Each of the nine phases of interprofessional EBP has its own characteristics involving mentor challenges, complexity of EBP and implementation science tasks, and team micro- and macro-contexts.	**Interprofessional EBP phases:** Interprofessional EBP phases are a collection of work tasks that result in completion of a step in EBP. **Phase characteristics:** Each step in EBP has unique team experiences and challenges as a result of the tasks and the contexts.	**Team member:** I already knew a lot about literature searches so could really provide a lot of help. I felt comfortable giving feedback on the grant. I did what I could to help with data collection; but I really was not able to do much because of my class schedule."
Tenet 3: The characteristics of the phases interact to influence the work output and work quality of the teams on their EBP projects.	**Work output:** Work output includes the tangible work products the team produces in each interprofessional EBP phase, such as a completed literature search, appraisals, synthesis charts, etc. **Work quality:** Work quality shows whether the work output meets acceptable standards for progression to the next interprofessional EBP phase.	**Team member:** "When the statistician was given our data, she was so surprised how carefully done and well organized everything was. Our mentor really guided us well and all the team members went over the data during each team meeting. The statistician told us she was impressed."

(continued)

TABLE 3-3 (CONTINUED)

THEORETICAL TENETS AND SUPPORTING DATA

TENET	DEFINITIONS	SUPPORTING DATA
Tenet 4: Mentor challenges indicate the team members' or the scholar's need for mentoring because of questions, barriers, disagreements, confusion, team relationship difficulties, and novel opportunities.	**Mentor challenges:** Mentor challenges include the potential or current impact of barriers, novel tasks, opportunities, and team behaviors on the work progression or timeline, work output, work quality, team outcome, and funding requirements.	**Team member:** "Some team members did not come to certain sessions. We were counting on them to have their work done. At times, this issue kept us from moving forward."
Tenet 5: The complexity of the interprofessional EBP and implementation science tasks creates demands on team performance and may create mentor challenges.	**EBP and implementation science task demands:** This is the way in which the work activities of the interprofessional EBP program tests the team and scholar in terms of their cognitive, emotional, and physical capacity. These tasks create a demand load continuum from low to high.	**Team member:** "We really had a handle on the research." **Team member:** "I really struggled with why we had to do the literature search the way we did."
Tenet 6: The micro-context arises from the team dynamics because of individual team member and mentor personalities and the kinds of expertise and experience of team members and mentors.	**Micro-context:** Micro-context is the most proximal environment of the team created from team interactions occurring as a result of team member personalities, communication styles, and previous experience and expertise.	**Team member:** "We had great camaraderie on our team. We were willing to take a step back and let somebody else take the leadership, too, when they wanted to do so." **Team member:** "The team dynamic at times was a little tough. One team member would completely ignore whatever I said."
Tenet 7: The macro-context involves the external environment (e.g., the health care policy environment), the culture of the health care organization and its units or divisions, and the mixing of this culture with the culture of the university.	**Macro-context:** Macro-context is the distal environments of the team arising from various aspects of the health care and university cultures, the health care organizational milieu and the broader health care circumstances.	**Team member:** "Working with our mentor was helpful as she was insightful about hospital politics and how that could affect our project."
Tenet 8: The interaction among mentor challenges, the interprofessional EBP and implementation science task demands, the phases of the work, and the micro- and macro-contexts prompts mentors to use specific techniques to mentor their teams and scholars.	**Mentor techniques:** Mentor techniques involve the strategies mentors use with their teams and scholars in response to a challenge to facilitate smooth team interactions and completion of work on time and on budget according to standards.	**Mentor:** "I worked with the team to create a work schedule. After that, we started getting the work done on time." **Team member:** "The mentor was an excellent facilitator and would really help us get through the tough parts."

(continued)

TABLE 3-3 (CONTINUED)		
THEORETICAL TENETS AND SUPPORTING DATA		
TENET	DEFINITIONS	SUPPORTING DATA
Tenet 9: Program coordinators use a variety of mentor supports to mentor the mentors and other team members.	**Mentor supports:** Mentor supports include the strategies program coordinators use in response to a challenge that assists the mentors and their teams to engage in smooth interactions and to complete work on time and on budget according to standards.	**Team member:** "The program coordinator always made us feel good about our contributions. She made everyone feel comfortable. When you feel comfortable in a group, you bring more."
Tenet 10: The outcome of the work of the teams and the evolving micro- and macro-contexts and project phases lead to additional mentor challenges, task demands, and subsequent need for mentoring techniques and supports.	**Work outcome:** Work outcome includes a combination of work quality, output, and team perception regarding the EBP phase and its tasks as being a positive or a negative experience.	**Team member:** "Being on the team was really satisfying. The student on our team kept the minutes and created meeting agenda. She really kept the team focused and moving."

Other mentors describe how they believed the synthesis forms were helpful but found they also needed to develop some other forms for their team to explore the intervention dosage more carefully. The program coordinator asked the mentors to share these additional forms with each other as a mentor technique they all could use.

The program coordinator who leads the mentor meeting needs to share his or her mentor meeting field notes with the other program coordinators during the weekly program meetings. The program coordinator leading the mentor meeting might describe to the other program coordinators that the mentors are all experiencing team communication problems. As a result, the program coordinators decide to focus the next mentoring workshop on team communication strategies as an additional mentor support. In addition, the program coordinators should also share with each other their participant observations of the teams and mentors from the interprofessional EBP workdays. When program coordinators discuss this information, they may discover, for instance, the need for additional educational sessions or the need for more work time for the teams before the next education session occurs. As a result, the program coordinators institute a slight schedule modification. Consequently, mentors and program coordinators are not only engaging in a reflective mentoring practice, but are progressing because of their dialogue to deliberative mentoring in order to enable positive consequences or outcomes of the teams' work and experiences.

Work Phases of the Teams (Tenets 2, 3, and 10)

Emerging from the data were nine phases (orienting, figuring it out, settling in, transitioning, designing, implementing, evaluating/analyzing, wrapping up, and disseminating) of the interprofessional EBP work of the team. These phases are the basis for organizing this book so that the reader will learn how to perform as a program coordinator, how to mentor an interprofessional team, or how to work successfully on an interprofessional EBP team during each phase. These EBP work phases incorporate a number of program events including mentor meetings, interprofessional EBP workdays, and extra team meetings (Figure 3-1).

Each of these phases has its own characteristics because of the way in which the team members focused their work (Table 3-4). In addition, the interaction of phase characteristics or dynamic factors influences the work output and work quality of the teams on their interprofessional EBP projects. These dynamic factors or characteristics include the following:

- Mentor challenges
- Interprofessional EBP and implementation science task demands
- Micro- and macro-contexts
- Mentor techniques
- Mentor supports

Developing Deliberative and Reflective Mentoring 49

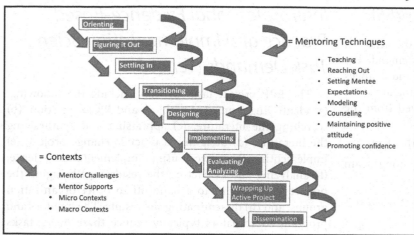

Figure 3-1. EBP team project phases.

	TABLE 3-4
	PHASE DESCRIPTIONS
Phase 1	**Orienting** involves team members learning about the interprofessional EBP program, their roles and that of the mentor, and their preferred leadership and work styles.
Phase 2	**Figuring it Out** is one of turmoil about the EBP process, as each team member further clarifies his or her roles in the project and struggles to delineate the project's scope.
Phase 3	**Settling In** involves team members falling into the rhythm of the program through completion of carefully designed initial EBP steps.
Phase 4	**Transitioning** captures the initial sense of lack of structure as a result of completing the defined literature appraisal and synthesis steps. Teams develop their own work processes to complete the remaining EBP steps involving designing and implementing their specific EBP projects.
Phase 5	**Designing** occurs when team members spend time determining the nature of the implementation science project, writing their institutional review board proposals, and submitting grant proposals.
Phase 6	**Implementing** includes conducting the practice projects and gathering outcomes data. Establishing fidelity of the intervention is emphasized.
Phase 7	**Evaluating** includes analyzing and interpreting the data.
Phase 8	**Wrapping Up** concludes the active aspects of the projects as teams make sure all tasks have been completed successfully, grant budgets are reconciled, and sustainability of the project is considered.
Phase 9	**Disseminating** often occurs after official EBP program completion with the teams writing and presenting their results and sharing the project and its results with the health care organization and the university, as well as other external organizations and groups.

Mentor challenges indicate the team members' or the scholar's need for mentoring because of questions, disagreements, confusion, barriers, novel tasks, team relationships, and opportunities. The complexity of the interprofessional EBP and implementation science tasks creates demands on team performance. The micro-context arises from the team dynamics because of individual team member and mentor personalities and the kinds of expertise and experience of team members and mentors. The macro-context, in addition to factors in the local and national health care system, involves the culture of the health care organization and its units or divisions, and the mixing of this culture with the culture of the university. This interaction among mentor challenges, the interprofessional EBP and implementation science task demands, the phases of the work, and the micro- and macro-contexts prompts mentors to use specific techniques to mentor their teams and scholars. These same factors prompt the program coordinators to use a variety of mentor supports to mentor the mentors and other team members when indicated. The outcomes of the teams and the evolving micro- and macro-contexts and project phases typically lead to additional mentor challenges, task demands, and subsequent need for mentoring techniques and supports.

Mentor Challenges (Tenets 4 and 5)

Mentor challenges indicate the team's or the scholar's need for mentoring in response to a task demand, the phase of the interprofessional EBP program, and changes in the micro- and macro-contexts. The following are some common mentor challenges inductively derived from the mentoring study:

- Keeping team members on track with the plan
- Addressing communication issues among team members
- Confronting unrealistic expectations that teams will perform in an ideal fashion
- Handling frustration and criticism of team members, of the mentor, and of each other
- Solving problems beyond the mentor's level of expertise
- Resolving time demands on the mentor and team members
- Reducing negative macro-contextual effects on the team
- Confronting negative behaviors of team members
- Holding team members accountable for task completion on time and within budget
- Encouraging team members to recognize and celebrate team successes

Whether a mentor perceives a mentor challenge as an obstacle is partially a function of the mentor's degree of optimism. Optimism is a positive, though realistic, perception of a situation as being an opportunity for the following:

- Trying something different
- Learning something new
- Gaining skills
- Having a unique experience
- Experimenting
- Meeting new people and developing relationships
- Gaining emotional maturity or feeling more deeply

Optimism is not the same as having the expectation that there will not be any challenges and that the experiences one will have will be ideal. Optimism is an understanding that challenges will happen, but that they will paradoxically bring many opportunities as well. Mentors who are more optimistic encourage team members to use an active problem-solving approach to address each challenge. Mentors who are less optimistic in their mentoring ability when faced with team problems require significantly more support from the program coordinators.

Interprofessional Evidence-Based Practice and Implementation Science Task Demands (Tenet 5)

The EBP project tasks broadly include the following: (a) identifying a practice problem and PICO question, (b) searching the literature, (c) appraising and synthesizing the literature, (d) designing a practice change project, (e) implementing the project using implementation science, (f) analyzing and evaluating the results, (g) bringing the project to a close or to a hand-off to other organization groups, and (h) disseminating the results. The mentors and program coordinators typically reduce these major tasks into manageable subtasks (Table 3-5).

These tasks and their subtasks vary in their type of task demand(s) (cognitive, emotional, interpersonal, and physical) and level of task load (low to high) on the team and its members. Task load broadly refers to the levels of difficulty an individual encounters when executing a task. Levels of difficulty impact the person cognitively, emotionally, and physically, as well as may create social expectations in terms of requisite interpersonal ability. Program coordinators and mentors should use Table 3-6 to guide strategies for modifying task demands to better match the capacities of team members. For instance, if the mentors are concerned about the complexity of the appraisal process in terms of the team members' knowledge of research and statistics, the appraisal task potentially has a high cognitive load. To reduce the cognitive load, mentors and program coordinators may have to modify the appraisal task by providing cognitive supports via education sessions, mentor education, and team coaching from experts.

The coordinators and mentors can maximize the way in which strengths of persons on the teams facilitate project completion. For example, the interprofessional teams should assign tasks with a high cognitive task load because of its complexity to a team member who has a higher capacity to handle complexity due to his or her education and experience. Because one of the important goals of the interprofessional EBP is that everyone learns, small groups of team members should work on tasks so those with less experience can learn from those with more experience. Mentors and program coordinators through deliberative and reflective mentoring facilitate matching of task demand with the physical, emotional, interpersonal, and cognitive capacity of team members. Matching task demand with capacity of team members occurs through the mentor offering mentor techniques (e.g., assigning the cognitively complex task to two team members, one with experience and one who wants to learn) and the program coordinator providing mentor supports (e.g., adding an educational session to explore the complex cognitive task in more depth).

TABLE 3-5

Example Evidence-Based Practice Sub-Tasks

PICO QUESTION	SEARCHING LITERATURE	APPRAISAL AND SYNTHESIS	PROJECT DESIGN	IMPLEMENT PROJECT	ANALYZE RESULTS	WRAP UP AND DISSEMINATE
Gather some information about topic	Determine search terms	Select appropriate appraisal tools	Determine intervention methods and parameters	Launch project and obtain consent	Enter data into spreadsheet	Develop dissemination plan
Narrow topic	Select databases	Appraise studies with appropriate tool	Receive stakeholder feedback on intervention	Monitor progress and problem solve as needed	Clean data for errors and locate missing data	Write report to grant source and to institutional review board
Write PICO question	Delineate inclusion criteria	Validate appraisal with others if needed	Write institutional review board proposal including precise procedures and analysis methods	Protect internal validity and intervention fidelity	Work with statistician	Present project to organizations
	Select research for appraisal	Synthesize level and quality of studies	Write grant	Gather and store data ensuring reliability and validity	Interpret results	Submit abstracts for professional presentation
	Eliminate irrelevant research	Identify what is known about intervention	Prepare equipment, supplies, and training	Manage budget		Write articles for publication
			Implement training	Manage volunteers and research assistants		Reconcile grant budgets
			Develop schedule of project implementation tasks			Plan for project sustainability

TABLE 3-6

TASK DEMANDS

TYPE OF TASK DEMAND	HIGH TASK LOAD	LOW TASK LOAD
Cognitive Demand		
Complexity	Difficult	Easy
Level of novelty	Novel	Routine
Learning	Abstract	Concrete
Attention	Focused	Short bursts of attention
Time	Long time frames	Short time frames
Models or patterns	None available	Exact model or pattern
Information available	Inadequate	Adequate
Instructions	Incomplete or not available	Complete
Flexibility of methods	Highly flexible	Structured
Repetition	Not repetitive	Highly repetitive
Outcomes	Unpredictable	Predictable
Experience	Vital	None needed
Physical Demand		
Tool use	Multiple tools	Few tools
Dexterity level	Intricate	Basic
Physicality	High	Low
Interpersonal Demand		
Use of people	Coordinated team(s)	Individual or few individuals
Relationships	Interdependent	Independence
Cooperation	High	Low
Emotional Demand		
Emotionality	High	Low
Rewards available	Intrinsic	Extrinsic
Barriers	Multiple	Few
Risks	High	Low

Developmental growth of the team in terms of becoming comfortable with team roles, communication strategies, interaction styles, and levels of trust with each other complicates the task demand or load. Earlier stages of team development may cause a team to experience a task as very demanding, but if the task was to occur at a later stage, the team members would find the task to be a low load or low task demand. If a team experiences a disruption in development because of chronic team member absence or nonparticipation, low-demand tasks could suddenly become much more demanding.

Team members respond to high task demands differently. Some might assume the challenge with interest and excitement and will readily engage in problem solving or will seek expertise. Teams sometimes display negative behaviors in response to high task load, such as spending too much time in discussion and debate, withdrawing, taking too long on a task, becoming confused, or feeling overworked. When negative behaviors occur, it is important for team members to help each other. If that does not automatically happen, mentors and/or program coordinators have to intervene at the right time in order to keep the team moving forward. The emotional load of the task is removed when mentors use mentor techniques and program coordinators use mentor supports to address barriers affecting team performance.

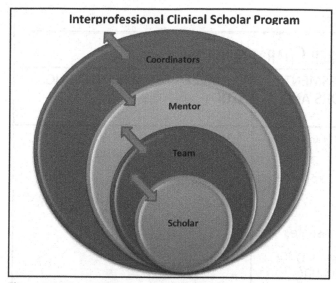

Figure 3-2. Micro-contexts.

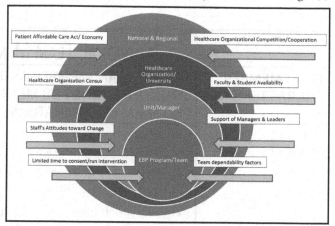

Figure 3-3. Macro-contexts.

Micro- and Macro-Contexts (Tenets 6 and 7)

Context includes not only physical space (built environments and geography), but also virtual, temporal, cultural, social, organizational, political, and economic environments. In addition, local, national, and global communities influence how each person behaves. Contexts are boundaries that influence observed phenomena. Context drives each individual's cognition, attitudes, and behaviors. Interactions among individuals and groups occur uniquely in a context. If the context changes for a project, the interactions among team members would change as well. Individuals and groups generate and shape the meaning of their team experience through interactions happening within multiple layers of dynamically changing contexts from the micro- to the macro-levels.

Mentoring occurs within rich and various micro-contexts. Like rippling circles, these contexts influence the interprofessional EBP process of each team. Circles of micro-contexts place the interprofessional EBP scholar or fellow at the center surrounded by team members of faculty and students, a mentor or mentors, program coordinators, and the elements of the program (Figure 3-2).

Each team member demonstrates individual characteristics that contribute to the micro-context in terms of ultimately forming a team identity (Table 3-7). These individual characteristics include skills and abilities, character traits, values and beliefs, interests, experience, knowledge, and competing responsibilities. Effective mentors and program coordinators assess their teams' strengths based on the characteristics of each team member and his or her corresponding interactions. These assessments are ongoing and occur through the team charter process, team meeting discussions and team debriefings, work sessions, the work

outputs and quality, and team member feedback to each other and to the mentors or program coordinators. Mentors and program coordinators learn to be aware of their teams' weaknesses and learning needs that require mentors to use mentor techniques and require program coordinators to use mentor supports.

Macro-contexts consist of layers affecting the previously described micro-contexts. To understand the phenomenon of mentoring, the program coordinators and mentors must be aware of and interpret the influence of macro-contexts on the interprofessional EBP program. Macro-contexts include the influence of specific units of the health care organization, the partner institutions as a whole, the local community, and national and global pressures on the interprofessional EBP projects (Figure 3-3).

Some macro-contexts facilitate the work of the team in the form of support (e.g., a nurse agreeing to encourage other staff on the unit and the rehabilitation staff of the health care organization to participate in the project) and of stakeholder involvement (e.g., an organizational manager, physician, and leaders in other disciplines helping the team design the project). The macro-contexts also create barriers to the work (e.g., the organization changes priorities). Each team member, the mentors, and the program coordinators should note any potential barriers to the interprofessional EBP project as soon as possible so that work plans will incorporate solutions right from the beginning (Table 3-8).

Mentor Techniques (Tenets 1 and 8)

Before discussing specific mentoring techniques, it is important to understand that the work of mentors also includes taking on some of the work tasks of the teams, preparing for team meetings, notifying the program coordinators when assistance is needed, reading and studying to prepare, attending mentor meetings, and learning about mentoring. In addition, an important aspect of mentoring work involves the intentional and deliberative use of mentoring techniques to assist team members. Mentor

TABLE 3-7

INDIVIDUAL TEAM MEMBER CHARACTERISTICS

TEAM MEMBER CHARACTERISTICS	SAMPLE TEAM MEMBER ASSESSMENT CONSIDERATIONS FOR MENTORS AND PROGRAM COORDINATORS	EXAMPLES FROM MENTORING STUDY
Skills and abilities, character traits	• What time of day works best for each team member to accomplish work? • How much structure and supervision does the team member need? • How much initiative to complete work does the team member demonstrate? • What is the team member's capacity for ambiguity and for problem solving? • How does the team member handle frustration?	"Scholar struggles with ability to anticipate activities outside regular meetings; waits for assignments from the mentor; needs clear directions...." (Program Coordinator Field Note, 7/16/12)
Values and beliefs	• Does the team member value EBP and research? • Does the team member believe he or she can learn EBP and eventually engage in EBP independently? • Does the team member value interprofessional team patient care processes? • How does the team member express the values of his or her respective organization?	"Difference between clinical setting/academia and practice environment were discussed. Good discussion and feedback. Bridging the differences." (Mentor Field Note, 2/2/12)
Interests	• Is the team member interested in the patient care EBP question? In research? In EBP? In interprofessional practice?	"She [mentor] noted that a faculty member identified interest in supervising students to help with securing patient consent for one project." (Program Coordinator Field Notes, 8/9/12)
Experience with EBP and implementation science	• Has the team member completed course work, continuing education, or independent learning in EBP and implementation science? • Has the team member ever engaged in any aspect of EBP and implementation science?	"The students do literature searching and want to support the team with their abilities." (Mentor Field Note, 1/26/12)
Experience with research	• Has the team member completed course work, continuing education, or independent learning in research? • Has the team member ever engaged in any aspect of research?	"All of the mentors are struggling with their teams because...their lack of knowledge about research makes it difficult to know how to best facilitate the teams. They are learning alongside of their team members." (Program Coordinator, Field Note, 2/9/12)

(continued)

TABLE 3-7 (CONTINUED)		
INDIVIDUAL TEAM MEMBER CHARACTERISTICS		
TEAM MEMBER CHARACTERISTICS	**SAMPLE TEAM MEMBER ASSESSMENT CONSIDERATIONS FOR MENTORS AND PROGRAM COORDINATORS**	**EXAMPLES FROM MENTORING STUDY**
Knowledge of patient care topic	• Has the team member completed course work, continuing education, or independent learning on the patient care topic? • Has the team member ever been involved in providing care for the patient population that the EBP question addresses? Is the team member currently providing care for this population?	"Faculty member is very helpful adding the perspective of another discipline and helping the team think about the spine and positioning." (Mentor Field Note, 1/26/12)
Communication style	• What is the preferred communication method of each team member? • What is the frequency and pattern of communication for each team member? • Is each team member comfortable asking questions, sharing opinions, and expressing feelings?	"I think the things that are working well that I've observed in the whole experience are the different perspectives, different questions, and the clarifications of vocabulary for example and the ability to clarify the issues is really good." (Mentor Interview, 8/10/12)
Experience with technologies	• Is the team member able to use computer programs, e-mail, and various communication technologies?	"Scholar is adept in using computers." (Mentor Field Note, 1/26/12)
Experience leading and working on an interprofessional team	• Has the team member ever worked on an interprofessional team? • Has the team member ever worked on any type of team? • Has the team member ever led a professional team of any type? • Has the team member ever led an interprofessional team?	"Mentor is frustrated with her team and feels they are not making progress and that they seem to be all 'over the place.'" (Program Coordinator Field Note, 2/16/12)
Experience in the discipline	• How long has the team member practiced, taught, or studied his or her discipline? Is the team member currently involved with some aspect of the work of his or her discipline?	"There was a lot of posturing...that was related to typical professional roles, but I do think that the OT piece could've been stronger but she was a student and seemed hesitant about her discipline knowledge." (First Mentor Interview, 10/23/12)
Competing workload, school, and family responsibilities	• How many days per week and hours per week is the team member working and/or going to school? • How does this work fit in with the faculty team members' course load, community service, and scholarship expectations of the university?	"Faculty and students have a different schedule during summer and are less available." (Program Coordinator Field Note, 7/26/12)

TABLE 3-8

MACRO-CONTEXTUAL SUPPORTS AND BARRIERS

MACRO-CONTEXT BARRIER	FIELD NOTE EXAMPLES	YOUR TEAM/ PROGRAM BARRIERS
Logistical problem	"Faculty and students have different schedule during summer and are less available." (Program Coordinator Field Note, Mentor Seminar, 7/26/12)	
Lack of support	"Need more respondents to complete the survey in order to have enough to analyze." (Program Coordinator Field Note, Team 4, 11/8/12)	
Lack of stakeholder involvement	"I [Program Coordinator] think there needs to be work about validating the problem, such as doing a larger chart audit, as well as a patient or staff survey." (Program Coordinator Field Note, Team 2, 5/14/12)	
Policy barrier	"Program coordinator reviewed the process for inserting an educational module on the e-learning platform. It needs to be reviewed by several persons before it is posted." (Program Coordinator Field Notes, Team 3, 6/28/12)	
Organizational change	"Mentor told team member about the uncertainty with emerging changes at the hospital-there is going to be a restructuring." (Program Coordinator Field Note, Team 3, 12/13/12)	
Cultural barrier	"Nurses on the unit found it hard to mentor their peers about the new intervention. It feels like, culturally, the staff members were not prepared to mentor." (Program Coordinator Field Note, Team 4, 12/13/12)	
Negative behaviors	"Negative responses include 'another study,' 'why do we have to decrease sedation,' and 'I'll have to be at the bedside more.'" (Program Coordinator Field Note, Team 3, 9/20/12)	
Knowledge issues	"Discussed need to increase the awareness of staff about the study." (Program Coordinator Field Note, Team 1, 7/26/12)	
Competing projects	"Scholar asked how her project would interface with the delirium study." (Program Coordinator Field Note, Team 3, 6/28/12)	

techniques include all of those strategies the mentors use in response to mentor challenges that result from the team's interaction with the task load, project phase, or micro- and macro-contexts. In addition, mentors do not always use mentor techniques just in response to a challenge. Mentors often use these same techniques as a part of facilitating the routine work of the team. An example of routine use of a mentor technique occurs when the mentor encourages the team to follow its plan without letting minor challenges create distractions. Mentor techniques have a particular focus in terms of targeting the team or targeting individual team members. The following is a list of mentoring techniques inductively derived from the mentoring study:

- Teaching
- Reaching out
- Setting expectations
- Anticipating what might happen
- Modeling key behaviors
- Counseling
- Maintaining a positive attitude
- Promoting confidence
- Providing resources
- Pushing team members to lead
- Providing structure
- Facilitating team interaction

Consider these mentor techniques as a way for the mentor to "be" with the team. For instance, a team member's need for learning may result in the mentor using teaching or modeling techniques. When a team member is frustrated, the mentor might engage in counseling, maintain a positive attitude, and promote self-confidence. The mentor could also encourage the team member's expression of frustration to the team through team dialogue and problem solving.

These ways of being during mentoring help team members change their behaviors. The implication is that the mentor selects one or more of the mentoring techniques as the best way of being in order to accomplish the objectives of the team. Adept use of mentor techniques requires the mentor to wield a strategy more likely to address the mentor challenge rather than using a technique that would only weakly address the challenge or that would not address it well in terms of achieving a positive outcome. In fact, mentor techniques highly matched to the mentor challenge produce more positive outcomes than those that do not match. For example, if a team was not staying on track with the plan, the mentor could quickly provide structure to address the mentor challenge. The risk in using this mentor technique is that the team continues to expect the mentor to solve its problems. If the mentor instead facilitates team discussion about how the team was not staying focused on the plan, the risk is that the discussion could fail to lead to a solution. Consequently, the better mentor technique is for the mentor to facilitate the team to devise strategies to stay focused.

There is an assumption in mentoring that all actions of the mentor are intentional and are part of a conscious deliberative mentoring plan. Deliberative mentoring does occur, but mentors cannot possibly know every aspect of their practice as mentors. In fact, a mentor may not be aware of several aspects of his or her mentoring practice, and without spending time in reflection, successive deliberative mentoring is less likely to occur.

There is an additional assumption undergirding the concept of a deliberative mentoring practice, that the mentors are able to accurately communicate or deliver the mentor techniques. For example, if a mentor chooses to motivate a team member to keep working through a problem, the mentor may inadvertently communicate a hidden belief that the team member does not really have the skills to proceed. Authentic mentoring occurs when the actions of the mentor are a reflection of the mentor's underlying values and beliefs.

Mentoring meetings, an important component of an interprofessional EBP program, are a safe and important space for mentors to reflect together with the program coordinators about their mentoring practices. Mentors share outcomes of mentoring techniques, practice new mentoring techniques and receive feedback, discuss their practices in relationship to the mentor challenges they face, and receive suggestions for additional mentoring techniques. Mentoring workshops or seminars, another important element of an interprofessional EBP program,

include more time for reflection on the important topic of team communication, a common mentor challenge for most mentors regardless of skill level. Within an interprofessional team communication workshop, mentors can use metaphors to describe their current and ideal team communication patterns. For example, a mentor might describe the current team communication as a tangled web in contrast to the ideal team communication being like a well-oiled machine. This reflection shows the mentors the discrepancy between the current situation and the ideal, and then discussion helps them identify the specific mentor techniques that should help the situation. Program coordinators can use "1-minute mentoring updates" or newsletters to promote mentor reflection on mentoring techniques and to suggest additional mentoring techniques as well.

Mentor Supports (Tenet 9)

Program coordinators use mentor supports or ways of being present with the mentors and teams during their work on the interprofessional EBP projects. These mentor supports derived partially from Darling's (1984) mentoring research include those that inspire, invest in, support, and teach mentors and team members. Table 3-9 provides detailed information about each mentor support inductively substantiated from the data. For example, a program coordinator inspires a mentor when celebrating the success of the work output with the mentor and team. Likewise, the program coordinator invests in the mentor when substituting for the mentor when he or she is absent from a team meeting due to work schedule conflicts, illness, or vacation.

Program coordinators engage in a deliberative mentoring strategy for the mentors and teams when selecting a mentor support. For instance, when choosing to teach and clarify the understanding of concepts, the program coordinators most likely notice confusion, misunderstandings, and struggles with new learning and processes of not only the mentors, but with team members as well. Mentors may need help determining the best way to facilitate the learning of all team members who vary in their skills and experience in interprofessional EBP. Becoming too focused on the inexperienced may lead the mentors to ignore the learning needs of the more experienced team members. Program coordinators helping mentors manage team problem behaviors is triggered when the relationship between the team and mentor has not gelled, when the mentor–team relationship is falling apart, or when the mentor has difficulty managing the behavior of some team members. Additionally, the program coordinators manage the workload of the mentors when they report feeling overwhelmed, when the mentor is having difficulty keeping the team on task and on deadline, and when the workload of the mentor in his or her job competes with the workload of the project. Workload issues motivate the program coordinators to find resources for the mentor in terms of volunteers to complete

TABLE 3-9	
PROGRAM COORDINATOR MENTOR SUPPORTS	
INSPIRE	**SUPPORT**
• Pointing out success of team and mentor • Facilitating commitment to project • Motivating perseverance • Celebrating team and mentor successes	• Keeping mentor engaged • Assisting with consistency • Helping with problem team behaviors • Developing mentor's team role and identity • Coping with frustrations and fostering patience
INVEST	**TEACH**
• Managing workload of mentor • Helping to adapt the work • Facilitating stakeholder involvement • Finding resources for mentor • Substituting for mentor when absent	• Developing mentor facilitation skills • Clarifying concepts • Growing team communication skills • Expanding ability to solve problems • Summarizing learning

labor-intensive tasks, such as data collection. Program coordinators inspire when the mentor is unaware of his or her successes or is losing energy and struggling with motivating the team.

When mentors use their mentoring techniques without mentor supports from the program coordinators, typically there are equal numbers of positive outcomes in terms of task completion or supportive team and scholar behaviors compared to when program coordinators provide mentor supports with and without the mentors using their techniques. However, when the mentor's mentoring techniques fail to produce a positive outcome or a high-quality output, program coordinators who add mentor supports are more likely to produce a positive change in team outcome and output. Program coordinators need to use mentor supports even when mentors use mentor techniques to address a negative outcome. Otherwise, without the mentor supports in addition to the mentor techniques, negative outcomes could continue. In addition, when the program coordinators add mentor supports after a positive outcome because of the mentor's mentor technique, the outcome is more likely to stay positive compared to when mentors continue with using their mentor techniques alone.

Putting It All Together (Tenets 1 and 10)

The design of the interprofessional EBP program helps the mentors and the program coordinators develop a deliberative and reflective mentoring practice where the field note process and the mentor and program coordinator meetings highlight micro- and macro-contexts, interprofessional EBP and implementation science task demands, and mentor challenges that occur in each project phase. During these meetings, the program coordinators and mentors recognize the need for mentor supports and mentor techniques, respectively. In the mentor meetings, the mentors listen to the successes and challenges of the other mentors and share possible techniques or strategies. The program coordinators devise mentor supports because of understanding gained from the mentor meetings. Therefore, the roles of the program coordinators and the mentors are interdependent in terms of enacting an iterative process for managing the experience of the teams and for ensuring productivity (Figure 3-4).

While an interprofessional team improves the likelihood of bringing greater expertise to the project, the team complicates the mentoring process. Because of the mentoring complexity, program coordinators are integral to the mentoring process through the provision of mentoring supports for the mentors and the teams. The program coordinators use mentor supports partially based on input from the mentors. Program coordinators also generate and offer supports as the result of their observations of mentor and team performance. The purpose of mentor supports is to facilitate mentor and team member engagement in an iterative process to prevent poor EBP and implementation science task results or outputs that ultimately could lead to little effect of the project on improving patient care.

Mentors have to reach out to less active team members, counsel the team about problem team behaviors, maintain a positive attitude, promote confidence, and facilitate team interaction. Mentoring involves reciprocity to achieve a more balanced give-and-take process of learning over time

Figure 3-4. Mentoring process.

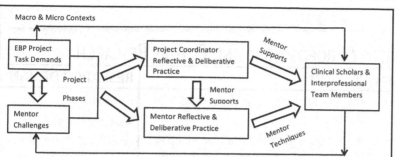

that benefits both the mentor and the team. In other words, the mentor needs to promote other team members leading the team according to their interest, expertise, and task assignments. Timing of this reciprocity is different among teams depending upon the capacity of team members to understand interprofessional EBP and implementation science, to take responsibility for the project's success, and to develop trust with their team members and mentor. There are situations in which the mentor is unable to achieve full reciprocity with the team due to multiple developmental and contextual issues the team experiences.

NEED FOR FURTHER RESEARCH

Although Darling's (1984) work on mentoring produced specific mentor roles, such as door opener, eye opener, teacher, and counselor (see Chapter 1, Figure 1-3), the data from this study did not produce different types of roles and instead identified the central phenomenon of the theory as reflective and deliberative mentoring practice. Mentors and project coordinators examined the task demands, the micro- and macro-contexts, and the mentor challenges of each EBP phase in order to determine the best use of mentor techniques and mentor supports that would help the team experience positive team outcomes and work outputs.

Future research is needed to verify the 10 tenets of the theory, particularly with increases in the EBP and implementation science skill levels of the mentors and of the team members. For example, would skilled mentors be less likely to need a supportive interprofessional EBP program structure to encourage reflective mentoring, or would they need as many mentor supports from the program coordinators? There were many propositional statements arising from the grounded theory mentor study described in this chapter that also could guide further research, such as that program coordinators adding mentor supports after a negative team outcome were more likely to produce a positive change in outcome and output compared to mentors using only their mentor techniques. See Table 3-10 for some of these propositions, sample research questions, and corresponding research designs.

SUMMARY

This chapter presented a mentoring theory developed inductively from a study of mentoring of program coordinators and of mentors during an interprofessional EBP program. Regardless of whether organizations are fortunate enough to have experienced interprofessional EBP mentors on staff or on faculty, any interprofessional EBP program should include processes for supporting the reflective and deliberative practice of their mentors. Potential mentors who are inexperienced in interprofessional EBP should at a minimum complete an advanced interprofessional EBP course prior to the start of the program. Ideally, it is better when mentors have had at least one interprofessional EBP project experience where they have received supervision from an experienced mentor. As the interprofessional EBP program continues, the program coordinators can tap members of previous teams to become mentors in subsequent years.

This chapter also raises the importance of assessing the macro- and micro-contexts. Readiness for interprofessional EBP in the organization is an important prerequisite to an interprofessional EBP program, as described in Chapter 2. Although organizational readiness of both organizational partners is determined prior to the launch of an interprofessional EBP program, readiness might not stay intact given that all organizations constantly change. Abrupt organizational change during the program, such as turnover of leadership, should not impede completion of the projects as long as the program coordinators have the resources and the support of remaining leaders in both organizations to provide more frequent mentor supports than what might occur in a stable leadership situation.

The next chapter (Chapter 4) further delineates mentor techniques with its focus on team performance and the manner in which mentors might use team enhancement tools throughout the nine phases of interprofessional EBP. Additionally, Chapter 5 as a further delineation of mentor techniques and mentor supports helps mentors and program coordinators examine ways to foster team communication, a seemingly intuitive approach, but is a necessary review given that most teams experience communication difficulties at some point during the EBP project.

TABLE 3-10

SAMPLE OF MENTORING THEORY PROPOSITIONS AND FUTURE RESEARCH

PROPOSITION	RESEARCH QUESTION	RESEARCH DESIGN
Mentor techniques matched to the mentor challenge produce more positive outcomes than those that do not match.	• How do mentors match mentor challenges with mentor techniques? • Do mentor techniques that are matched to the mentor challenge produce more positive team outcomes in comparison to mentor techniques that are not matched to the challenge?	Case study Experimental Quasi-experimental
Mentor techniques of the mentor help team members change their behaviors.	• With skilled mentoring does each team member improve performance?	Experimental Quasi-experimental Case control Mixed methods
Effective mentors assess their teams' strengths based on the characteristics of each team member and his or her corresponding interactions.	• How do mentors assess the strengths and weaknesses of their teams? • How do mentors use this assessment to select the best mentor techniques?	Case study
Mentors who are more optimistic encourage team members to use an active problem solving approach to address each challenge.	• Are optimistic mentors more likely to use active problem solving to address mentor challenges as compared to mentors with less optimism?	Experimental Quasi-experimental Case control
The complexity of the interprofessional EBP and implementation science tasks creates demands on team performance.	• Does the functioning of the team differ when presented with a complex EBP task demand compared to a less complex EBP task demand?	Experimental Quasi-experimental
If a team experiences a disruption in development because of chronic team member absence or nonparticipation, low-demand tasks could suddenly become much more demanding.	• Do teams with members who are chronically absent produce fewer outputs and have negative outcomes in comparison to teams whose members attend regularly?	Experimental Quasi-experimental Case control Mixed methods

REFLECTION QUESTIONS

1. Identify mentoring reflection strategies and describe how you would use them to develop your mentoring techniques. (For example, how would you use a journal to inform your mentoring practice?)

2. The most common mentor challenge is team communication. Identify key communication mentoring techniques in which you would need the most development and outline learning strategies for developing these communication techniques.

REFERENCES

Abdullah, G., Rossy, D., Ploeg, J., Davies, B., Higuchi, K., Sikora, L., & Stacey, D. (2014). Measuring the effectiveness of mentoring as a knowledge translation intervention for implementing empirical evidence: A systematic review. *Worldviews on Evidence-Based Nursing, 11*(5), 284-300. doi:10.1111/wvn.12060

Darling L. A. (1984). What do nurses want in a mentor? *The Journal of Nursing Administration,* Oct, 42-44. doi:10.1097/00005110-198410000-00009

Haas, S. (2008). Resourcing evidence-based practice in ambulatory care nursing. *Nursing Economics, 26,* 319-322.

Interprofessional Education Collaborative Expert Panel. (2011). *Core competencies for interprofessional collaborative practice: Report of an expert panel.* Washington, DC: Interprofessional Education Collaborative.

Melnyk, B. M. (2007). The evidence-based practice mentor: A promising strategy for implementing and sustaining EBP in healthcare systems (Editorial). *Worldview Evidence Based Nursing, 4*(3), 123-125. doi:10.1111/j.1741-6787.2007.00094.x

Melnyk B. M., & Fineout-Overholt, E. (2002). Putting research into practice. Reflections on nursing Leadership/Sigma Theta Tau International. *Honor Society of Nursing 28*(2), 22-25.

Melnyk, B. M., & Fineout-Overholt, E. (2012). The state of evidence-based practice in US nurses: Critical implications for nurse leaders and educators. *Journal of Nursing Administration, 42,* 410-417.

Melnyk, B. M., Fineout-Overholt, E., Feinstein, N. F., Li, H., Small, L., Wilcox, L., & Kraus, R. (2004). Nurses' perceived knowledge, beliefs, skills, and needs regarding evidence-based practice: Implications for accelerating the paradigm shift. *Worldviews on Evidence-Based Nursing, 1*(3), 185-193. doi:10.1111/j.1524-475X.2004.04024.x

Moyers, P. A., Finch Guthrie, P. L., Swan, A. R., & Sathe, L. A. (2014). Interprofessional evidence-based clinical scholar program: Learning to work together. *American Journal of Occupational Therapy, 68,* S23-S31. doi:10.5014/ajot.2014.012609

Novak, I., & McIntyre, S. (2010). The effect of education with workplace supports on practitioners' evidence-based practice knowledge and implementation behaviors. *Australian Occupational Therapy Journal, 57,* 386-393. doi:10.1111/j.1440-1630.2010.00861.x

Strauss, A. L. (1987). *Qualitative Analysis for Social Scientists.* New York, NY: Cambridge University Press.

Strauss, A. L., & Corbin, J. M. (1998). *Basics of qualitative research: Techniques and procedures for developing grounded theory.* Thousand Oaks, CA: Sage.

Wallen, G. R., Mitchell, S. A., Melnyk, B., Fineout-Overholt, E., Yates, J., & Hastings, C. (2010). Implementing evidence-based practice: effectiveness of a structured multifaceted mentorship programme. *Journal of Advanced Nursing, 66*(12): 2761-2771. doi:10.1111/j.1365-2648.2010.05442.x

Supplemental materials for this chapter are available online.
Please refer to the sticker in the front of the book and enter the access code provided.

Forming Interprofessional Teams and Clarifying Roles

Janet Benz, DNP, RN and Patricia L. Finch-Guthrie, PhD, RN

CHAPTER TOPICS

- Interprofessional team philosophy
- Interprofessional team definition and framework
- Interprofessional team structures
- Interprofessional team competencies, skills, and techniques
- Mentor challenges
- Mentor techniques and supports

PERFORMANCE OBJECTIVES

Following completion of this chapter, the interprofessional program coordinators and leaders will be able to do the following:

1. Develop a team philosophy to ensure teamwork through development of interprofessional competencies.

2. Use the TeamSTEPPS® (TeamSTEPPS, 2014) model of leadership, communication, situation monitoring, and mutual support as a framework for an interprofessional evidence-based practice program.

3. Use strategies to promote interprofessional collaboration and team cohesion.

4. Anticipate, prevent, and resolve team issues related to evidence-based practice.

Once leaders in a health care organization and a university have established a partnership, assessed readiness for engaging in interprofessional evidence-based practice (EBP), selected an EBP model, and determined program goals for improving patient care and the patient/family experience (Chapters 1 through 3), the next step is to establish teams that work together throughout the interprofessional EBP program. There is increasing evidence that highly performing teams are an essential part of an effective health care delivery system (Mitchell et al., 2012). Specifically, the Institute of Medicine (IOM; 2001) report *Crossing the Quality Chasm* found that, to improve quality

Moyers, P. A., & Finch-Guthrie, P. L.
Interprofessional Evidence-Based Practice:
A Workbook for Health Professionals (pp 63-78).
© 2016 Taylor and Francis Group.

in health care, clinicians and institutional leaders should actively work together to coordinate care and engage in evidence-based decision making. In response to a growing need to improve health care, the World Health Care Organization (WHO, 2010) identified that it is essential that interprofessional health care teams learn how to use each team member's skills, share case management activities, and work in collaboration to provide better care.

Contributions of professionals from a variety of disciplines, because of the extensive experience and perspectives that each provides, are critical to the success of solving practice problems. Organizations providing opportunities for various practitioners and clinicians to come together for shared learning are effective in improving patient and family outcomes (Baker, Day, & Salas, 2006; Riley, Davis, Miller, & McCullough, 2010). However, Kvarnström (2008) reported that, while there are great hopes that interprofessional collaboration will improve the quality of health care, interprofessional teams experience difficulties related to team dynamics. Thus, when establishing interprofessional EBP teams, leaders of the program must provide learning opportunities and strategies that improve team performance. Therefore, the purpose of this chapter is to provide information about developing highly performing interprofessional EBP teams.

INTERPROFESSIONAL TEAM PHILOSOPHY

Every individual on the interprofessional team contributes his or her unique knowledge and skill to the process of EBP. Successful interprofessional EBP teams have a shared philosophy, such as that every team member works to contribute to the project, teaches others, and learns from the team (Moyers, Finch Guthrie, Swan, & Anderson, 2013). This philosophy stems from the idea that "interprofessional education occurs when two or more professions learn with, from, and about each other to improve collaboration and the quality of care" (Centre for the Advancement of Interprofessional Education [CAIPE], 2002). Adopting this definition of interprofessional education (IPE) for an interprofessional EBP program gives team members the understanding that team learning is interactive.

Establishing a team philosophy prior to initiating an interprofessional EBP program develops the esprit de corps necessary for effective teamwork. A team philosophy is especially important when team members have different levels of experience and knowledge (e.g., students and practicing clinicians). Freeman, Miller, and Ross (2000), in a case study with six interprofessional teams, found that team members had individual team philosophies, which led to different meanings and perceptions about teamwork and performance. For example, the directive philosophy for teamwork aligned with organizational power and status. Team members with this team philosophy often assumed those in formal organizational leadership positions would automatically provide team leadership and have the primary responsibility for decision making. In contrast, team members with an integrative philosophy believed the work and contributions of all team members had equal value and also thought that distributed leadership responsibilities based on the needed expertise and experience was the best approach to high performance. Unless a team philosophy is articulated, team members function from their own individual philosophy, which has the potential to create conflict and poor collaboration. However, adopting a team philosophy alone is not enough for developing highly performing teams as part of an interprofessional EBP program.

INTERPROFESSIONAL TEAM DEFINITION AND FRAMEWORK

To understand the nature of teams in the interprofessional EBP program, it is helpful to examine some basic definitions of teams. Specifically, Salas, DiazGranados, Weaver, and King (2008) define a team as "two or more individuals who must interact and adapt to achieve specified, shared, and valued objectives" (p. 1003). From this definition, it is clear that team members have shared goals, they are interdependent, and they learn to work together to meet objectives. This definition is similar to the description of Dyer, Dyer, and Dyer (2013) about highly performing teams as having "members whose skills, attitudes, and competencies enable them to achieve team goals. These team members set goals, make decisions, communicate, manage conflict, and solve problems in a supportive, trusting atmosphere in order to accomplish their objectives" (p. 13). The difference between the two definitions is that Dyer et al. stated that highly performing teams have special skills, attitudes, and competencies and that these teams function best within a team environment supportive of achieving team goals.

In an interprofessional EBP program, the charge to the team is specific to improving practice as a result of appraising and synthesizing evidence. Thus, taking the other definitions of teams into account, a team in an interprofessional EBP program is *a group of individuals from various disciplines who have unique and complementary expertise important to the interprofessional EBP process, as well as have the team skills of working interdependently and establishing mutual accountability.* This interprofessional EBP team definition organizes major concepts as a foundation for an interprofessional EBP team framework. These concepts include unique and complimentary expertise, team skills, interdependence, and mutual accountability as all being necessary for interprofessional EBP.

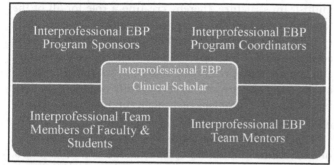

Figure 4-1. Interprofessional EBP team model.

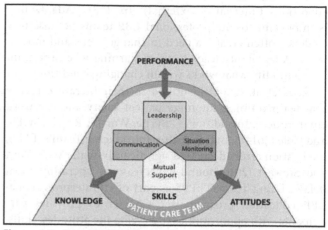

Figure 4-2. TeamSTEPPS framework: team strategies and tools to enhance performance and patient safety. (Reprinted with the permission of the Agency for Healthcare Research and Quality; Rockville, MD.)

The interprofessional EBP team definition also indicates the relationship between team performance in applying these interprofessional team concepts and the team's success in discerning and implementing the ultimate solution for a practice problem. As discussed in Chapter 1, an aspect of the interprofessional team framework is driven through the EBP model that the interprofessional EBP program adopts. The EBP practice model used within this book is the Iowa model (Titler et al., 2001), which provided a framework for the way the interprofessional teams were formed and for the major team decision points in the EBP phases (see Chapter 1, Figure 1-2). In an interprofessional EBP program, practitioners and clinicians submit practice problems for review. The health care organization selects the clinical scholars based on whether their application addresses a priority problem for the organization (see Chapter 6). The health care organization in collaboration with a university partner further selects team membership to include a mentor and interprofessional faculty and students. Figure 4-1 illustrates the interprofessional EBP team model that supports progression through the decision points in the EBP model. The interprofessional EBP team model requires the health care organization and university sponsors, team members, and mentor to surround and support the clinical scholar in addressing his or her identified clinical question.

While other EBP models also involve interprofessional teams in the EBP process (Dearholt & Dang, 2012; Goode, Fink, Krugman, Oman, & Traditi, 2011; Melnyk, 2012; Rycroft-Malone, 2004), few outline methods for ensuring team performance. Teamwork and collaboration is not an intuitive process but requires team education. Using a structured framework or model that describes essential elements of teamwork, skills for facilitating interaction, and processes for team integration and cohesiveness is critical for developing highly performing teams (Ateah et al., 2011; D'Amour & Oandasan, 2005; Robben et al., 2012).

The Agency for Healthcare Research and Quality (AHRQ), in collaboration with the Department of Defense, (http://teamstepps.ahrq.gov/) developed TeamSTEPPS, which is an evidence-based team approach designed to improve patient safety through team communication and teamwork skills. The four skills in the model are

appropriate for all types of teams, including interprofessional EBP teams (Figure 4-2). The AHRQ website for TeamSTEPPS includes a well-designed, structured curriculum that includes teamwork principles and materials that interprofessional EBP program coordinators can adapt for an interprofessional EBP program.

At the core of the TeamSTEPPS framework are the essential skills for highly performing teams, which include leadership, communication, mutual support, and situation monitoring (see Figure 4-2). The TeamSTEPPS model focuses on the team-related outcomes of greater knowledge, improved attitudes, and the exemplary team performance necessary to reach the objectives for assigned work. The knowledge outcome for TeamSTEPPS occurs when teams have a shared understanding of the work or a shared mental model (McComb & Simpson, 2013; Wilson, Burke, Priest, & Salas, 2005). Baker et al. (2006) defined mental models as "an organizing knowledge structure of the relationships between the task in which the team is engaged in and how the team members will interact" (p. 1582). With clearly outlined objectives, strategies, and team member assignments, teams are more likely to understand the nature of the work, the responsibilities for each member, and the need for interdependence. Misunderstandings are less likely when shared mental models exist (Westli, Johnsen, Eid, Rasten, & Brattebo, 2010; Wilson et al., 2005).

The TeamSTEPPS outcome related to team attitudes occurs when teams develop mutual trust and a team orientation that leads to a team commitment (Bandow, 2001; Molyneux, 2001; Webber, 2002). Optimal team performance occurs when team members become adaptable, efficient, productive, and accurate with the quality of the work. Baker et al. (2006) defined *team adaptability* as the "ability to adjust strategies based on information gathered from the environment through the use of compensatory behavior and reallocation of intrateam resources, altering a course of action or team repertoire in response to changing conditions (internal or external)" (p. 1581). Adaptability is important to interprofessional EBP teams because new evidence often creates a need to change focus and modify work. Adaptability leads to team learning when the team has to modify what works within changing conditions.

Salas et al. (2008) identified in their literature review that team training improves patient safety and the work environment. In addition, O'Byrne, Worthy, Ravelo, Webb, and Cole (2014) found that after introducing TeamSTEPPS, medication errors decreased significantly, while Wolf, Way, and Stewart (2010) found a decrease in operating room delays. Using TeamSTEPPS as part of an interprofessional EBP education program (see Chapter 6) provides participants with opportunities to develop the attitudes, skills, and competencies for effective collaboration in order to prevent unnecessary time delays and to reduce reworking because of recognizing upfront potential pitfalls in the EBP process.

INTERPROFESSIONAL TEAM STRUCTURES

An important understanding for successful formation of an interprofessional EBP team is recognition of the various functions of specific types of teams. Mosser and Begun (2014) discussed different types of health care teams as including clinical and project teams, which have differences in responsibilities, capabilities, and limitations. Interprofessional EBP teams are project teams because they have specific goals and are time limited. However, according to Mosser and Begun, project teams like clinical teams still need an appropriate team composition, effective leadership, well-described tasks, autonomy, education, and solid intra-organizational relationships (p. 29).

In TeamSTEPPS, team structure includes the coordinating activities of a multi-team system in which the teams work in concert to support patient safety (Pocket Guide, TeamSTEPPS, 2014). To illustrate the multi-team system, core teams offer essential direct care, coordinating teams facilitate the work of core teams, other teams may provide patient care but take a more supportive role in relationship to the core team, and administrative teams arrange overall direction and provide resources for the teams.

The design of an interprofessional EPB program also includes a multi-team system, consisting of the core interprofessional EBP teams, an administrative team, and a coordinating team. The administrative team includes the program sponsors and coordinators who work together to develop the interprofessional EBP program and provide overall direction. The coordinating team includes all of the team mentors and program coordinators working to meet the needs specific to each interprofessional EBP team. Continuous improvement is a goal within the EBP

multi-team structure, thereby creating a role for all of the teams in ensuring the interprofessional EBP process leads to successful team and project outcomes. For example, the administrative team continuously monitors the program and makes appropriate adaptations to substantiate teams are learning and are able to successfully negotiate the EBP process to take advantage of available opportunities regardless of barriers.

The structure of the teams also involves consideration of size, team composition, systems for communication, and processes for completing tasks and meeting the team objectives. Some studies identify that smaller teams have greater engagement and effectiveness compared to larger teams (Molyneux, 2001; Rutherford & McArthur, 2004; Shortell et al., 2014). However, multiple factors affect team function, such as team capacity, tasks, demands, processes for completing work, and level of interdependence (Funke, Knott, Salas, Pavlas, & Strang, 2012). Thus, team composition regarding EBP knowledge and skills is a critical consideration given the high task demands and cognitive load associated with EBP (see Chapter 3). The goal for team member selection is to create a balance of team membership with those who have expertise and skills to offset the lack of skill of some of the members in each EBP phase. Given that there is such a broad range of skills and expertise needed to accomplish the nine EBP phases, teams made up of members who have varied skills and expertise have an advantage compared to teams whose members have similar experiences and expertise. This similarity of team member expertise and skills might, as a result, be overly focused in only a few of the phases, leaving the team more reliant on outside experts.

Composition of the interprofessional teams may comprise various disciplines, such as nursing, occupational and physical therapy, social work, respiratory care, dietetics and nutrition science, pharmacy, medicine, physician assisting, holistic health, public health, exercise science, and library science. The nature of the clinical problem and needed expertise determines to some degree the disciplines to include on a team. Borrill, West, Shapiro, and Rees (2001) identified that occupational diversity not only improves team effectiveness, but also supports innovation. Greater team diversity often facilitates a generation of radical ideas that dramatically improve patient care and care delivery. Thus, selecting some team members without clear connections with the EBP problem may stimulate creativity because of different perspectives and paradigms. Individuals with limited knowledge and experience about the problem often ask critical questions that those steeped in the problem avoid, do not consider, or miss.

Two additional criteria essential for selecting team members include the level of commitment for the project and desire to collaborate with other disciplines (Molyneux, 2001). As members from different disciplines and organizations are brought together to participate on an interprofessional EBP team, it is crucial that transparency exist with the selection process. Transparency provides the foundation for trust, improves relationships among professions, and demonstrates the integrity of program sponsors (Mitchell et al., 2012). Having selection criteria prepares team members for their roles and needed contributions. Chapter 6 provides recommendations for selecting members of an interprofessional EBP team based on clear criteria.

Interprofessional Team Competencies, Skills, and Techniques

Different professional groups and various authors have described team competencies. For example, the 2003 IOM report includes a description of essential processes for teams including communication, cooperation, coordination, and collaboration; however, the report did not outline specific competencies for these processes. The 2003 IOM report does include competencies for health care professionals that involve working on interprofessional teams, providing patient-centered care, applying quality improvement, employing EBP, and using informatics. MacDonald et al. (2010) identified six team competencies that include communication, strength in one's professional role, knowledge of the roles of other discipline, leadership, team functioning, and conflict resolution (pp. 239-240). Mosser and Begun (2014) classify competencies for teams according to the team's focus on patients or projects, team orientation, collaboration, and team management (pp. 113-123).

The Interprofessional Education Collaborative (IPEC) Expert Panel (2011) that included pharmacy, nursing, osteopathic medicine, medicine, public health professionals, and dentists identified competency domains valuable for educating health care students and for developing interprofessional practice teams. The competency domains in the IPEC document include team roles and responsibilities, communication, values and ethics, and teamwork and team practice. Each domain has eight to 11 competencies. Because communication is often at the root of negative team outcomes, this book devotes a separate chapter (see Chapter 5) exclusively to this domain and its competencies.

However, communication is also a critical skill outlined in TeamSTEPPS, and communication is defined as "a structured process by which information is clearly and accurately exchanged among team members" (Pocket Guide, TeamSTEPPS, 2014, p. 5). The TeamSTEPPS approach (Table 4-1) includes several communication techniques that interprofessional EBP teams may find helpful, such as ensuring closed-loop communication (check back) and a standardized communication method about problems (i.e.,

situation, background, assessment, and recommendations [SBAR]). Specifically, closed-loop communication involves team members repeating back crucial information during a team meeting in order to validate understanding. The standard communication tool of SBAR is useful for the purpose of facilitating the team in making decisions and taking action as the result of presenting information and recommendations about a situation to the team, stakeholders, or project sponsors. This chapter focuses on the IPEC domains of value and ethics, roles and responsibilities, and teamwork and team practice.

Team Values and Ethics

The IPEC (2011) competencies for value and ethics (Table 4-2) focus the team's work on patients, families, and communities, as well as the related responsibilities for team members and each team member's individual practice as a professional. When team members are patient centered, the team has a shared purpose for improving patient safety, effectiveness, and efficiency of care. Meeting the value and ethic competencies assists with creating a team orientation and commitment. Each team member in the interprofessional EBP program has professional accountability for using evidence to improve patient care and team functioning. The value and ethics competencies highlight the importance of respect, trust, personal integrity, cultural diversity, and cooperation, as well as managing ethical dilemmas and maintaining professional competence.

Mitchell et al. (2012), in their exploration of core principles and values of effective team-based care, identified that teams first consist of individuals. Thus, establishing team values starts with identifying effective personal values that improve team performance. In reviewing the literature and through interviews, they identified five personal values, including honest and transparent communication, discipline in carrying out team roles and responsibilities, creativity and a desire to improve practice, humility regarding the value of everyone's contribution, and a curiosity and dedication to team learning. Including information about team values in orientation is important in setting the stage for highly performing interprofessional EBP teams.

Leadership Roles and Responsibilities

Team leaders who work with teams to create goals, establish clear expectations, and opportunities for regular communication, in addition to providing space, time, and support, will more likely have highly performing teams (Salas et al., 2008). The needs of the interprofessional EBP team should determine the most appropriate leader or leaders rather than the program directors or mentors automatically assigning someone on the team as the leader who has a formal leadership position in one of the partnering organizations. Interprofessional EBP teams may need

	TABLE 4-1	
	**HOW TO INCORPORATE TeamSTEPPS INTO AN INTERPROFESSIONAL EVIDENCE-BASED PRACTICE PROGRAM**	
SKILLS	**TEAMSTEPPS TOOLS/STRATEGY—USED IN AN INTERPROFESSIONAL EBP PROGRAM**	**EVIDENCE SOURCES**
Leadership: Mentors and program coordinators use tools to structure and coordinate the work of the team.	Briefings: A planning process that occurs at the beginning of the interprofessional team meeting to identify meeting goals, assignment of work, and potential issues for solving. Program coordinators also use briefings at the end of EBP learning sessions with all teams in attendance to provide guidance for next steps before teams convene their individual team meetings.	Phadnis & Templeton-Ward, 2015; Salas, DiazGranados, Weaver, & King, 2008
	Debriefings: A quality improvement strategy that occurs at the end of the interprofessional EBP team meeting to review accomplishments, identify what went well and what did not go well, plan for the next meeting, and identify next steps.	Salas et al., 2008
	Huddles: Ad hoc problem solving meetings that the interprofessional EBP teams call in between regular meetings to finalize submission of grants and internal review board applications, and address an implementation or data collection issue or a timeline or budget concern.	Shunk, Dulay, Chou, Janson, & O'Brien, 2014; Pocket Guide, TeamSTEPPS, 2014
Communication: Mentors and program coordinators promote the use of standards, routines, and methods for communication to ensure an accurate exchange of information.	The SBAR (i.e., situation, background, assessment, and recommendations) structure for communication may serve as a clear method for describing team information about a problem.	Martin & Ciurzynski, 2015
	Closed loop communication involves exchange of clear and concise information (check back). A team member communicates essential information, the team makes any necessary clarification and states the information back, and the sender acknowledge the team's correct understanding of the information.	Salas et al., 2008; Wilson et al., 2005; Pocket Guide, TeamSTEPPS, 2014
Mutual support: Mentors use mentor techniques and program coordinators provide mentor supports.	The interprofessional EBP team philosophy of everyone works, teaches, and learns promotes mutual trust and task assistance where team members are expected to ask for assistance and provide support to other members. The team climate is one of team commitment through good working relationships.	Brock et al., 2013; Wilson et al., 2005

(continued)

different leadership during specific EBP phases based on needed knowledge, expertise, and experience that the task demands require.

For example, the clinical scholar may be the best person to lead the team because of his or her familiarity with the practice area. However, at the beginning of the project, the mentor of the team is often the most logical team leader because of the clinical scholar's inexperience in conducting EBP. The mentor should develop the clinical scholar's

leadership skills and work toward transferring leadership to the clinical scholar. It is also possible that a faculty member is the best leader for submitting a grant application or an article for publication. A student may be the best leader during selection and training in communication technologies or in searching the literature.

Carson, Tesluk, and Marrone (2007) found that shared leadership is effective only when a positive team environment exists, the team has a shared purpose, social support

TABLE 4-1 (CONTINUED)		
HOW TO INCORPORATE TEAMSTEPPS INTO AN INTERPROFESSIONAL EVIDENCE-BASED PRACTICE PROGRAM		
SKILLS	**TEAMSTEPPS TOOLS/STRATEGY—USED IN AN INTERPROFESSIONAL EBP PROGRAM**	**EVIDENCE SOURCES**
Mutual support: Mentors use mentor techniques and program coordinators provide mentor supports.	Providing and encouraging timely feedback is a team expectation. Methods that the team can use for managing concerns are as follows: • Advocacy and assertion—used when there is a team disagreement. Make an opening, state the concern, make a suggestion, and obtain an agreement. • Two challenge rule—state the concern two times and ensure acknowledgement, ask for coordinator support as needed. • CUS—I am Concerned; I am Uncomfortable; there is a Safety issue. • DESC script—Describe the specific situation, Express how the situation impacts you, Suggest different ways to handle the situation, reach an agreement, and identify Consequences related to the project and team goals.	Pocket Guide, TeamSTEPPS, 2014
Situation monitoring: Mentors and program coordinators routinely assess and scan the situation that may affect the EBP project and team environment. Mentors and coordinators role model the process of situation monitoring and the importance of maintaining awareness to the team.	The team learns to cross-monitor each other's actions and work; is alert to potential errors, oversights, or misinterpretation of evidence; and creates an environment where the team easily identifies the potential for mistakes. The team creates a climate where everyone is looking out for the other team member.	Fioratou, Flin, Glavin, & Patey, 2010; Wilson et al., 2005
	Uses STEP process to monitor the situation in which the team determines the status of the project; team member involvement in each aspect of the project, their workload, and need for assistance; environment, ensuring that team members have what they need to do the work; and team progress in meeting project goals.	Pocket Guide, TeamSTEPPS, 2014
TeamSTEPPS® 2.0: Core Curriculum. March 2014. Agency for Healthcare Research and Quality, Rockville, MD. http://www.ahrq.gov/professionals/education/curriculum-tools/teamstepps/instructor/index.html		

is present for using multiple leaders, and the team receives external coaching to transfer leadership and improve performance. Thus, the interprofessional EBP program coordinators and team mentors facilitate having the best leaders at the right time. Coaching should include encouraging and recognizing the leadership that each member provides and assisting teams during times of conflict. Carson et al. also found that shared leadership can occur even when the team has a designated leader who acts more like a facilitator. TeamSTEPPS has a clear description of the role of a team leader applicable to the interprofessional EBP program, which includes the following (Pocket Guide, TeamSTEPPS, 2014, p. 15):

• Creating a team learning culture
• Role-modeling effective teamwork
• Organizing the team for the work of the interprofessional EBP project
• Assisting with establishing team goals for the EBP project
• Developing a plan with the team that includes ongoing monitoring and evaluation
• Ensuring the team assigns tasks for completing the EBP project
• Fostering communication and information sharing

TABLE 4-2

VALUE AND ETHICS

DESCRIPTION	SPECIFIC COMPETENCIES
General competency statement: Work with individuals of other professions to maintain a climate of mutual respect and shared values.	• Place the interests of patients and populations at the center of interprofessional health care delivery. • Respect the dignity and privacy of patients while maintaining confidentiality in the delivery of team-based care. • Embrace the cultural diversity and individual differences that characterize patients, populations, and the health care team. • Respect the unique cultures, values, roles/responsibilities, and expertise of other health professions. • Work in cooperation with those who receive care, those who provide care, and others who contribute to or support the delivery of prevention and health services. • Develop a trusting relationship with patients, families, and other team members (CIHC, 2010). • Demonstrate high standards of ethical conduct and quality of care in one's contributions to team-based care. • Manage ethical dilemmas specific to interprofessional patient-/population-centered care situations. • Act with honesty and integrity in relationships with patients, families, and other team members. • Maintain competence in one's own profession appropriate to scope of practice.

Interprofessional Education Collaborative Expert Panel. (2011). Core competencies for interprofessional collaborative practice: Report of an expert panel. Washington, DC: Interprofessional Education Collaborative. Reprinted with permission from American Association of Medical Colleges (AAMC).

• Managing the needed resources with the team

• Facilitating team evaluation, effective feedback, and conflict resolution

TeamSTEPPS methods also include strategies that program coordinators, mentors, and other team leaders of an interprofessional EBP team can use to coordinate the team, such as briefings, debriefings, and huddles (see Table 4-1). Program coordinators incorporate briefings at the end of each EBP learning session to outline expectations for the subsequent interprofessional team meeting occurring after the education activities. These briefings are short and stem from the specific learning session. For example, following a learning session about appraising the literature, a general briefing to all of the teams may include instructions for assigning evidence to each team member for an initial appraisal, identifying a process for collecting and sharing completed appraisals, and practicing the appraisal process jointly through examination of a team-selected study. At individual team meetings, the designated leader briefs the team regarding specific decisions and goals for the meeting that relate to the general briefing that the program coordinators provided.

The program coordinators and the team leaders use debriefings to evaluate the effectiveness of learning sessions and meetings. Debriefing questions include the following: (a) what went well, (b) what did not go well, and (c) what actions, resources, and education are needed. The mentors and program coordinators address the information generated from the debriefings at the program coordinating and administrative team meetings. Program coordinators, mentors, and team leaders use huddles to address issues that need immediate action. Huddles may occur virtually or face-to-face, depending on the issue. A team might use a virtual huddle, for example, when a deadline for submitting to a grant funder is actually earlier than originally planned. Consequently, there needs to be an immediate change in plans that cannot wait for the team discussion at the next formal meeting. The huddle would determine if and how the interprofessional EBP team would complete the funding proposal for on-time submission to the grant funder.

Team Roles and Responsibilities

In addition to developing the role of the team leaders, the roles and responsibilities of each team member also

TABLE 4-3	
ROLES AND RESPONSIBILITIES	
DESCRIPTION	**SPECIFIC COMPETENCIES**
General competency statement: Use the knowledge of one's own role and those of other professions to appropriately assess and address the health care needs of the patients and populations served.	• Communicate one's roles and responsibilities clearly to patients, families, and other professionals. • Recognize one's limitations in skills, knowledge, and abilities. • Engage diverse health care professionals who complement one's own professional expertise, as well as associated resources, to develop strategies to meet specific patient care needs. • Explain the roles and responsibilities of other care providers and how the team works together to provide care. • Use the full scope of knowledge, skills, and abilities of available health professionals and health care workers to provide care that is safe, timely, efficient, effective, and equitable. • Communicate with team members to clarify each member's responsibility in executing components of a treatment plan or public health intervention. • Forge interdependent relationships with other professions to improve care and advance learning. • Engage in continuous professional and interprofessional development to enhance team performance. • Use unique and complementary abilities of all members of the team to optimize patient care.

Interprofessional Education Collaborative Expert Panel. (2011). Core competencies for interprofessional collaborative practice: Report of an expert panel. Washington, DC: Interprofessional Education Collaborative. Reprinted with permission from American Association of Medical Colleges (AAMC).

need clarification in order to create highly performing interprofessional EBP teams. The IPEC (2011) competencies also delineate roles and responsibilities appropriate for EBP interprofessional teams (Table 4-3). The competencies most relevant for interprofessional EBP team members are those that create expectations to routinely share information about the disciplinary role, engage in team development that enhances team performance, understand limitations of each team member, and use the full scope of each member's knowledge, skills, and abilities for creating an effective EBP project. Knowing what team members do best is critical for developing a high-performing team. Often, interprofessional EBP teams forget to examine the strengths the students on the team possess and tend to focus primarily on their learning needs. Without addressing the students' strengths as an asset to the team, the risk of marginalizing the student is higher.

According to Buckingham (2007) when leading the effort with the Gallup organization to identify the core characteristics of great managers and workplaces, the survey item regarding employee satisfaction that showed the strongest correlation with organizational performance was "I have the opportunity to do what I do best every day at work." Maximizing each team member's contribution also applies to the interprofessional EBP program. Specifically, it is important that interprofessional teams cultivate an understanding and respect for the unique roles, responsibilities, and knowledge of each discipline represented on the team. The way in which the team assigns work to each team member should be partially based on each member's expertise, personal strengths, interests, and learning goals.

Multiple roles and responsibilities exist for each member of the interprofessional EBP team, with some responsibilities serving to maintain team processes (e.g., setting up meetings and writing agendas) or advance the EBP process (e.g., conducting literature searches and appraising literature), while others are specific to project management (e.g., working with stakeholders and developing staff education). Important team member responsibilities that support team processes may include but are not limited to the following:

• Providing leadership in area of expertise

• Contributing to and taking responsibility for aspects of the team work plan

• Facilitating team discussions

• Keeping track of time in relation to meeting goals

TABLE 4-4	
TEAM AND TEAMWORK	
DESCRIPTION	**SPECIFIC COMPETENCIES**
General competency statement: Apply relationship-building values and the principles of team dynamics to perform effectively in different team roles to plan and deliver patient-/population-centered care that is safe, timely, efficient, effective, and equitable.	• Describe the process of team development and the roles and practices of effective teams. • Develop consensus on the ethical principles to guide all aspects of patient care and team work. • Engage other health professionals—appropriate to the specific care situation—in shared patient-centered problem solving. • Integrate the knowledge and experience of other professions—appropriate to the specific care situation—to inform care decisions, while respecting patient and community values and priorities/preferences for care. • Apply leadership practices that support collaborative practice and team effectiveness. • Engage self and others to constructively manage disagreements about values, roles, goals, and actions that arise among health care professionals and with patients and families. • Share accountability with other professions, patients, and communities for outcomes relevant to prevention and health care. • Reflect on individual and team performance for individual, as well as team, performance improvement. • Use process improvement strategies to increase the effectiveness of interprofessional teamwork and team-based care. • Use available evidence to inform effective teamwork and team-based practices. • Perform effectively on teams and in different team roles in a variety of settings.

Interprofessional Education Collaborative Expert Panel. (2011). Core competencies for interprofessional collaborative practice: Report of an expert panel. Washington, DC: Interprofessional Education Collaborative. Reprinted with permission from American Association of Medical Colleges (AAMC).

- Recording minutes and agreements and keeping track of team documents

- Securing needed team resources

The team should assign routine tasks in a manner that balances team needs, considers the goals of the project, and uses available resources. Teams should identify appropriate responsibilities for each team member; rotating responsibilities creates a sense of ownership and facilitates commitment to the team. Creating a work plan that identifies work for conducting each phase of the EBP process, identifying timelines for completing the work, and assigning team members specific responsibilities ensure clear expectations.

Team and Teamwork

The IPEC competencies regarding team and teamwork focus on team dynamics and relationship building (Table 4-4). The interprofessional EBP teams need to have a philosophical orientation supportive of placing team goals before the goals of each individual on the team (Mosser & Begun, 2014; Salas et al., 2008). The essential TeamSTEPPS strategies for improving team dynamics include situation monitoring and providing mutual support (see Figure 4-1 and Table 4-1). Interprofessional EBP team members support the team when maintaining awareness about the progress of the project, problems that team member's face, issues that may occur, and the resources needed. The STEP (i.e., status, team, environment, and progress) process is one method to maintain a high degree of situation awareness (see Table 4-1) (Pocket Guide, TeamSTEPPS, 2014). At meetings, the mentor and team leaders ask about the status of the project, how well team members are doing in completing assignments, issues or barriers that exist, and strategies needed to maintain progress.

Mutual support is about team members asking for task assistance when needed and for fellow team members to provide the requested assistance (see Table 4-1) (Pocket Guide, TeamSTEPPS, 2014). Team members protect each

	TABLE 4-5	
	CREATING THE TEAM CHARTER	
ELEMENT	**DESCRIPTION**	
Team name	How does the team refer to itself?	
Team purpose	What is the team's reason for being?	
Strategic alignment	How does the team's work support and relate to organizational goals?	
Key stakeholders	Who are the team's internal and external stakeholders?	
Team objectives and priorities	What are the team's primary objectives and how are they prioritized?	
Team leader and mentor	Who is the team leader and who is the mentor?	
Key deliverables	What are the team's key deliverables or tangible work products?	
Team member roles and responsibilities	Who are the team members and what are their roles and responsibilities?	
EBP project time commitments	What time commitments are expected for all team members?	
Team communication plan	What are the communication rules and strategies for the team?	

other from undue workload and provide effective feedback and guidance that promotes growth and development. Mutual support also occurs when team members are assertive, making the team aware of individual concerns and the seriousness of specific problems. Assertiveness prevents the team from making mistakes. Table 4-1 covers the TeamSTEPPS strategies for mutual support, such as advocacy and assertion, and the two-challenge rule for addressing concerns.

An initial step for fostering each member to put the team first is for the interprofessional EBP team to create a team charter during the program orientation. A team charter is a document that the interprofessional team develops together to facilitate consensus building and sharing fundamental information that creates team identity (Brownlee, 2012). The team charter is a dynamic document evolving with changes in team composition, processes, organization, or other factors that affect the team and the project. According to Brownlee (2012), team charters typically have common elements as outlined in Table 4-5. The team norms outlined in the charter provide a frame of reference in which the team operates effectively. The team revisits these initial norms in order to revise the norms to reflect the interprofessional team's growth in understanding and experience with the EBP process. Additional elements of the charter for interprofessional EBP teams may include a plan for dissemination of the work once completed, such as the type of papers and presentations that will occur. While the team can complete this aspect of the charter later when the team has developed a project plan, it is critical that the team identifies authorship and agrees to the dissemination plan and products (see Chapter 14). Two common mistakes that many teams make in creating the team charter are as follows:

1. The team rushes to complete the document in order to move on to what is perceived as more important work, and therefore the team has not created a strong basis for functioning.

2. The team forgets about the existence of the team charter after its completion. The most successful teams review the team charter regularly in order to revise it as needed.

MENTORING CHALLENGES

Teams often have problems with collaboration, communication, and coordination because of strong professional cultures that keep disciplinary groups separated. Specifically, Ginsburg and Tregunno (2005) identified that each profession has established roles and functions, specific disciplinary competencies, and definitive professional cultures. Well-defined scopes of practice and professional boundaries, while necessary for single-disciplinary practice, create barriers for team practice often resulting in territorialism, misperceptions, and stereotypical beliefs. A team member may develop not only a stereotypical belief about his or her own discipline, but about other disciplines as well (Oandasan & Reeves, 2005). Differences in entry-level education (e.g., baccalaureate vs. graduate level) may also contribute to the perceptions one discipline has about another. Oandasan and Reeves also found that faculty may have negative attitudes toward other professions as well, which can affect IPE.

Other common problems affecting teamwork include social loafing, freeloading, production blocking, and diminished creativity. According to Schmidt, Montoya-Weiss, and Massey (2001), there is a tendency for teams to conform or agree, which limits creativity. Production blocking also decreases creativity because it reduces information exchange between members of the team. Production blocking occurs when team members are interrupted and do not completely communicate their ideas and thoughts or when individuals withhold information out of anxiety or fear about how others may perceive what they say.

Mosser and Begun (2014) identified social loafing as the most common risk for teams, and it often occurs when teams have more than one person who can perform an assigned task. Thus, it is tempting for team members to stand by while someone else does the work. The work involved in interprofessional EBP comprises more than coming to meetings and exchanging information, such as how to appraise studies, when the real need is to complete appraisals on time. Perceptions about what members believe they are providing versus their actual contributions and the perceptions of other members may be at odds.

Differences in power also exist within a team. Nugus, Greenfield, Travaglia, Westbrook, and Braithwaite (2010) revealed the existence of both "competitive power" and "collaborative power" within health care systems. Competitive power involves one or more clinicians from one profession dominating team members from other disciplines. Collaborative power involves interdependent participation and decision making, as well as each member having a team orientation rather than a discipline orientation.

Interprofessional relations in the EBP program depend on how well environments support team function and collaboration. Therefore, it is important to identify time periods throughout the program at which the interprofessional teams evaluate how well they are performing as a team. Table 4-6 provides a description of team instruments available for evaluating teams. Periodic evaluation of team performance provides opportunities for interprofessional teams to address problems, make changes to the team charter, and increase the likelihood of achieving team goals.

MENTOR TECHNIQUES AND MENTOR SUPPORTS

The mentor facilitates teamwork, promotes positive relationships among team members, responds to team member's concerns, identifies challenges that impede the team's progress, removes barriers, and consults with appropriate experts who can assist with challenges (Heale, Mossey, LaFoley, & Gorham, 2009). To assure success of the EBP projects, program coordinators, team mentors, and team members need to revisit and redefine team roles throughout the project and develop leaders within the project team. Team roles frequently change, which is especially true when

new members come onto the team or when other members finish their commitments.

According to Turaga (2013), assuring clarity in roles has a positive effect on the performance of the team. Team members need to feel they have a specific role, defined work, and responsibilities. Role clarity makes team members more comfortable, which helps them trust the process and their team members. The mentors and team leaders should assess and rotate certain roles to alleviate frustration or feelings that any team member is providing more support or work in comparison to other members.

Mentors should assist teams in clarifying time commitments and schedules to ensure attendance and engagement during project meetings. Consistent team meetings and interactions among team leaders, the mentor, and team members help to ensure transparency and a sense of belonging. Incorporating tools such as meeting polls to obtain input from team members regarding the best times for meetings helps to ensure an inclusive process and communicates the value placed on all team members. Consistent use of briefings, huddles, and debriefing helps to keep the teams coordinated. Engaging the team in ongoing improvement of team performance through facilitating feedback and formal evaluation assists with providing effective leadership, ensuring closed-loop communication, situation awareness, and mutual support.

SUMMARY

Creating highly performing teams is a deliberate process in which the leaders of the interprofessional EBP program plans for and intentionally includes team processes into the program. A clear selection process helps team members begin to understand their team roles and the expertise they can provide. Establishing a team philosophy, such as that everyone works, learns, and teaches prior to starting an interprofessional EBP program, assists in creating a shared vision for how team members will interact. Various team members may provide leadership at different times, depending on the step in the EBP process.

Because many clinicians have not received formal team education, interprofessional competencies are useful to focus on team values and ethics, roles and responsibilities, communication, and teamwork and team practice (CAIPE, 2002). An important team framework is TeamSTEPPS, which describes the importance of shared leadership, communication, mutual support, and situation monitoring to promote team cohesiveness and collaboration. Important team strategies include using a team charter, briefings, debriefings, and huddles to coordinate the teams. The role of mentors includes supporting the team, role-modeling collaboration, encouraging the use of effective team strategies, and developing team leaders.

		TABLE 4-6

TEAM ASSESSMENT INSTRUMENTS

	INSTRUMENT	SOURCE	DESCRIPTION
1	Assessment of Interprofessional Team Collaboration Scale (AITCS)	Orchard, King, Khalili, & Bezzina, 2012	**Team Collaboration** The AITCS is a 47-item instrument, using a 5-point Likert scale that includes four subscales 1. Partnership 2. Cooperation 3. Coordination 4. Shared decision making for team collaboration
2	TeamSTEPPS Teamwork Perceptions Questionnaire (T-TPQ)	The American Institute of Research, 2010	**Team Skills and Behaviors** The T-TPQ tool measures team members' perceptions of their team's skills and behavior. The questionnaire is based on TeamSTEPPS. A Likert scale addresses team structure, leadership, communication, mutual support, and situation monitoring.
3	Team Diagnostics Survey (TDS)	Wageman, Hackman, & Lehman, 2005	**Team Behavior and Performance** The TDS instrument measures strengths and weaknesses regarding team behavior and performance. The conceptual model for the instrument identifies five elements that increase the likelihood of high team performance: 1. A real team versus in name only 2. Clear direction for the assigned work 3. Appropriate team structure 4. Organizational support for the work of the team 5. Coaching that assist team members in the work of the team
4	Communication and Teamwork Skills (CATS)	Frankel, Gardner, Maynard, & Kelly, 2007	**Team Communication and Team Skills** Team skills are organized in the instrument's four areas: coordination, cooperation, situational awareness, and communication. The scoring of the instrument is based on the actual occurrence and quality of the team behaviors.
5	Safety Attitudes Questionnaire (SAQ)	Sexton et al., 2006	**Teamwork Climate** The SAQ examines attitudes of caregivers, using six factors that stem from the following: 1. Teamwork climate 2. Safety climate 3. Job satisfaction 4. Perceptions of management 5. Working conditions 6. Stress recognition

(continued)

TABLE 4-6 (CONTINUED)		
TEAM ASSESSMENT INSTRUMENTS		
INSTRUMENT	**SOURCE**	**DESCRIPTION**
6 Comprehensive Assessment of Team Member Effectiveness (CATME)	Loughry, Ohland, & Moore, 2007	**Team Member Effectiveness** The CATME instrument includes 39 items that measure 29 different types of team member contributions grouped into five categories: 1. Contributing to the team's work 2. Interacting with other team members 3. Keeping the team on track 4. Expecting quality 5. Having relevant knowledge, skills, and abilities

REFLECTION QUESTIONS

1. Think about your attitude, skills, knowledge, and readiness to be part of an interprofessional EBP team. What are your strengths? Identify areas in which you need further development. What kinds of professional contribution, resources, and leadership can you bring to the team? Where do your knowledge and skills overlap with other disciplines?

2. After reading this chapter, what stands out to you and excites you about teamwork? What observations and insights can you bring to the team?

REFERENCES

Ateah, C. A., Snow, W., Wener, P., MacDonald, L., Metge, C., Davis, P., ... Anderson, J. (2011). Stereotyping as a barrier to collaboration: Does interprofessional education make a difference? *Nurse Education Today, 31*(2), 208-213.

Baker, D. P., Day, R., & Salas, E. (2006). Teamwork as an essential component of high-reliability organizations. *Health Services Research, 41*(4), 1576-1598.

Bandow, D. (2001). Time to create sound teamwork. *The Journal for Quality and Participation, 24*(2), 41-47.

Borrill, C., West, M., Shapiro, D., & Rees, A. (2000). Team working and effectiveness in health care. *British Journal of Health Care Management 6*(8), 364-371.

Brock, D., Abu-Rish, E., Chiu, C. R., Hammer, D., Wilson, S., Vorvick, L., ... Zierler, B. (2013). Interprofessional education in team communication: Working together to improve patient safety. *Postgraduate Medical Journal, 89*(1057), 642-651.

Brownlee, D. (2012). Team charter: Get your team back on track. *Leadership Excellence.* Vol. 15.

Buckingham, M. (2007). *Go put your strengths to work.* New York, NY: One Thing Productions.

CAIPE. (2002). *Interprofessional education: A definition.* Retrieved December 8, 2014, at http://caipe.org.uk/about-us/defining-ipe/.

Canadian Interprofessional Health Collaborative. (2010). A national interprofessional competency framework. Retrieved from http://www.cihc.ca/resources/publications

Carson, J. B., Tesluk, P. E., & Marrone, J. A. (2007). Shared leadership in teams: An investigation of antecedent conditions and performance. *Academy of Management Journal, 50*(5), 1217-1234.

Centre for the Advancement of Interprofessional Education. (2002). The definition and principles of interprofessional education. Retrieved from http://caipe.org.uk/about-us/the-definition-and-principles-of-interprofessional-education/

D'amour, D., & Oandasan, I. (2005). Interprofessionality as the field of interprofessional practice and interprofessional education: An emerging concept. *Journal of Interprofessional Care, 19,* Supplement 1, 8-20.

Dearholt, S. L., & Dang, D. (2012). *Johns Hopkins nursing evidence-based practice: Model and guidelines* (2nd Ed.). Indianapolis, ID: Sigma Theta Tau International Honor Society of Nursing.

Dyer, W. G., Dyer, J. H., & Dyer, W. G. (2013). *Team building: Proven strategies for improving team performance,* San Francisco, CA: Jossey-Bass.

Fioratou, E., Flin, R., Glavin, R., & Patey, R. (2010). Beyond monitoring: Distributed situation awareness in anesthesia. *British Journal of Anaesthesia, 105*(1), 83-90.

Frankel, A., Gardner, R., Maynard, L. & Kelly, A. (2007). Using the Communication and Teamwork Skills (CATS) Assessment to Measure Health Care Team Performance. *The Joint Commission Journal on Quality and Patient Safety, 33*(9), 549-558.

Freeman, M., Miller, C., & Ross, N. (2000). The impact of individual philosophies of teamwork on multi-professional practice and the implications for education. *Journal of Interprofessional Care, 14*(3), 237-247.

Funke, G. J., Knott, B. A., Salas, E., Pavlas, D., & Strang, A. J. (2012). Conceptualization and measurement of team workload: A critical need. *Human Factors, 54*(1), 36-51.

Ginsburg, L., & Tregunno, D. (2005). New approaches to interprofessional education and collaborative practice: Lessons from the organizational change literature. *Journal of Interprofessional Care, 19, Supp* (1), 177-187.

Goode, C. J., Fink, R. M., Krugman, M., Oman, K. S., & Traditi, L. K. (2011). The Colorado patient-centered interprofessional evidence-based practice model: A framework for transformation. *Worldviews on Evidence-Based Nursing, 8*(2), 96-105.

Heale, R., Mossey, S., LaFoley, B., & Gorham, R. (2009). Identification of facilitators and barriers to the role of a mentor in the clinical setting. *Journal of Interprofessional Care. 23*(4), 369-379.

Institute of Medicine. (2001). *Crossing the quality chasm: A new health system for the 21st century.* Washington, DC: National Academy Press.

Institute of Medicine. (2003). *Health professions education: A bridge to quality.* Washington, DC: The National Academies Press.

Interprofessional Education Collaborative Expert Panel. (2011). *Core competencies for interprofessional collaborative practice: Report of an expert panel.* Washington, DC: Interprofessional Education Collaborative.

Kvarnström, S. (2008). Difficulties in collaboration: A critical incident study of interprofessional teamwork. *Journal of Interprofessional Care, 22*(2). 191-203.

Loughry, M., Ohland, M., & Moore, D. (2007). Development of a theory-based assessment of team member effectiveness. *Educational and Psychological Measurement, 67*(3), 505-524.

MacDonald, M., Bally, J., Ferguson, L, Murray, B., Fowler-Kerry, S., & Anonson, J. (2010). Knowledge of the professional roles of others: A key interprofessional competency. *Nurse Education in Practice, Vol. 10*(4), 238-242.

Martin, H., & Ciurzynski, S. (2015). Situation, background, assessment, and recommendations improve communication and teamwork in the emergency department. *Journal of Emergency Nursing, 41*(6), 484-488.

McComb, S., & Simpson, V. (2013). The concept of shared mental models in healthcare collaboration. *Journal of Advanced Nursing, 70*(7), 1479-1488.

Melnyk, B. M. (2012). Achieving a high-reliability organization through implementation of the ARCC model for systemwide sustainability of evidence-based practice. *Nursing Administration Quarterly, 36*(2), 127-135.

Mitchell, P., Wynia, W., Golden, R., McNellis, B., Okun, S., Webb, C.E., ... Von Kohorn, I. (2012). Core principles & values of effective team based health care. *Institute of Medicine.* Retrieved at http://nam.edu/perspectives-2012-core-principles-values-of-effective-team-based-health-care/.

Molyneux, J. (2001). Interprofessional teamworking: what makes a team work well? *Journal of Interprofessional Care,15*(1), 29-35.

Mosser, G., & Begun, J. (2014). *Understanding teamwork in health care.* New York, NY: McGraw Hill Education.

Moyers, P., Finch Guthrie, P., Swan, A., & Anderson, S. (2013). Interprofessional evidence-based clinical scholar program: Learning to work together. *American Journal of Occupational Therapy, 68,* S23-S31.

Moyers, P., Finch Guthrie, P., Swan, A., & Swanson, S. (2013). *Interprofessional evidence-based clinical scholar program: learning to work together.* St Paul, MN: St. Catherine University; 1-25.

Nugus, P., Greenfield, D., Travaglia, J., Westbrook, J., & Braithwaite, J. (2010). How and where clinicians exercise power: Interprofessional relations in health care. *Social Science & Medicine, 71*(5), 898-909.

O'Byrne, N., Worthy, K., Ravelo, A., Webb, M. & Cole, A. (2014). Stepping forward for patient safety: Using TeamSTEPPS concepts to reduce medication errors in a surgical intensive care unit. *Critical Care Nurse, 34*(2), e28.

Oandasan, I. & Reeves, S. (2005). Key elements of interprofessional education. Part 2: Factors, processes and outcomes. *Journal of Interprofessional Care, 19*(s1), 39-48.

Orchard, C., King, G., Khalili, H., & Bezzina, M. (2012). Assessment of Interprofessional Team Collaboration Scale (AITCS): Development and testing of the instrument. *Journal of Continuing Education in the Health Professions. 32*(1), 58-67.

Phadnis, J. & Templeton-Ward, O. (2015). Inadequate preoperative team briefings lead to more intraoperative adverse events. *Journal of Patient Safety, April 22,* published ahead of print. doi:10.1097/PTS.0000000000000181

Pocket Guide, TeamSTEPPS. January 2014. Agency for Healthcare Research and Quality, Rockville, MD. http://www.ahrq.gov/professionals/education/curriculum-tools/teamstepps/instructor/essentials/pocketguide.html

Riley, W., Davis, S. E., Miller, K. K., & McCullough, M. (2010). A model of developing high-reliability teams. *Journal of Nursing Management, 18*(5), 556-563.

Robben, S., Perry, M., van Nieuwenhuljzen, L., van Achterberg, T., Rikkert, M.O., Shers, H., ... Melis, R. (2012). Impact of interprofessional education on collaboration attitudes, skills, and behavior among primary care professionals. *Journal of Continuing Education in the Health Professions, 32*(3), 196-204.

Rycroft-Malone, J. (2004) The PARIHS framework—A framework for guiding the implementation of evidence-based practice. *Journal of Nursing Care Quality 19*(4), 297-304.

Rutherford, J., & McArthur, M., (2004). A qualitative account of the factors affecting team-learning in primary care. *Education for Primary Care, 15*(3), 352-360.

Salas, E., DiazGranados, D., Weaver, S., & King, H. (2008). Does team training work? Principles for health care. *Academic Emergency Medicine, 15*(11), 1002-1009.

Schmidt, J. B., Montoya-Weiss, M. M., & Massey, A. P. (2001). New product development decision-making effectiveness: Comparing individuals, face-to-face teams, and virtual teams. *Decision Sciences, 32*(4), 575-600.

Sexton, J., Helmreich, R., Neilands, T., Rowan, K., Vella, K., Boyden, J.,...Thomas, E. (2006). The Safety Attitudes Questionnaire: psychometric properties, benchmarking data, and emerging research. *BMC Health Services Research, 6*(1), 44.

Shortell, S., Marsteller, J. A., Lin, M., Pearson, M. L, Wu, S. Y., Mendel, P., ...Shunk, R., Dulay, M., Chou, C., Janson, S., & O'Brien, B. (2014). Huddle-coaching: A dynamic Intervention for trainees and staff to support team-based care. *Academic Medicine, 89*(2), 244-250.

TeamSTEPPS® 2.0: Core Curriculum. March 2014. Agency for Healthcare Research and Quality, Rockville, MD. http://www.ahrq.gov/professionals/education/curriculum-tools/teamstepps/instructor/index.html

The American Institute of Research. (2010). *TeamSTEPPS® Teamwork Perceptions Questionnaire (T-TPQ) Manual.* Washington D.C. American Institute for Research. Retrieved at http://teamstepps.ahrq.gov/Teamwork_Perception_Questionnaire.pdf.

Titler, M., Kleiber, C., Steelman, V., Rakel, B., Budreau, G., Everett, L.,...Goode, C. (2001). The Iowa model of evidence-based practice to promote quality care. *Critical Care Nursing Clinics of North America. 13*(4), 497-509.

Turaga, R. (2013). Building trust in teams: A leader's role. *The IUP Journal of Soft Skills, VII*(2), 3-31.

Wageman, R., Hackman, J. & Lehman, E. (2005). Team diagnostic survey: Development of an instrument. *The Journal of Applied Behavioral Science. 41*,(4) 373-398.

Webber, S.S. (2002). Leadership and trust facilitating cross-functional team success, *Journal of Management Development, 21*(3), 201-214.

Westli, H. K., Johnsen, B. H., Eid, J., Rasten, I., & Brattebo, G. (2010). Teamwork skills, shared mental models, and performance in simulated trauma teams: An independent group design. *Scandinavian Journal of Trauma, Resuscitation and Emergency Medicine, 18*(47), 2-8.

Wilson, K. A., Burke, C. S., Priest, H. A., & Salas, E. (2005). Promoting health care safety through training high reliability teams. *Quality and Safety in Health Care, 14*(4), 303-309.

Wolf, F., Way, L., & Stewart, L. (2010). The efficacy of medical team training: Improved team performance and decreased operating room delays: A detailed analysis of 4863 cases. *Annals of Surgery, 252*(3), 477-485.

World Health Organization Health Professions Networks Nursing & Midwifery Human Resources for Health. (2010). Framework for action on interprofessional education & collaborative practice. World Health Organization, Department of Human Resources for Health, CH-1211 Geneva 27, Switzerland. http://www.who.int/hrh/nursing_midwifery/en/

Supplemental materials for this chapter are available online.
Please refer to the sticker in the front of the book and enter the access code provided.

Facilitating Effective Interprofessional Team Communication

Therese Whalen Dlugosch, MA, OTR/L and Penelope A. Moyers, EdD, OT/L, FAOTA

CHAPTER TOPICS

- Barriers to communication
- Evidence supporting the need for better team communication
- Interprofessional communication competencies
- Communication strategies creating a highly effective team
- Assessments of team communication
- Mentor challenges
- Mentor techniques and supports

PERFORMANCE OBJECTIVES

By the end of the chapter, program coordinators, team members, and mentors should be able to do the following:

1. Create and implement a communication plan for the interprofessional team to use during the evidence-based project.
2. Identify core interprofessional communication competencies for further team development.
3. Identify strategies to improve communication within the interprofessional team.

Communication is essential to building a highly effective interprofessional team. Communication is "the act or process of using words, sounds, signs, or behaviors to express or exchange information" (Communication, Merriam-Webster Online Dictionary, n.d.). This definition does not reflect the complicated nature of interprofessional communication in terms of the team's skill in decision making and affective competencies (e.g., mutual respect), cultural factors influencing communication, and contextual structure that supports good communication (Sargeant, Loney, & Murphy, 2008). All team members, even those with experience working with several kinds of teams, have to continually improve their communication skills due to the ebb and flow of mutual understanding that occurs over the course of the team's interactions (Quinlan & Robertson, 2013). Mutual understanding is not permanent because

Moyers, P. A., & Finch-Guthrie, P. L.
*Interprofessional Evidence-Based Practice:
A Workbook for Health Professionals* (pp 79-92).
© 2016 Taylor and Francis Group.

BOX 5-1. A STUDENT'S PERCEPTION OF COMMUNICATION

As a student on the project, I thought we all had well-developed communication skills. After all, everyone on the team was very experienced. I was a graduate student and had been in the workforce for a period of time after getting my undergraduate degree. I wondered, "Why is communication an emphasis for learning in this program? It seemed obvious to me that communication is important." However, during the beginning of the project we were not communicating as a team. Consequently, our timeline suffered as did the quality of work. I quickly learned the time our group eventually spent on a communication plan made a huge difference in our project in that we started making significant progress.

---

teamwork contributes to knowledge exchange that leads team members to challenge their previously held assumptions. Even though new information is learned, team members paradoxically begin to question what they know and understand, thereby temporarily decreasing mutual understanding.

Teams may vacillate from stability to instability unless the mentors, program coordinators, and team members undertake strategies that support effective team functioning throughout periods of intensive knowledge exchange in which instability is likely (Quinlan & Robertson, 2013). Mentors function in a role that Quinlan and Robertson described as boundary spanning when coordinating knowledge exchange among the different professions on the team in a way that does not destabilize the team's functioning.

In forming an interprofessional evidence-based practice (EBP) team, an initial step is to identify the leader and assign team roles and to document these decisions in an interprofessional EBP team charter (see Chapters 4 and 6). To ensure that the interprofessional EBP project stays on track with budget and timeline, key elements in interprofessional communication (i.e., briefing, debriefing, and feedback) are operationalized as consistent team processes. Recall from Chapter 4 that briefing and debriefing are leadership coordination communication strategies and that feedback is a method for establishing mutual support. Consequently, teams need to establish these expectations for communication early in the interprofessional EBP project so that habits of engagement will serve the team well throughout the project (Box 5-1). Teams that do not pay attention to communication problems suffer the consequences of a greater number of conflicts, misunderstandings, and inability to move forward on the project (Schyve, 2009, p. v).

BARRIERS TO COMMUNICATION

The EBP mentor study conducted with North Memorial Hospital and St. Catherine University (see Chapter 3) indicated that interprofessional team communication was the most frequent and most difficult mentor challenge for the mentors and program directors. Factors impacting communication in the mentor study of interprofessional EBP as well as those cited in the literature (Novak & McIntyre,

2010) include the availability of team members to meet due to varied schedules, productivity requirements of team members that inadvertently reduced their time for team activities, and whether the organization allows team members to work on team assignments during work hours or during relevant courses in the case of students.

Each team member and the mentor bring their unique experiences, cultures, generational differences, learning paths, and communication styles to an interprofessional team. It is evident that team members from different professions have each been socialized into a professional culture that includes a set of values, beliefs, and approaches to problem solving that may be unique to a specific discipline (Hall, 2005; Khalili, Orchard, Laschinger, & Farah, 2013). At times, members from the same interprofessional team have very different viewpoints about a situation, causing each to see different aspects of the same problem, which technically should be expected given the differences in disciplines. Consequently, each team member might recommend a different problem-solving approach that may not be understood by others on the team (Hall, 2005).

Turf wars reduce the cohesiveness of the team and impact the interprofessional EBP process and the final result of the team project. According to Khalili et al. (2013), turf wars or turf protection is rooted in standard health profession education that does not include interprofessional experiences. Without better understanding of the roles of professionals in other disciplines, there is a tendency for team members to use common stereotypes about another discipline to inform their own attitudes and behaviors. In addition to turf protection issues, some team members may not believe they share project responsibility or may not voice their opinion due to power differentials in perceived status commonly associated with various professions or due to being in the student role.

EVIDENCE SUPPORTING THE NEED FOR BETTER TEAM COMMUNICATION

Communication problems, whether silence or miscommunication, create medical errors and unsafe practices (Maxfield, Grenny, Lavandero, & Groah, 2011; O'Daniel

& Rosenstein, 2008). These communication errors influence patient care, the team of providers, and potentially the entire organization. Maxfield et al. (2011) identified three themes impacting patient care: dangerous shortcuts, incompetence, and disrespect. Dangerous shortcuts lead to risky consequences that ultimately impact the patient. In terms of the interprofessional EBP project, shortcuts in the work of the team could lead to addressing the wrong problem, selecting an intervention that is not feasible, and creating a weak practice change plan. Incompetence typically arises when staff members have not been appropriately trained for their responsibilities. The program coordinators and mentors have to make sure the interprofessional team is well trained in interprofessional EBP and that the team carefully trains other staff in the health care organization about how to implement the practice change the team has designed.

Lastly, disrespect impacts coworkers, department morale, patient care, and patient satisfaction depending on the environment in which the disrespect occurred. Power dynamics creating disrespect can influence whether another team member decides in a strategic or defensive manner to speak up, avoids responding to questioning, or speaks quietly (Gardezi et al., 2009). Garon (2011) highlighted the personal factors that promote silence in practice, such as learned behavior associated with a negative or positive value for assertiveness, level of support within one's culture for women to speak up, and amount of confidence in professional knowledge. In addition, there is often strong organizational pressure that encourages silence through peer pressure of colleagues and through managers who take system feedback personally or who view vocal employees as self-serving. An interprofessional EBP team that does not pay attention to creating a supportive and respectful team environment may have difficulty contending with many personal and organizational factors that eventually become barriers to communication, thereby leading to a poorly designed interprofessional EBP project if these barriers are not addressed.

INTERPROFESSIONAL COMMUNICATION COMPETENCIES

The Interprofessional Education Collaborative Expert Panel (2011) outlined the *Core Competencies for Interprofessional Collaborative Practice* in which communication is a core domain for any interprofessional team (see Chapter 4). The competencies for communication include choosing effective communication tools and techniques, speaking in a common language, listening and encouraging team members to participate, providing timely feedback, and valuing the experience and expertise each team member brings to the team. Juggling all of these

aspects of communication is often challenging for any team. See Table 5-1 for strategies to develop communication competencies.

Choosing Effective Communication Tools

There is some research (Papadimitriou & Cott, 2015; Pentland, 2012) indicating the most effective form of communication occurs when individuals interact face-to-face. Face-to-face communication is not always possible due to the interprofessional teams having members from two different organizations where each member most likely has conflicting schedules at some point during the interprofessional EBP project. Consequently, mentors should view their teams as dispersed teams. Dispersed teams have members located locally, nationally, or internationally who are connected via communication technology, thereby having limited face-to-face contact (Allen & Vakalahi, 2013). The technologies a dispersed team uses may be synchronous where everyone interacts together in real time, may be asynchronous where team members communicate within their own time frames, or may include a combination of synchronous and asynchronous approaches. There are many communication technologies available including conference calls, video conferencing, email, learning platforms, and Google documents and chats.

Dispersed teams are like traditional teams in that team members experience mutual dependency in accomplishing tasks, have needs for continuous communication regarding team strategies, and desire involvement in decision making (Allen & Vakalahi, 2013). Communication technology can provide the avenue for the team to set clear objectives and goals, establish norms, have regular meetings, and provide feedback and management of milestones for the interprofessional EBP project.

Regardless of the similarities that dispersed teams have with face-to-face teams, there are differences that the mentor should realize (Allen & Vakalahi, 2013). Because of the characteristics of the tool or method of communication the team chooses, time is required to ensure that all team members receive training and become proficient with the technology, as well as to ensure all team members have access to the chosen tool. Dispersed teams also require ways to establish quick trust among team members, which means providing more time to establish sound group norms in terms of expressing respect and for engaging actively and regularly, meeting the need for strong and inclusive leadership to make sure everyone on the team follows the norms of the group, and creating structured work processes in advance of making assignments in order to avoid confusion. Norms associated with establishment of quick trust include the following: a team orientation that reviews how work will occur when using the technology; well-developed communication processes that match the capability of the

TABLE 5-1

STRATEGIES FOR COMMUNICATION COMPETENCIES

INTERPROFESSIONAL COMMUNICATION COMPETENCY	STRATEGY
Choose effective communication tools and techniques, including information systems and communication technologies, to facilitate discussions and interactions that enhance team function.	• Communication planning and continuous modification • Communication technology orientation, ensuring team member access, and ongoing assessment of usefulness • Dispersed team methods of establishing quick trust
Organize and communicate information with patients, families, and health care team members in a form that is understandable, avoiding discipline-specific terminology when possible.	• Awareness of language differences amongst professions and within organizational cultures • Creation of team common language • Clarifying understanding • Use of inclusive language and formal and informal communication • Briefings
Express one's knowledge and opinions to team members involved in patient care with confidence, clarity, and respect, working to ensure a common understanding of information and treatment and care decisions.	• Establishing and reviewing team values focused on improving patient care, interprofessional EBP, and creating the common understanding characteristic of interprofessional team behavior • Distribution and approval of minutes
Listen actively and encourage the ideas and opinions of other team members.	• Clarifying team roles and team norms • Appreciating expertise of other professions • Structure agenda to encourage participation
Give timely, sensitive, instructive feedback to others about their performance on the team, responding respectfully as a team member to feedback from others.	• Debriefing • Crucial conversations • Crew resource management • Team Communication Assessments
Use respectful language appropriate for a given difficult situation, crucial conversation, or interprofessional conflict.	• Crucial conversations • Crew resource management • Supportive micro-context for observable candor
Recognize how one's own uniqueness, including experience level, expertise, culture, power, and hierarchy within the health care team, contributes to effective communication, conflict resolution, and positive interprofessional working relationships (University of Toronto, 2008).	• Team charter • "No fault" or "no blame" team attitude • Reduction of threats to professional identity • Prevention of disciplinary polarization • Diminution of power differentials
Communicate consistently the importance of teamwork in patient-centered and community-focused care.	• Promoting shared responsibility among team members • Develop team identity • Articulate patient-centered team goals • Assign interdependent team tasks • Use tactical communication

Interprofessional Education Collaborative Expert Panel. (2011). Core competencies for interprofessional collaborative practice: Report of an expert panel. Washington, DC: Interprofessional Education Collaborative. Reprinted with permission from American Association of Medical Colleges (AAMC).

BOX 5-2. COMMON LANGUAGE

For the project I was on as a graduate student in occupational therapy, the team asked certain nurses on one of the units to become trained mentors for other nurses in how to address a patient's chronic pain. The term *mentor* was not something with which the nurses were comfortable, as they tended to associate the term with a long-term role involving a high level of expertise. Therefore, we spent additional time explaining the time-limited aspects of the role and the specific knowledge needed, causing the participant recruitment process to be extended beyond the original timeline. If we had used the word *champion*, this process of recruiting nurses to coach others would have gone much smoother. We would have used language familiar to them because of their experience with other practice change projects. We should have asked the stakeholders what they would have named the process for teaching other nurses about chronic pain.

technology; cultural awareness regarding attitudes and familiarity with communication technologies; and conflict resolution that is timely and specific and that moves the team to action (Smith & Blanck, 2002).

Speaking in a Common Language

Interprofessional team members come from a variety of professions in which terminology may differ from one profession to another. Creating an atmosphere in which there is a foundation of transparency, trust, and common language benefits all team members and enhances team learning (Hewitt, Sims, & Harris, 2015). Common language is created when team members do not assume they understand terminology used in other professions that may seem similar to the terminology in one's own discipline (Sheehan, Robertson, & Ormond, 2007). Thus, creating a common language early in the interprofessional EBP process reduces the occurrence of misunderstandings, particularly when members from different organizations also use language common within an organizational culture. When there are differences in using the same terms, the team members need to agree about how they plan to use the term within the interprofessional EBP project (Box 5-2).

Listening and Encouraging Participation

Sheehan et al. (2007) observed differences in communication between interprofessional and multidisciplinary teams. Multidisciplinary team members work within their particular scope of practice, are more likely to work in parallel, and tend to interact formally with each other. In contrast, interprofessional team members are comfortable with overlapping professional roles and are therefore experienced in using both formal and informal communication to share problem solving on behalf of the patient. According to Sheehan et al., differences in team member participation and communication appeared to correlate with the definitional distinctions between multidisciplinary and interprofessional teams as reported in the literature. They discovered that interprofessional teams used inclusive

language to promote the continual sharing of information in order to create a collaborative approach to patient care. Multidisciplinary team members drew information from each other; however, they did so in a way that did not lead to a common understanding of the needs of the patient.

Interprofessional team research (Suter et al., 2009) shows that teams are more effective when the team members have well-defined roles and when they appreciate explicitly the expertise that each team member brings to facilitate the work. Numerous authors (Hewitt et al., 2015; McCaffrey et al., 2011; O'Daniel & Rosenstein, 2008; Suter et al., 2009) highlight that clear and open communication involving careful listening to promote trust and to foster respectful collaboration among team members affects the delivery of high-quality care and patient outcomes. Additionally, team members working in highly effective teams form stronger interprofessional relationships that are more likely to be sustained over time (Sinclair, Lingard, & Mohabeer, 2009). These positive interprofessional relationships influence job satisfaction for each team member. Students who have the opportunity to participate on a highly effective interprofessional team learn how to become excellent team members, which supports their development as a new health care professional (Suter et al., 2009).

Providing Timely Feedback

Feedback is a team communication approach that improves the team process, reduces uncertainty, assists in problem solving, builds trust among team members, and creates mutual support as described in Chapter 4. Feedback does not automatically happen and is more apt to occur within a supportive micro-context where team members are comfortable with sharing opinions, ideas, and concerns. Ferrazzi (2012) describes *observable candor* as characteristic of highly effective teams. While it may be easier to avoid tough conversations, doing so typically prevents the team from making progress and impacts team satisfaction.

Crucial conversations are a way to communicate with the end goal of striving for action and changes in behavior when opinions vary, the stakes are high, and emotions are charged (Patterson, Grenny, McMillan, & Switzler, 2012). In some cases, a crucial conversation is necessary to rescue the

BOX 5-3. STUDENT STATUS

When my professor asked me to join an interprofessional EBP project with a local hospital, I jumped at the chance to build upon what I was learning in my occupational therapy curriculum. I quickly discovered that, while I knew the roles and language of an occupational therapist, I needed to understand the knowledge and viewpoints of the others in the group. Each team member, from nursing, holistic health, and faculty in occupational therapy, had their unique perspective and made interesting contributions to the group. It was truly a gift to sit at the table with highly respected team members; however, it was also intimidating at times. I learned to ask questions, use new communication tools, and avoid making assumptions. To increase my participation on the team, I volunteered to oversee certain aspects of the practice change project. In fact, I recruited student volunteers to go through the student onboarding process at the hospital so that they could help me collect data from the electronic medical record. As our project evolved, I took opportunities to learn from the other members while also finding ways to use my strengths within the group. As the result of open dialogue and respect for each other's professional roles and contributions, there was a mutual benefit to understand how the team together could impact patient care. Now that I am no longer a student, this experience changed how I communicate and work with other professionals in acute care where I now work. I seek to collaborate with those who care for the patients assigned to me. In the end, not only does the patient benefit, but collaboration also brings me greater job satisfaction.

interprofessional EBP project when stalled or spiraling out of control in terms of budget, workload or complexity, and deadlines. Patterson et al. outlined a framework in which to conduct these crucial conversations involving the following: (a) starting with the heart or examining motivations for the conversation, (b) learning to become aware of when a crucial conversation is needed, (c) making it safe or establishing respect, (d) mastering the story or separating interpretation of the circumstance from the facts, (e) stating the path or making it clear why the conversation is occurring, (f) exploring the path of others or asking questions to learn the other person's perspective, and (g) moving to action or deciding how to resolve the situation and plan to follow up. Mentors may find this structured approach to a difficult conversation useful with a team member whose behavior needs to change or to assist team members in working with difficult stakeholders.

Patient safety has partially been an issue as a result of fear of reprisal and conflict avoidance, especially involving followers of more powerful team leaders. Methods for enhancing assertive communication among team members, particularly in high-risk patient situations, involve crew resource management (CRM), which was derived from the airline industry for application in health care (Dunn et al., 2007). CRM describes *followership* as the ability of team members to use critical thinking and to assume shared responsibility for team decisions. Team members learn to be active through the delivery of direct and concise feedback to decision makers. This feedback is referred to as the three *W*s and include: *what* one has seen, *what* one is concerned with, or *what* one wants to see happen instead. Assertive communication occurs when a team member makes a timely statement of concern, offers solutions, and poses questions. Mentors may want to introduce these basic CRM techniques that are based on an attitude of "no fault

or blame" so that problems are prevented, learned from, and corrected immediately from a systems perspective.

Valuing Experience and Expertise

Respectful communication fosters effective team collaboration early on in the project and promotes development of a supportive micro-context for the team. Professional identity may be construed as being threatened when there is a perceived risk of the marginalization or devaluation of the profession's role or expertise (McNeil, Mitchell, & Parker, 2013). Threats to professional identity include such factors as differential treatment of professional groups, professions holding differing values, expecting professionals from other disciplines to act the same as one does in one's own discipline, insulting or humiliating action, and simple contact with other professional groups without recognizing polarization may occur. Polarization occurs when professionals within a single discipline seem to unite against members in other disciplines. An example of simple contact occurs when groups of disciplines may take a course together. Often in this situation, the professionals from like disciplines tend to sit together rather than intermixing automatically. The facilitator of the course needs to be aware of this tendency and should ask people to sit with professionals from another discipline. Otherwise, polarization of viewpoints could occur when disciplines are segregated in this way from each other.

The team needs to value the diversity, knowledge, and skills that each team member brings regardless of his or her job title or current status as a student (Box 5-3). The following strategies reduce the polarization among disciplines serving on an interprofessional team:

- Remaining aware of differences in power so that mentors strive to minimize the power differential among team members, especially on behalf of students

- Encouraging faculty to create a collaborative relationship with students on the team rather than a traditional teacher/student relationship

- Developing a strong team identity to reduce the likelihood that teams divide into conflicting subgroups (Jehn & Bezrukova, 2010)

- Emphasizing patient-centered team goals when professional identities are also respected relieves intergroup tensions (Callan et al., 2007; Mitchell, Parker, & Giles, 2011)

- Assigning team members to work on interdependent tasks that necessitate the acquisition of new knowledge as a way to alleviate professional identity threat (van Dick, van Knippenberg, Hägele, Guillaume, & Brodbeck, 2008)

- Facilitating team leaders to think about and challenge norms of medical dominance and differential treatment of medical and nonmedical practitioners (Long, Forsyth, Iedema, & Carroll, 2006)

- Fostering awareness of the team members from the dominant professional group to be aware of professional identity threat triggers (Chrobot-Mason, Ruderman, Weber, & Ernst, 2009)

COMMUNICATION STRATEGIES CREATING A HIGHLY EFFECTIVE TEAM

Currently, there is a lack of precise understanding of the concrete communication processes linked to improvements in collaborative care (Lingard et al., 2006). Hewitt et al. (2015) conducted a qualitative synthesis of the literature to identify the interprofessional team contexts that trigger particular team communication mechanisms or strategies and the outcomes subsequently produced in the team's work. These authors labeled this relationship among the communication-related variables as the context–mechanism–outcome (CMO) configuration (p. 100). Context is the antecedent facilitating the type of communication that occurs. Context and the communication mechanisms tend to lead to a specific team performance outcome. The synthesis identified four broad groups of mechanisms related to communication, including the following: (a) efficient, open, and equitable communication; (b) tactical communication; (c) shared responsibility and influence; and (d) team behavioral norms. It is helpful for mentors and team members to review the definitions of these mechanism categories and to use them as achievable goals for interprofessional communication (Table 5-2).

Hewitt et al. (2015) found that only two of the mechanism categories (i.e., efficient, open, and equitable communication and tactical communication) were supported regularly in the literature with descriptions of the complete configuration (i.e., CMO). The interprofessional team literature indicated the need for the mechanism of shared responsibility and influence but was not clear regarding the contexts leading to this mechanism and the outcomes attributable to the complete configuration. The same was true of the team behavioral norms for communication. Descriptions of the context that lead to setting behavioral norms were not described in the literature. Likewise, there was a lack of discussion in the literature about the outcomes of team performance when a team sets these norms.

Mentors should pay close attention to achieving all of the broad mechanism categories that Hewitt et al. (2015) identified as goals for communication. Mentors might want to give greater emphasis to shared responsibility and influence and the team behavioral norms. These broad communication mechanisms may be harder to establish within a variety of contexts in order to produce the desired teamwork outcomes. Shared responsibility between two organizations is complicated, especially since the practice change is obviously beneficial to the health care organization. Mentors may have to encourage faculty and students to reflect on and discuss the benefits to them and the university that occur when each team member actively owns and influences the interprofessional EBP project. Establishing team norms for communication and sharing responsibility happens when the interprofessional EBP team uses specific techniques to foster development of these two broad mechanism categories. Discussion of team values fosters the creation of team norms. Engaging in careful communication planning, team communication assessments, and common-sense communication strategies promote shared responsibility (Hewitt et al., 2015).

Value Sharing as Communication

Conflicts among professional groups on the team tend to arise during times when the team's identity is at issue because of disagreement about the values the group has established (Tagliaventi & Mattarelli, 2006) (see Chapter 4). Conflict signals to the team that it is important to revisit the values as a conduit for untangling disagreements. For example, perhaps the team is discussing evidence that initially seems diametrically opposed to what a particular discipline normally does in practice. If the evidence for this practice change is strong and is of high quality, the team members have to verbally remind themselves of the ultimate goal of the interprofessional EBP project as improving the outcomes for the patient. Team members view conflict as an opportunity to respectfully help the individual team member objecting to the new information to examine his or her thinking through a focus on the evidence rather than on

TABLE 5-2

COMMUNICATION CONFIGURATIONS

COMMUNICATION GOALS	DEFINITION (HEWITT ET AL., 2015)	CONTEXT	COMMUNICATION MECHANISM	TEAMWORK OUTCOME
Efficient, open, and equitable communication	"All members of a team offer their opinion, constructively challenge one another and mutually resolve disagreements, regardless of perceived professional status, and each member's contribution is given due consideration" (p. 101).	Team has finished their EBP literature review to answer their foreground question. Team has assigned each team member two appraisals to complete before the next meeting.	Agenda for meetings scheduled each team member to present two appraisals for feedback and input. Completed appraisals were posted on Google docs in advance of meetings so everyone could read them ahead of time.	All the appraisals were reviewed in two 2-hour meetings as scheduled according to timeline. Each team member participated.
Tactical communication	"Team members consciously control the amount or type of information they share with others in order to achieve outcomes that are to their own advantage or what they perceive to be their patient's advantage" (p. 102).	Team scheduled meeting with stakeholders to determine their support of the proposed practice change.	Team met to determine the materials to give to stakeholders in advance of the stakeholder meeting. The goal was to share how the intervention for a practice change was selected in terms of evidence appraisal and synthesis.	Stakeholders agreed the intervention looked promising and wanted to participate in designing the practice change.
Shared responsibility and influence	"All team members can influence team decisions and share responsibility for those decisions and their outcomes" (p. 102).	Team charter identified which team members were skilled in particular areas related to the interprofessional EBP process.	The team created a schedule of team leadership at the beginning of each EBP phase that matched team expertise and allowed the team member to prepare in advance for leadership.	Student on the team successfully led the team meeting where communication technology training occurred.
Team behavioral norms	"Teams share behavioral 'norms' or rules which govern how they are expected to communicate and work together" (p. 103).	Team wanted to decide how to stay on track with their timeline.	Team developed a Gantt chart to track time needed for each EBP task. The Gantt chart was reviewed at each meeting. Timeline was adjusted when needed so team knew where they were on the project and the time available before completion.	Team members understood completing tasks on time was a value and asked for help if the task was taking longer than expected.

TABLE 5-3

DOCUMENTING TEAM COMMUNICATION DECISIONS

WHAT IS THE PURPOSE OF THE COMMUNICA-TION?	WHAT WILL THE TEAM COMMUNI-CATE?	WHEN WILL THE TEAM COMMUNI-CATE? (DEADLINE)	WHERE/HOW DOES COMMUNI-CATION NEED TO OCCUR?	WHO IS RESPON-SIBLE FOR COM-MUNICATING TO WHOM?
Information Utility				
Provision of information				
Identifying problems or ambiguities				
Functional Utility				
Decision making				
Planning				
Follow-up actions				

what may appear to be an attack on a particular discipline. The team should see this conflict as a chance to bring forward other evidence that may support the individual team member's disciplinary point of view as well. In this way, the team is letting the strength and quality of the evidence lead the team toward a particular decision or direction because of their value for EBP as a vehicle for ultimately improving the lives of patients.

Mentors act as brokers of this new knowledge arising from the team's work and intense sharing and discussion of disciplinary-related knowledge throughout the tasks that occur during each interprofessional EBP phase (Tagliaventi & Mattarelli, 2006). Effective mentors understand their role in establishing the team's value for sharing and discussing knowledge that crosses disciplinary boundaries in order to create the new knowledge the team needs for changing practice. The broker role involves the mentor encouraging team members to carefully listen to disciplinary-specific knowledge in order to explore how this knowledge may be relevant to the interprofessional EBP problem (Tagliaventi & Mattarelli, 2006). The mentor is facilitating the team to initiate communication pathways for the transferal of knowledge from one discipline to another as a way to address the shared value of improving patient care.

Communication Planning

Mentors should prompt the interprofessional team to develop a communication plan, using who, what, and where questions in order to delineate specific communication strategies (McComb, Schroeder, Kennedy, & Vozdolska, 2012) and to promote team member responsibility for participating in and leading these communication efforts.

Lingard et al. (2006) described the common purposes of team communication as being of two major types of utility, defined as "the visible impact of communication on team awareness and behavior" (p. 471). Informational utility is communication designed to provide new information, confirmation of what is known, and reminders of details. An example of an information utility communication plan is to determine what is currently known about the selected intervention for a practice change, what needs to be learned, who needs to learn about the intervention, how the team and other stakeholders will learn the information, and the timing of the learning. Functional utility is communication designed to produce specific work actions, such as planning. A functional utility communication plan would determine who will lead the planning of the practice change, when this planning needs to occur, what decisions need to be made, what stakeholders should engage with the team in the planning, and what follow-up actions are needed to vet the proposed plan. View Table 5-3 for communication plan questions combined with utility purposes that aid in documenting the communication decisions the team makes.

ASSESSMENTS OF TEAM COMMUNICATION

Another mechanism for enhancing team communication is assessing the quality of the team's and each team member's communication. Prior to assessment, the mentor helps the team develop the value for functioning as a highly effective team because of the critical effect on the

TABLE 5-4

TEAM MEMBER SELF-ASSESSMENT OF COMMUNICATION

NAME OF TEAM MEMBER:

DATE OF RATING:

ASSESSMENT ITEM	SELF-ASSESSMENT RATING ON A SCALE OF 0 TO 5, WITH 5 BEING THE HIGHEST SCORE	COMMENTS	PEER ASSESSMENT RATING ON A SCALE OF 0 TO 5, WITH 5 BEING THE HIGHEST SCORE	COMMENTS
Produces quality in assigned work.				
Demonstrates timeliness and consistency in meeting deadlines.				
Listens to others and asks clarifying questions.				
Provides respectful and helpful feedback to the team and individual team members.				
Asks for feedback or help when needed in a timely manner.				
Explains unfamiliar terminology.				
Helps the team remain focused.				
Attends team meetings and team work group sessions.				
Other				

central value of improving patient care. Assessments help each team member understand his or her responsibility for the team improvement necessary for successfully completing the interprofessional EBP project phases. Mentors need to determine the team support for engagement in assessment. Asking each member about how they want to be assessed, when they want the assessments, and the way the assessments' results should be communicated are key questions that can be decided upon as a part of the team charter. Other questions to resolve include whether team members want to concentrate on self-assessment, whether team members also want to assess each other, and whether the team wants to evaluate team functioning to determine progress over time.

For the interprofessional EBP program at North Memorial Medical Center, the program coordinators created a self-assessment for use throughout the entire project that targets the communication performance of the team as one focus (Table 5-4). Teams may decide other elements to include on the assessment as a way to target specific issues of communication that seem to affect the team the most. In this way, the team achieves buy-in from everyone about what to assess due to the importance in upholding the team's core values.

Another interprofessional self-assessment that addresses communication and teamwork is the Interprofessional Collaborator Assessment Rubric (Curran et al., 2010) (http://www.med.mun.ca/CCHPE/Faculty-Resources/Interprofessional-Collaborator-Assessment-Rubric.aspx).

BOX 5-4. TEAM MEETING TIP

Make sure to provide an opportunity for each team member to present his or her literature search results with an agreed upon method decided at previous meetings. For example, the team may decide to post articles on the learning platform prior to the meeting. At the meeting, according to a clear agenda, each team member verbally presents the literature search to the team. On the team I was on when I was an occupational therapy student, another student member's library search results were not discussed at the meeting and, consequently, the individual did not feel valued and respected by the team. Ultimately, the student left the team without explaining her reasoning for leaving or discussing her negative experience. Everyone's contributions are critical to the success of the team. Overlooking the work of someone who has worked hard defeats teamwork. The team must be careful to bring the work of students and other less powerful team members forward to the team for discussion. By involving these team members, power differentials are diminished.

A rubric is a scoring guideline and, in this case, addresses team members' competencies for collaboration. The rubric was designed for use across a variety of health profession educational programs and was not originally designed for use with interprofessional EBP teams. The team should review this rubric to determine its usefulness as a summative assessment in stimulating suggestions for each team member's improvement. The team decides who completes the rubric for each person, more than likely considering the value of each team member, completing one for every member on the team.

The rubric is composed of a series of dimensions, which are statements of behavior associated with the competency. For instance, the dimensions for the communication competency include respectful communication and communication strategies. Each dimension is associated with a set of behavioral indicators. A scale of 1 (indicating minimal performance) to 5 (being mastery) rates achievement on each dimension of the collaborator competencies. For the communication strategies dimension, for example, statements on which one is rated with the numerical scale include being able to use verbal and nonverbal communication strategies according to the situation, communicating in a logical and structured manner, explaining discipline-specific jargon or terminology, and communicating appropriately with anyone with specific impairments. Feedback provided to the team member involves his or her level of demonstrated competence with a numerical value on a dimension and a space for evaluators to provide comments and concrete examples of the observed behaviors. There is also a space for indicating the dimension was not observed, which is useful in situations when team members have been interacting more with specific individuals and not as much with other team members.

The Style Under Stress Quiz (available at https://www.vitalsmarts.com/styleunderstress/) assists team members in identifying their communication style during difficult situations in order to develop crucial conversation skills as described previously. The resulting self-awareness helps the team member modify his or her more negative communications as quickly as possible through the process of thinking about a relationship with a team member, mentor, or program coordinator. The team member is instructed to think of a difficult situation that occurred in the relationship with the person about whom the team member is thinking. To complete the quiz, the team member responds with true or false regarding statements such as, "Rather than tell people exactly what I think, sometimes I rely on jokes, sarcasm, or snide remarks to let them know I'm frustrated." Regardless of the communication assessment tools selected, the team goal is to help each other improve within a supportive and respectful context while avoiding overly harsh criticism that potentially leads to damaged relationships.

Common-Sense Team Communication Strategies

There are common-sense team strategies for enhancing team communication involving the development of meeting agendas, thorough construction and distribution of minutes, the scheduling of meetings in advance, and the monitoring of team meeting attendance. An agenda helps organize the meeting where the team begins with a briefing so that members can report progress on assigned tasks, introduce new topics, and identify the decisions to be made (Box 5-4). The meeting ends with setting a preliminary agenda, making assignments for the next meeting, and debriefing regarding the success of the meeting in accomplishing the goals for the meeting.

Meeting minutes are an important way to document the subjects addressed within the agenda (Box 5-5). Scheduling meetings is often challenging given the work schedules of team members and the class and work schedules of students. Team members may need to change the times of the meetings to accommodate the schedules of team members, which for faculty and students, may change every semester. Faculty members should schedule an additional meeting with the students to ensure questions are answered and the students have a plan for their assignments. The faculty member's role is to support all students on the team. When a meeting absence is expected, the team member should let everyone know in advance so that the team can adjust

---

BOX 5-5. STUDENT TIP

Students should consider volunteering to take the meeting minutes. Taking minutes is a good way for the student to be engaged, ask questions, and use expertise in technology tools to ensure the meeting proceedings are documented. However, if you volunteer for this role, remember this is an important vehicle for team communication. Minutes must be thorough while at the same time should record only what is necessary. Asking team members to approve your chosen minute-taking method is beneficial so that the team can make any changes prior to taking minutes. Responsibility for taking minutes is an important role and requires consistency in completing the minutes on time. Be sure to ask for another minute taker if you plan to be absent.

---

the upcoming agenda as needed. Teams should expect team members to submit their work even when missing the meeting, especially when the team needs the material for conducting the meeting.

Some team members may display a pattern of absenteeism and tardiness. Often these team members also do not notify the team leader, mentor, and fellow team members of the pending absences or a reason for missing meetings. These absent team members may also fail to submit their assignments for the meeting or provide consistent updates on task progress. The team leader, mentor, or program coordinators need to talk to these habitually absent team members, asking them to begin regular attendance. Sometimes the team member will resolve attendance problems or he or she will withdraw from the team. The program coordinator may need to draft another team member for the team, especially if the team has few members. A larger team may elect not to replace the member who has withdrawn participation. The mentor will then have to orient the new team member to help him or her catch up with the current work of the team. If the clinical scholar is the one demonstrating an attendance problem, the mentor and program coordinator will need to work with the clinical scholar, the immediate supervisor of the clinical scholar, and the program sponsor to determine the best way to address the problem.

MENTOR CHALLENGES

As noted previously, each stage of the project requires extensive collaboration among team members, mentors, program coordinators, and stakeholders. Team members join the group with various levels of developed communication skills. The mentor needs to capitalize on the strengths in communication of each team member. In this way, each team member is able to use his or her unique set of communication skills and style of communicating to facilitate interprofessional EBP task completion. If the team is a distributed team, members have to thoughtfully choose effective technology for communication. However, team members may need additional education for some of the selected communication technology. The mentor should not forget that students also grow with leadership opportunities and may have extensive knowledge about communication

technologies. The student could assume the task of teaching the team about the use of the communication technology.

MENTOR TECHNIQUES AND SUPPORTS

This chapter described a variety of mentor techniques, such as CRM, crucial conversations, awareness and management of polarization triggers, the use of communication technology for distributed teams, discussions of team values, communication planning, team communication assessments, and the use of common-sense communication tools. In conclusion, mentors and program coordinators should remember the following communication strategies, which require mentors and team members to:

- Help create a team whose members are open and aware of biases and are willing to work through them (i.e., a supportive micro-context)
- Respect the expertise and opinions of all team members
- Monitor those who demonstrate a consistent pattern of silence and uncover the reason a member's participation is limited, or help the more reticent team members to develop comfort with the team and confidence in their abilities
- Establish team accountability for commitments and identify early when these commitments require adjustment
- Develop thorough communication plans throughout the interprofessional EBP project
- Encourage team members to ask for help in a timely way
- Identify communication issues when they arise
- Use communication technologies for distributed teams
- Ask questions to clarify communication challenges
- Give careful and effective feedback
- Promote belief that the goals of the project are worthwhile and feasible

SUMMARY

As mentioned throughout the chapter, effective team communication is central for team progress and for on-time task production where the outcomes of the work are of high quality. Spending time working on team communication prior to beginning the interprofessional EBP project not only assists in the development of rapport among the team members and the mentor, but promotes the communication necessary to proceed through each of the nine phases of the interprofessional EBP project. This chapter discussed the processes of creating a communication plan, using IPE core communication competencies, developing meeting agendas, and taking minutes. Use of communication technologies are helpful to keep the team engaged. The team decides which technology to use when developing a communication plan that the team revises when needed, particularly when communication is ineffective. Team assessments are important in determining the effectiveness of team communication in order to devise solutions to strengthen team communication processes. Methods for providing helpful feedback include conducting the crucial conversations necessary to change an individual team member's performance or communication style and frequency.

REFLECTION QUESTIONS

1. What are your strengths and areas of development in communication that should be included in the team communication plan?

2. After deciding on the communication plan, how will you learn new technology before the next meeting?

REFERENCES

Allen, S., & Vakalahi, H. F. O. (2013). My team members are everywhere! A critical analysis of the emerging literature on dispersed teams. *Administration in Social Work, 37,* 486-493. doi:10.1080/03643107.2013.828002

Callan, V. J., Gallois, C., Mayhew, M. G., Grice, T. A., Tluchowska, M., & Boyce, R. (2007). Restructuring the multi-professional organization: Professional identity and adjustment to change in a public hospital. *Journal of Health and Human Services Administration, 29*(4), 448-477.

Chrobot-Mason, D., Ruderman, M. N., Weber, T. J., & Ernst, C. (2009). The challenge of leading on unstable ground: Triggers that activate social identity faultlines. *Human Relations, 62*(11), 1763-1794. doi:10.1177/0018726709346376

Communication [Def. 1]. (n.d.). *Merriam-Webster Online.* In Merriam-Webster. Retrieved from http://www.merriam-webster.com/dictionary/communication.

Curran, V., Hollett, A., Casimiro, L. M., McCarthy, P., Banfield, V., Hall, P., ...Wagner, S. (2011). Development and validation of the interprofessional collaborator assessment rubric (ICAR). *Journal of Interprofessional Care, 25*(5), 339-344. doi:10.3109/13561820.2011.589542

Dunn, E. J., Mills, P. D., Neily, J., Crittenden, M. D., Carmack, A. L., & Bagian, J. P. (2007). Medical team training: Applying crew resource management in veterans' health administration. *The Joint Commission Journal on Quality and Safety, 33,* 317-325.

Ferrazzi, K. (2012). Candor, criticism, teamwork. *Harvard Business Review, 90*(1-2), 40.

Gardezi, F., Lingard, L., Espin, S., Whyte, S., Orser, B., & Baker, G. R. (2009). Silence, power and communication in the operating room. *Journal Of Advanced Nursing, 65*(7), 1390-1399. doi:10.1111/j.1365-2648.2009.04994.x

Garon, M. (2011). Speaking up, being heard: registered nurses' perceptions of workplace communication. *Journal of Nursing Management, 20,* 461-371. doi:10.1111/j.1365-2834.2011.01296.x

Hall, P. (2005). Interprofessional teamwork: professional cultures as barriers. *Journal Of Interprofessional Care, 19,* 188-196. doi:10.1080/13561820500081745

Hewitt, G., Sims, S., & Harris, R. (2015). Evidence of communication, influence and behavioural norms in interprofessional teams: a realist synthesis. *Journal Of Interprofessional Care, 29*(2), 100-105. doi:10.3109/13561820.2014.941458

Interprofessional Education Collaborative Expert Panel. (2011). *Core competencies for interprofessional collaborative practice: Report of an expert panel.* Washington, DC: Interprofessional Education Collaborative.

Jehn, K. A., & Bezrukova, K. (2010). The faultline activation process and the effects of activated faultlines on coalition formation, conflict, and group outcomes. *Organizational Behavior and Human Decision Processes, 112*(1), 24-42. doi:10.1016/j.obhdp.2009.11.008

Khalili, H., Orchard, C., Spence Laschinger, H. K., & Farah, R. (2013). An interprofessional socialization framework for developing an interprofessional identity among health professions students. *Journal Of Interprofessional Care, 27* (6), 448-453. doi:10.3109/13561820.2013.804042

Lingard, L., Whyte, S., Espin, S., Baker, G. R., Orser, B., & Doran, D. (2006). Towards safer interprofessional communication: Constructing a model of "utility" from preoperative team briefings. *Journal of Interprofessional Care, 20*(5), 471-483. doi:10.1080/13561820600921865

Long, D., Forsyth, R., Iedema, R., & Carroll, K. (2006). The (im) possibilities of clinical democracy. *Health Sociology Review, 15*(5), 506-519. doi:10.5172/hesr.2006.15.5.506

Maxfield, D., Grenny, K., Lavandero, R., & Groah, L. (2011). The silent treatment: why safety tools and checklist aren't enough to save lives. *Patient Safety and Quality Healthcare, 14,* 48.

McCaffrey, R., Hayes, R. M., Cassell, A., Miller-Reyes, S., Donaldson, A., & Ferrell, C. (2012). The effect of an educational programme on attitudes of nurses and medical residents towards the benefits of positive communication and collaboration. *Journal of Advanced Nursing, 68*(2), 293-301. doi:10.1111/j.1365-2648.2011.05736.x

McComb, S., Schroeder, A., Kennedy, D., & Vozdolska, R., (2012). The five Ws of team communication. *Industrial Management, 54*(5), 10.

McNeil, K. A., Mitchell, R. J., & Parker, V. (2013). Interprofessional practice and professional identity threat. *Health Sociology Review, 22*(3), 291-307. doi:10.5172/hesr.2013.22.3.291

Mitchell, R., Parker, V., & Giles, M. (2011). When do interprofessional teams succeed? Investigating the moderating roles of team and professional identity in interprofessional effectiveness. *Human Relations, 64*(10), 1321-1343. doi:10.1177/0018726711416872

Novak, I., & McIntyre, S. (2010). The effect of education with workplace supports on practitioners' evidence-based practice knowledge and implementation behaviors. *Australian Occupational Therapy Journal, 57*(6), 386393. doi:10.1111/j.1440-1630.2010.00861.x

O'Daniel, M., & Rosenstein, A. H. (2008). Professional communication and team collaboration. In R. G. Hughes (Ed.), *Patient safety and quality: An evidence-based handbook for nurses* (pp. 801-814). Rockville, MD: Agency for Healthcare Research and Quality (US).

Papadimitriou, C., & Cott, C. (2015). Client-centered practices and work in inpatient rehabilitation teams: results from four case studies. *Disability & Rehabilitation, 37*(13), 1135-1143. doi:10.3109/09638288.2014.955138

Patterson, K., Grenny, J., McMillan, R., Switzler, A. (2012) *Crucial conversations: Tools for talking when the stakes are high.* New York, NY; McGraw Hill.

Pentland, A. (2012). The New Science of Building Great Teams. *Harvard Business Review, 90*(4), 60-70.

Quinlan, E., & Robertson, S. (2013). The communicative power of nurse practitioners in multidisciplinary primary health-care teams. *Journal of the American Association of Nurse Practitioners, 25*, 91-102. doi:10.1111/j.1745-7599.2012.00768.x

Sargeant, J., Loney, E., & Murphy, G. (2008). Effective interprofessional teams: 'Contact is not enough' to build a team. *Journal of Continuing Education In The Health Professions, 28*, 228-234. doi:10.1002/chp.189

Schyve, P. (2009). Foreword. In I. J. Chatman (Ed.), *The Joint Commission guide to improving staff communication* (2nd ed.) (p. v). Oakbrook Terrace, IL: Joint Commission on Accreditation of Healthcare Organizations.

Sheehan, D., Robertson, L., & Ormond, T. (2007). Comparison of language used and patterns of communication in interprofessional and multidisciplinary teams. *Journal of Interprofessional Care, 21*(1), 17-30. doi:10.1080/13561820601025336

Smith, P. G., & Blanck, E. L. (2002). From experience: Leading dispersed teams. *Journal of Product Innovation Management, 19*, 294-304. doi:10.1111/1540-5885.1940294

Sinclair, L. B., Lingard, L. A., & Mohabeer, R. N. (2009). What's so great about rehabilitation teams? An enthnographic study of interprofessional collaboration in a rehabilitation unit. *Archives of Physical Medicine and Rehabilitation, 90*, 1196-1201. doi:10.1016/j.apmr.2009.01.021

Suter, E., Arndt, J., Arthur, N., Parboosingh, J., Taylor, E., & Deutschlander, S. (2009). Role understanding and effective communication as core competencies for collaborative practice. *Journal Of Interprofessional Care, 23*(1), 41-51. doi:10.1080/13561820802338579

Tagliaventi, M. R., & Mattarelli, E. (2006). The role of networks of practice, value sharing, and operational proximity in knowledge flows between professional groups. *Human Relations, 59*(3), 291-319. doi:10.1177/0018726706064175.

University of Toronto. (2008). Advancing the interprofessional education curriculum 2009. Curriculum overview. Competency framework. Toronto: University of Toronto, Office of Interprofessional Education. Retrieved from http://www.interprofessional education.utoronto. ca/std/docs/Core%20Competencies%20 Diagram%202010.pdf

Van Dick, R., van Knippenberg, D., Hägele, S., Guillaume, Y. R. F., & Brodbeck, F. C. (2008). Group diversity and group identification: The moderating role of diversity beliefs. *Human Relations, 61*(10), 1463-1492. doi: 10.1177/0018726708095711

Supplemental materials for this chapter are available online.
Please refer to the sticker in the front of the book and enter the access code provided.

Section II

- Preparation for an Interprofessional Evidence-Based Practice Program

  Section I

- Immersion Into the Evidence

  Section II

- Completion and Dissemination of the Interprofessional Evidence-Based Project

  Section III

Chapter 6	Orienting the Interprofessional Team and Addressing Program Logistics	What is the right way to launch an interprofessional evidence-based practice program?
Chapter 7	Figuring Out the Problem and Getting Focused	What does the interprofessional team need to know about the EBP problem?
Chapter 8	Settling Into the Rhythm of the Interprofessional Evidence-Based Practice Process	What are the best team strategies for conducting and documenting a literature search to answer the PICO question?
Chapter 9	Transitioning Into Interprofessional Evidence-Based Practitioners	How do you develop the appraisal and synthesis skills of the interprofessional EBP team?

6

Orienting the Interprofessional Team and Addressing Program Logistics

Sue E. Sendelbach, PhD, APRN CNS, FAHA, FAAN and Patricia L. Finch-Guthrie, PhD, RN

CHAPTER TOPICS

- Selecting an evidence-based practice model
- Selecting participants
- Developing an orientation for the interprofessional evidence-based practice program
- Elements of the ongoing interprofessional evidence-based practice program
- Mentor challenges
- Mentor techniques and supports

PERFORMANCE OBJECTIVES

At the conclusion of this chapter, the leadership of the health care organization and the university will be able to do the following:

1. Develop the process for selecting the coordinators of the interprofessional evidence-based practice program.
2. Develop the process for selecting the mentors and the interprofessional team members.
3. Develop the educational and team building resources for the interprofessional evidence-based practice program.

Previous chapters of this book provide the context for developing an interprofessional evidence-based practice (EBP) program. Chapter 1 provides information about EBP, programs and models for EBP, and the elements of an interprofessional EBP program. This chapter covers the process for developing an interprofessional EBP program after a health care organization and a university have initiated a partnership as outlined in Chapter 2. Understanding the theory of mentoring from Chapter 3 and the importance of an effective team that excels at communication described from Chapters 4 and 5 is necessary for developing the elements of an actual program. The purpose of this chapter is to describe the high-impact educational approach, planning process, and participant selection methodology for interprofessional EBP program coordinators, clinical scholars, mentors, and team members. In addition, the chapter carefully addresses the program logistics necessary for implementing an interprofessional EBP program.

Moyers, P. A., & Finch-Guthrie, P. L.
Interprofessional Evidence-Based Practice:
A Workbook for Health Professionals (pp 95-108).
© 2016 Taylor and Francis Group.

The literature often does not cover these types of details, and the discussion in this chapter represents the authors' experience from conducting successful interprofessional scholar programs. Program planning and specifics are necessary to maintain the benefits of programs, institutionalize a program within settings, and build capacity for sustaining programs (Brownson, Colditz, & Proctor, 2012; Shediac-Rizkallah & Bone, 1998).

Selecting program coordinators, mentors, and program participants sets the tone for the interprofessional EBP program, which is distinctive in that team members come from a health care organization and a university. Each organization has a culture that contributes to the macro-context within which the interprofessional team learns to collaborate in order to complete the project. The interprofessional team functions best within this dynamic context when remaining flexible, open to new ideas, and supportive of team members.

The first step in planning the interprofessional EBP program is to develop clear learning goals and outcomes that fit an interprofessional perspective. Traditional EBP education generally stems from a silo approach often planned from a single discipline's perspective. Interprofessional education (IPE) uses a different framework that focuses on the interprofessional knowledge and abilities necessary to work with others (Pardue, 2015). Specifically, an interprofessional EBP program, while covering the traditional steps of EBP, modifies these same steps with the lens of interprofessionality. According to D'Amour and Oandasan (2005), interprofessionality is "the development of a cohesive practice between professionals from different disciplines. It is the process by which professionals reflect on and develop ways of practicing that provides an integrated and cohesive answer to the needs of the client/family/population" (p. 9). In an interprofessional EBP program, it is common for participants (staff, students, and faculty) to have limited or no previous experience with IPE. However, experienced clinicians and faculty have an in-depth understanding of their discipline and the unique contributions they make to patient care, which often makes them more comfortable sharing and conversing with others about patient care issues.

When planning an orientation for an interprofessional program, it is important to understand the learning needs of the team regarding EBP, interprofessional EBP, and interprofessional teamwork. Because IPE is a relatively new concept, it is important to start with a clear definition. The Center for the Advancement of Interprofessional Education (CAIPE) (2002) definition of IPE described in Chapter 1 is the basis for the interprofessional EBP program, which means that "interprofessional education occurs when two or more professions learn with, from and about each other to improve collaboration and the quality of care" (Defining IPE, para. 1). While EBP is a major focus for team learning, the interprofessional EBP program includes education about collaboration and melds together EBP approaches from a variety of disciplines to solve shared practice

problems. The knowledge exchange, negotiation, and integration of information from multiple disciplines are what makes interprofessional EBP different from traditional EBP approaches and creates stronger EBP projects. Clearly articulating the expectations for the interprofessional EBP program to all team members and providing an organized, structured program creates the micro-context that supports success.

SELECTING AN EVIDENCE-BASED PRACTICE MODEL

The overarching goal of the interprofessional EBP program is to promote an evidence-based approach for answering practice questions and developing clinical scholars and the interprofessional team to become champions of interprofessional EBP. Innovative models of infusing EBP into clinical practice include primarily discipline-specific models from nursing (Albert & Siedlecki, 2008; Brewer, Brewer, & Schultz, 2009; Cullen & Titler, 2004; Gawlinski, 2008; Graner, Sendelbach, Boland, & Koehn, 2011; Schultz, 2005), physical therapy (Schreiber, Downey, & Traister, 2009; Wojciechowski, 2009), and occupational therapy (Crist, Muñoz, Hansen, Benson, & Provident, 2005). Although EBP scholar-like programs most often cited in the literature involve an academic and hospital setting, other partnerships with universities described in the literature include those with community sites, such as a daycare center in an underserved community, a homeless shelter for women, and a county jail (Crist et al., 2005). Many programs focus only on providing education about EBP without an experiential component (Austin, Richter, & Frese, 2009; Dizon, Grimmer-Somers, & Kumar, 2012; Schreiber et al., 2009). However, a variety of disciplines provide paid time for clinicians as a strategy to support integrating EBP into practice (Caldwell, Whitehead, Fleming, & Moes, 2008; Newhouse, Dearholt, Poe, Pugh, & White, 2005; Schultz, 2005).

A literature search produced only two descriptions of interprofessional EBP programs. One description is from a case study of the interprofessional EBP program implemented at North Memorial Medical Center from the editors of this book (Moyers, Finch Guthrie, Swan, & Sathe, 2014) that brought together a variety of disciplines to work together on practice problems. Disciplines included in the program were not necessarily used to working together, such as those from exercise science and holistic health. The second was an interprofessional community scholar program using physical therapists and occupational therapists as preceptors, who represent disciplines with members who commonly collaborate (Richardson et al., 2010). Interprofessional EBP programs may strengthen existing professional relationships or expand working relationships to include other professions.

TABLE 6-1

USING AN EVIDENCE-BASED PRACTICE MODEL TO SELECT CONTENT FOR THE INTERPROFESSIONAL EVIDENCE-BASED PRACTICE PROGRAM

UNIVERSITY OF IOWA EBP TO PROMOTE QUALITY CARE (TITLER ET AL., 2001)	ABBOTT NORTHWESTERN HOSPITAL EDUCATION CONTENT
Problem and knowledge focused triggers	Overview of EBP The clinical question: PICO
Form a team	Mentor orientation: TeamSTEPPS and tools for mentoring
Assemble relevant research and related literature	Searching the literature
Critique and synthesize research for use in practice	Appraisal I: Levels of evidence Appraisal II: Levels of evidence
Pilot the change in practice	Project design and measurement Translational and implementation science Project management Project evaluation and analysis
Base practice on other types of evidence	Appraisal I: Levels of evidence Appraisal II: Levels of evidence
Conduct research	Institutional review board Project design and measurement Project management Project evaluation and analysis
Dissemination	Publishing and dissemination

Both Abbott Northwestern Hospital in Minneapolis, Minnesota, and North Memorial Medical Center in Robbinsdale, Minnesota, developed interprofessional EBP programs based on the Iowa model described in Chapter 1 (Titler et al., 2001). Table 6-1 illustrates connections between elements in the Iowa model and planned education sessions that the program coordinators for Abbott Northwestern Hospital's interprofessional EBP program designed. Some education topics depicted in the table cover more than one element of the model.

SELECTING PARTICIPANTS

Program Coordinators

Starting an interprofessional EBP program requires careful selection of participants, including program coordinators. Program coordinators develop, manage, and have overall accountability to the program sponsors for the program. While some programs identified the project coordinator as being a part of the interprofessional team, they did not elaborate on the function of the role

(Wojciechowski, 2009). Other authors clearly identify that the role was to promote the program and develop the partnerships between the academic and clinical sites (Crist et al., 2005) (see Table 6-2 for a checklist of program coordinator responsibilities).

Program coordinators might not initially develop the EBP program but instead modify an existing program to include interprofessional teams. The interprofessional EBP program should have at least two coordinators: one from the health care organization and one from the university. Numbers of actual program coordinators depend on the number of interprofessional teams, partners, and the logistics that require ongoing management (e.g., use of learning technology, arranging guest expert speakers, obtaining and maintaining continuing education [CE] credits, and ensuring program communication). Ideally, program coordinators from a health care organization are researchers with doctoral preparation who have experience translating evidence into practice using implementation science and dissemination research. However, program coordinators with master's degrees and a strong background in EBP, quality improvement, or research paired with a faculty member with doctoral preparation, research, and EBP experience

	TABLE 6-2

CHECKLIST FOR THE RESPONSIBILITY OF PROGRAM COORDINATORS

√	
	Develop and attend bimonthly interprofessional EBP team classes, obtain CE credits for the program
	Schedule rooms for classes and other meetings
	Ongoing communication with the interprofessional EBP teams, creating and distributing agendas for interprofessional EBP team meetings and classes
	Develop and maintain the electronic platform housing the educational site for the interprofessional EBP program
	Liaison between the university and the health care organization
	Facilitate and support EBP research with assigned clinical scholar team
	Attend bimonthly meetings with the interprofessional team and clinical scholar mentors
	Develop and distribute resources for interprofessional team and clinical scholar mentors
	Participate in weekly program coordinator conference calls between the health care organization and university
	Evaluate progress of the interprofessional teams on their EBP projects
	Address issues and concerns and develop strategies for continuous improvement

is an effective strategy as well. Characteristics of program coordinators are as follows:

- A track record of project completion
- Ability to work with interprofessional teams
- Respect from colleagues both internally and externally
- Ability to mentor and to mentor the mentors
- Expertise in EBP and research
- Ability to mitigate potential and actual barriers
- History of professional publications and presentations
- Ability to influence (i.e., informal and expert power)
- Experience in using change theory, implementation and dissemination science
- Flexibility in problem solving and adoption of approaches and solutions
- Good communication skills
- Commitment to the success of the EBP program

Mentors

Documented EBP programs have included using mentors, describing their role as helping the team to identify the clinical question, conduct a literature review, appraise the evidence, make recommendations for practice, and facilitate the change into practice (Brewer et al., 2009; Newhouse et al., 2005; Rosswurm & Larrabee, 1999). Some

authors also refer to mentors as EBP champions (Caldwell et al., 2008, p. 81).

Program coordinators may select mentors in the early years of EBP program delivery. Later, as more EBP mentors become available in the health care organization, it is best to provide a list of possible EBP mentors to potential clinical scholars. Ideally, the scholar seeks support from a mentor, and then, in writing, identifies his or her mentor as a part of the application to become a clinical scholar. In this way, mentors and clinical scholars who already have a relationship enter the program together. Barker (2006) determined that compatibility between the mentor and clinical scholar is essential to make the project work. Although the mentor role is a volunteer position and participation is paid for by the health care organization, once a mentor has agreed to participate in the program, a work agreement completed with the scholar assists in creating clear expectations for the relationship.

The majority of information about the role and process of mentoring in clinical scholar programs comes from the nursing literature in which advanced practice nurses (APRNs) serve as mentors to clinical scholars who are nurses. Specifically, Gerrish et al. (2012) found that expertise in EBP, clinical credibility in practice, and leadership styles were factors for the ability of APRNs to promote EBP. Clinical nurse specialists, one of the four types of APRNs often referred to as *knowledge brokers for clinical practice* (Fineout-Overholt, Levin, & Melnyk, 2004), tend to have a strong EBP knowledge base because of their formal role for supporting EBP within the health care organization and often serve as EBP mentors (Wallen et al., 2010). Health care practitioners from various disciplines and roles (e.g., physical and occupational therapy, pharmacology, and medicine) successfully serve as mentors in EBP programs (Caldwell et al., 2008; Crist, 2005; Richardson et al., 2010; Wojciechowski, 2009), so the role is not confined to a single discipline. However, the literature does not specifically describe the mentoring process for interprofessional EBP in which the mentor not only mentors the scholar but the team itself.

Physician involvement in the EBP program may occur as an organizational sponsor for the project, a mentor, a team member, or a stakeholder. However, because of schedules, physicians may have limited ability to attend the EBP program when serving as part of the team. Consequently, the mentor facilitates and ensures that the clinical scholar and the team stay connected with the physician team member. However, when physicians are sponsoring the team or are stakeholders in the project (see Chapter 12), the mentor with the clinical scholar establishes ongoing communication with the physicians and seeks their formal support and approval as needed for the project.

Implementation of an EBP project requires a systems approach; therefore, mentors assist the clinical scholar and team members to navigate the health care organization. In addition, the mentor socializes the EBP clinical scholar to his or her new role as a change agent (Greene & Puetzer, 2002). Factors to consider when selecting mentors include the following:

- Expertise related to the practice question
- Demonstrated leadership in working with interprofessional colleagues
- Knowledge of EBP and change theory
- Project management skills
- Ability to mentor, provide support, and delegate to interprofessional team members
- Support from administration for the mentor's time devoted to the EBP project
- Strong communication skills
- Flexibility in problem solving and openness to new ideas

Clinical Scholars

Clinical scholar programs in acute care settings have primarily included staff nurses as the scholar or fellow (Gawlinski, 2008; Gawlinski & Miller, 2011; Newhouse et al., 2005; Rosswurm & Larrabee, 1999; Schultz, 2005). Potential reasons that acute care health care organizations primarily use nurses as scholars is because nursing departments are often the largest department, are more likely to have the capacity to cover shifts of the scholar, and have other sources of funding for developing staff nurses

to cover program expenses. Most importantly, chief nursing officers (CNOs) support nursing clinical scholar programs often in the organization's quest to obtain Magnet certification, which is a prestigious designation from the American Nurses Credentialing Center (Lundmark, 2008) that requires evidence that nurses are using research to change practice. Research does identify the CNO as a key leader for EBP, both as a role model and as the driver of the strategic vision for EBP in nursing (Stetler, Ritchie, Rycroft-Malone, Schultz, & Charns, 2009).

Along with a greater focus on EBP, interprofessional team-based practice as a method for improving care and services is also growing in emphasis. Consequently, senior leaders of health care organizations, including acute care institutions, need to examine ways to sponsor clinicians and practitioners from all disciplines to participate in an interprofessional EBP program as a clinical scholar. The interaction between scholars from a variety of disciplines will only expand the interprofessional learning opportunities and serve to create new or deeper working relationships within an organization.

Clinical scholar characteristics include clinicians and practitioners in all disciplines who are curious, use critical thinking skills, are engaged in ongoing learning, reflect on practice, use a variety of resources, use evidence to improve effectiveness of care, and routinely ask "why" type of questions (Schultz, 2005; Sigma Theta Tau International, 1999; Strout, Lancaster, & Schultz, 2009). Clinical scholars are the out-of-the-box thinkers who question practice and are knowledge-based as opposed to rule-based (Breweret al., 2009; Schultz, 2005). These clinicians and practitioners from multiple disciplines should have strong skills in observation, an ability to analyze and synthesize different forms of information, the drive to implement results to change practice, and a desire to disseminate results (Brewer et al., 2009; Schultz, 2005; Sigma Theta Tau International, 1999) (see Table 6-3 checklist for eligibility requirements for selecting clinical scholars).

Clinical Scholars at Abbott Northwestern Hospital

Abbott Northwestern Hospital in Minneapolis, Minnesota, is a Magnet-certified hospital that started an EBP fellowship program in 2008, which became an interprofessional scholar program in 2014. The fellows or the clinical scholars are staff nurses practicing in the hospital who are on a team with faculty and students from a variety of disciplines. The coordinator of the EBP fellowship program publicized the program internally at the hospital through announcing the program at nursing council meetings, posting announcements on the nursing website of Abbott Northwestern, and including the EBP program information in the CNO's weekly email communication to nursing staff. A program brochure distributed to nursing

TABLE 6-3	
CHECKLIST FOR ELIGIBILITY REQUIREMENTS FOR SELECTING CLINICAL SCHOLARS	
√	
	Level of education: Baccalaureate degree or higher
	Work agreement: Works part-time or full-time; unit or department is able to accommodate time in the program
	Years at the organization: Sufficient hours worked within the organization as a practitioner or clinician; 1 to 2 years ensures that the practitioner has developed an understanding of the practice area and has developed relationships with other practitioners and clinicians
	Characteristics: Informal leader among peers, knowledge-based as opposed to rule-bound, strong observational skills, critical thinking, continuous learner, high level of curiosity, never stops asking "why?"
	Clinical question: Identifies a practice relevant question that is feasible to investigate and address
	Commitment: Will stay at the health care organization until the project is completed, participates fully until completion, and works to disseminate results

staff provided an overview of the program, including criteria for application and a commitment agreement. In addition, previous EBP fellows act as champions to help advertise the program and its effect on practice and professional development. Balakas, Sparks, Steurer, and Bryant (2013) found that previous clinical scholars significantly contribute to sustaining the EBP momentum within an organization, as well as enculturating others into the practice of using evidence to solve problems. Thus, incorporating past scholars into the process is an important strategy.

Staff nurses exploring the program receive application materials that provide an overview of the mission and vision of the hospital, define EBP, identify the interprofessional team as a program strategy, and outline program objectives and eligibility criteria and requirements. The committee selecting clinical scholars includes representatives active in the hospital's shared governance structure, a past clinical scholar, as well as the director of nursing research. The application requires the potential clinical scholar to pose a relevant practice question. Alignment of the practice question with a patient need that a front-line practitioner identifies is associated with successful EBP projects (Dogherty, Harrison, Graham, Vandyk, & Keeping-Burke, 2013; Harrison & Graham, 2012). However, potential scholars are not required to pose the initial practice question using the problem/patient population, intervention, comparison group, and outcome (PICO) format because it is unusual for nurses first learning EBP to know how to formulate EBP questions. The interprofessional team assists the nurse in refining the PICO question once the program starts (Harrison & Graham, 2012).

The checklist in Table 6-3 includes elements from the Abbott Northwestern interprofessional EBP program for selecting clinical scholars and may assist with facilitating the process for other programs as well. The application process may include the following:

- A multifaceted approach to advertise the interprofessional EBP program, which includes using online and face-to-face methods, such as newsletters, brochures, and announcements during new staff orientation

- A simple online or paper application process that includes identifying a practice-relevant question or topic, securing a mentor with whom to partner on the project, and obtaining letters of recommendation (one from a peer and one from a health care manager who can attest to the applicant's abilities)

- A letter of support from the prospective mentor who can address the relevance of the project, the feasibility of completion of the project within a defined time frame, and a possible design for the project

- A signed agreement between the practitioner and his or her mentor. The signed agreement should clearly state that if selected, both the clinical scholar and the mentor will comply with the terms and conditions of the program. Those agreements should include the following terms:
  - Attending all classroom sessions
  - Meeting regularly with the manager of the practice area
  - Meeting and working regularly with the mentor and the EBP team
  - Completing the project within a designated time frame
  - Disseminating the results to colleagues at the health care organization and the university
  - Disseminating the work to professional audiences

Faculty and Students

Selecting faculty and students is important not only to provide depth for the project and resources to the clinical scholar and mentor, but also for building strong partnerships between the health care organization and the university. The goal for the health care organization is to select faculty and students who will enhance the work and facilitate the timely completion of the project, while at the same time bring an interprofessional perspective. The partnership is a venue for the university to offer faculty and students opportunities to change practice and begin a line of scholarship addressing a variety of practice issues. Faculty selection for the interprofessional EBP teams includes evaluating the resource needs for the identified projects in order to bring a variety of expertise to the interprofessional EBP program. Some potential selection considerations for faculty may include the following:

- Project fit with the faculty member's profession or interests
- Practice and subject matter expertise
- Research and EBP experience and expertise
- Experience with grant writing and management
- Publication experience
- Skills in partnering and collaborating
- Project management skills
- Time to commit to the team and project
- Positive student relationships
- Effective communication skills
- Desire for scholarship opportunities within a health care organization

Faculty members do not need to fulfill all identified selection considerations and the project does not have to fit directly with the faculty member's discipline, background, or experience. Faculty with strong research and EBP backgrounds are important for all of the teams regardless of project focus. In addition, faculty expertise for a specific topic is not always readily apparent. The program coordinators may not have a complete understanding of the scope of practice for a variety of disciplines and may not fully realize areas of expertise shared across disciplines.

Students add significant value to interprofessional teams and have an opportunity to engage in a rich, real-world learning experience. Faculty members who join the interprofessional EBP program are critical for identifying students who will benefit and contribute to the team's EBP project. Just like faculty, students should come from a variety of disciplines and diverse experiences. Selection criteria for students may include the following:

- Junior or senior baccalaureate students or master's or clinical doctoral degree students in a health care profession educational program or a library science program
- High performance demonstrated by quality of didactic and clinical work
- Willingness to use the EBP project as the capstone, master's degree, or clinical doctoral project
- Time to commit to the team and project above the current class load or as a portion of a clinical practicum or internship
- Demonstrated professionalism, reliability, and interpersonal skills
- Faculty support and recommendations from the program directors of the health professions educational program or library science program

In general, identifying faculty and student participants once the health care organization has selected frontline practitioners for the clinical scholar positions facilitates an opportunity for faculty members and students to learn about specific projects before deciding to become involved. Thus, the program coordinators create a program timeline, which allows for obtaining the right faculty support and student involvement, taking into consideration when faculty are on contract and when students are available to contact.

Prior to selecting clinical scholars, it is important to discuss potential opportunities and requirements with faculty and students to increase awareness of the program. The program coordinator from the university and other academic leaders sponsoring the program may want to meet with potential faculty to determine the best fit or as a mechanism to recruit outstanding faculty. Once program coordinators select faculty, it is beneficial for the program coordinators and university leaders to spend time with faculty to clarify roles and expectations.

Student selection should involve those faculty selected to participate in the interprofessional EBP program and program directors or chairs of various academic departments. Faculty members who are planning to participate are often in the best position to identify appropriate students from their classes; however, it is not necessary that participating faculty personally know selected students. Faculty roles for the interprofessional EBP program include mentoring and developing all students on the team regardless of the student's program of study. The interprofessional EBP program coordinators should then meet with students and prepare them for participation, clarifying expectations, outlining opportunities, and addressing logistical concern (e.g., scheduling challenges).

Academic program directors and chairs identify additional students and assist with facilitating students' use of the experience in meeting educational expectations within their program of study (e.g., master's degree projects, capstone experiences, internships). When the EBP program becomes a part of the student's course expectations, faculty members and students on the team work with the academic program faculty of the students as well as the members of the team to devise specific tasks, responsibilities, and deliverables for students. These student EBP project assignments are not only worthy of academic credit but also address the learning goals of the student, including methods of determining whether the student met the learning outcomes.

DEVELOPING AN ORIENTATION FOR THE INTERPROFESSIONAL EVIDENCE-BASED PRACTICE PROGRAM

Two different program orientations need to take place in an interprofessional EBP program, one designed for mentors and another for the clinical scholars and their interprofessional teams. A structured orientation program for the participants of the interprofessional EBP program ensures a positive start and ultimately saves time in terms of preventing team confusion about how to develop the projects (Wallen et al., 2010).

Mentor Orientation

The program coordinators should ground the orientation for mentors in the evidence about effective mentoring. The goal of the mentor orientation is to offer a useful approach for leading and managing interprofessional teams engaged in EBP. Based on previous work described in Chapter 3, it is clear that a mentoring theoretical framework is helpful when creating a mentor program. Specifically, key principles identified in that chapter that assist with developing a mentor orientation are as follows:

- Mentoring challenges and EBP task demands vary in type, occurrence, and difficulty across the EBP project phases.

- Micro- and macro-contexts affect EBP task demands in a way that could create mentor challenges on a continuum of difficulty.

- Mentors match the best mentoring techniques with the nature of the mentoring challenges and the complexity of the EBP task demands to ensure successful progress of the team on the EBP project.

- Mentors select the best mentoring technique as a part of a reflective and deliberative mentoring practice.

- Team and team member characteristics, or the micro-context, impact effectiveness of mentoring.

- Interprofessional EBP program coordinators mentor not only the mentors of the clinical scholar, but mentor all of the interprofessional team members.

- Interprofessional EBP program coordinators use mentor supports to inspire, support, teach, and invest in the mentors.

- Phases of a project require different amounts and types of mentoring for team members.

The interprofessional EBP program coordinators can use the checklist in Table 6-4 for developing a mentor orientation program.

Orientation for Clinical Scholars and Interprofessional Team Members

Effective implementation of a practice change that has strong evidence for its use requires clinicians and practitioners to understand and value EBP (Brewer et al., 2009). EBP is a movement away from a task orientation to one of inquiry, reflection, and critical thinking (Clinical Scholarship Task Force of Sigma Theta Tau International, 1999). The orientation can be the clinical scholar's and interprofessional team members' first introduction to interprofessional EBP.

The program coordinators develop an orientation program that creates a culture of support, encouragement, and a sense of belonging that prepares the interprofessional team for functioning throughout the program. The quality of the orientation program is a factor in preventing team members from becoming overwhelmed and in preventing early attrition from the program. The content is designed to provide an overview of the program, but also generate excitement and enthusiasm for the upcoming work. Presentations should involve interaction through discussion and interspersed with specific team activities. Creating a team identity early in the process facilitates a successful program and prevents members from feeling isolated. The orientation, which is the first meeting of the teams, should have well-designed curricula that includes the following:

- Introduction of team members to their teams, mentors, and the practice problem that:

  o Includes time for the clinical scholar to tell the story of identifying the problem, his or her perspective about the importance to practice, and any expectations

  o Provides an opportunity for team members to discuss their interest, where they think they can assist with the project, and their expectations

- Overview of the syllabus that includes the details of the program: course description, learning objectives, meeting dates, times, locations, faculty for the EBP educational sessions, disclosures of conflict of interest, accreditation, course text and readings, and course schedules

- Identifying the best location for all those involved in the program is essential for preventing attrition

	TABLE 6-4
	CHECKLIST FOR DEVELOPING A MENTOR ORIENTATION PROGRAM AND SUPPORT

√	
	Course description: Provide mentors with an overview of the interprofessional EBP program, the orientation program for the clinical scholars and interprofessional team members, and the elements of the mentor orientation program
	Course prerequisite: To improve the understanding of the mentors about their role and participation in the program, provide mentors the interprofessional program education syllabus to review and access helpful articles about mentoring and leading interprofessional teams
	Logistics: Date/time/place of the orientation for the mentors and ongoing mentoring meetings, resources for the mentors, and access to the education learning platform for the interprofessional EPB program
	Program Coordinators: "Mentors for the mentors," assign the program coordinators to support each team and provide time for the program coordinators to meet with their assigned mentor
	Accreditation: Obtain approval from the local Board of Nursing, American Nurses Credentialing Center, and other professional organizations for mentors of various disciplines for CE credits
	Learning objectives: Identify clear understanding regarding what the participant will be able to do upon completion of the mentoring course
	Course text and other readings: Select an EBP text to which mentors and the interprofessional team can refer throughout the interprofessional EBP process
	Design the content and discussion: Dialogue about the reflective and deliberative mentoring process; discuss the mentoring challenges that occur, describe partnership responsibilities between the university and the health care organization, describe the effect of macro- and micro-contexts on changing practice, and discuss the mentor techniques for leading interprofessional teams

from the program. Alternating sites between the partnering organizations is an effective strategy to consider.

- Introduction to the program and the partnership, discussing the vision, and the benefits to both organizations

- Interprofessional EBP project phases

- Team framework for organizing the teams, team roles, and mentoring

- Program tools, materials, and resources

- Communication strategies, training, and practice on the technology for communication, such as learning platforms (see Chapter 5)

ELEMENTS OF THE ONGOING INTERPROFESSIONAL EVIDENCE-BASED PRACTICE PROGRAM

The ongoing program requires as much planning as the orientation of mentors and the interprofessional teams and should focus on the education needs identified in the readiness assessment described in Chapter 2. Teams will function more consistently when there is a set process or rhythm to the program that the teams can count on occurring. The goal is to ensure the interprofessional teams complete their work at a high-quality level. Before the program begins, the program coordinators develop an overall structure for the program. Figure 6-1 illustrates the essential elements of an interprofessional scholar program. Included in a possible structure are the following elements:

- *Education Sessions:* EBP learning opportunities created for the interprofessional teams focus on each phase of interprofessional EBP. These educational sessions provide an opportunity for the teams to learn together. See Chapter 1 for potential course content (e.g., overview of EBP, developing a PICO question, searching the literature, appraisal, implementation, evaluation, leadership and EBP, and dissemination). The two organizations identify individuals with expertise in the content to provide education (see the book's website for EBP educational PowerPoint slide presentations).

- *Educational EBP Materials:* The program coordinators may want to identify an EBP textbook as the basis for the educational program. Prior to the program, tools are identified that will facilitate

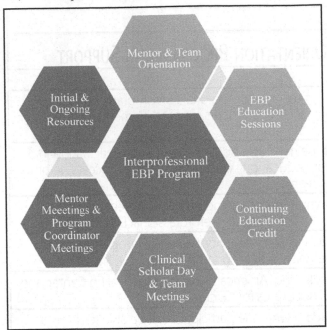

Figure 6-1. Structure for the interprofessional EBP program.

different aspects of the program, such as evidence appraisal, synthesis, and project management tools (see the book's website for tools).

- *CE Credit:* Obtaining authorization for offering CE credit for specific disciplines attending the program supports disciplines in maintaining their licenses and certification, brings value to the program, and serves as an additional incentive for the interprofessional team to attend the EBP education course sessions. Included in the CE requirements is the use of course evaluations that assist with making course corrections and identifying additional learning needs.

- *Clinical Scholar Day:* Budgeted time for the clinical scholar, such as an 8-hour day for the clinical scholar to work on the project (e.g., the first and third Thursday of every month) with approximately one of those 8 hours devoted to attending EBP education and another hour for the interprofessional team meeting.

- *Interprofessional Team Meetings:* Generally held on the same day as the clinical scholar day, the team negotiates the best time for the team to meet based on each member's schedule. The team may elect to use communication technologies for meetings (see Chapter 5).

- *Check-In Meetings:* Check-in sessions help the interprofessional EBP program coordinators assess the progress of the teams and give opportunities for all of the teams to dialogue together, sharing ideas and strategies. These sessions occur in between course

content sessions. The timing of the course content should correspond to when the teams will most likely address the next phase in the EBP process. Thus, there is time to schedule check-in sessions in place of educational content in order to spread out the learning sessions.

- *Mentor Meetings:* An hour meeting (e.g., every other week opposite the Thursday of the interprofessional EBP clinical scholar day) to share progress, address mentor challenges, select and develop skills in mentoring techniques, and request mentor supports from program coordinators.

- *Coordinator Meetings:* Thirty-minute weekly meetings for planning and addressing logistics and mentor challenges, and to determine and devise needed mentor supports (see Chapter 3).

- *Team Charters:* The interprofessional team charter is instrumental in ensuring a cohesive team. Time is provided during orientation to initiate the charter. The charter is then used during team meetings to continually clarify the roles of the team members and the corresponding expectations (see Chapter 4).

- *Team Communication Methods:* Setting up systems for communication is important (see Chapter 5). A university might offer its education platform system as a site for the program and for individual teams to dialogue and meet virtually. The program should also discuss using document-sharing systems (e.g., Google Docs).

- *Initial Resources:* The program coordinators identify resources that include space for classes and meetings, computers and printers, EBP books for participants, Internet access, and library support. Having access to a librarian who can assist with searching for evidence is an identified factor in facilitating EBP (Dogherty et al., 2013).

- *Ongoing Resources:* The coordinators also identify additional resources and supports throughout the program that are specific to the projects of each interprofessional team. For example, if the EBP question for a project leads to using quality improvement methods for evaluating the project outcomes, the interprofessional team may need support from quality improvement experts. If the project includes conducting research, the interprofessional team may need the support of a statistician.

Securing Leader Support

Throughout the development of an interprofessional EBP program, the program coordinators manage the macro-context when they work with top leaders in both the university, such as deans and the chief academic officer or provost, and from the health care organization, such as CNOs, chief medical officers (CMOs), and vice presidents of other service divisions. Deans of health profession programs are important for ensuring faculty and student participation, providing resources, communicating the importance of the program, and developing positive relationships with health care organizations. CNOs often reflect their support for EBP by incorporating statements about EBP within their division's vision and strategic plan (Titler, Cullen, & Ardery, 2002; Titler & Everett, 2006). The program coordinators should not underestimate the support a CNO, a CMO, or vice presidents of divisions can offer the interprofessional EBP program, especially given the empowerment and leadership they provide for nurses, physicians, rehabilitation professionals, and other disciplines within their health care organizations (Sredl et al., 2011; Titler et al., 2002). Physicians, managers, and leaders from occupational and physical therapy as well as many other disciplines are sometimes both facilitators and a major barrier for implementing EBP. Consequently, the importance of these leaders in the interprofessional EBP process as advocates for EBP resources and infrastructure cannot be overestimated (Gifford, Davies, Edwards, Griffin, & Lybanon, 2007; Jenkins, Sredl, Hsueh, & Ding, 2007; Melnyk et al., 2004; Melnyk, Fineout-Overholt, Gallagher-Ford, & Kaplan, 2012).

MENTOR CHALLENGES

Mentors from the health care organization are extremely busy and may struggle with spending time attending the orientation and learning sessions for the interprofessional EBP program. Because mentors have significant influence on achieving a successful EBP project, they may need support from the organization as well as information about the value their attendance has for maintaining and sustaining the program. Because mentors have a background in EBP, they may want to use the time to complete other work requirements, not recognizing that their presence, engagement, and knowledge sharing is critical for a successful EBP project. Mentors bring to the program their discipline-specific knowledge of EBP, their knowledge of the evidence-to-practice gaps that exist within their organization, and their understanding of the organizational culture and systems. The orientation and learning program also provides an opportunity for mentors to learn more about EBP from an interprofessional perspective and to remain current with the emerging and evolving techniques, methods, and processes for interprofessional EBP. In addition, mentors, clinical scholars, and the interprofessional team need time for establishing relationships and developing a team identity, which starts with the orientation programs.

The interprofessional EBP program should develop the interprofessional competencies related to team values and ethics, roles and responsibilities, communication, and teamwork and team practice (Interprofessional Education Collaborative Expert Panel, 2011). A major challenge in

developing EBP-ready practitioners and clinicians is to prepare them also to conduct EBP within a team (Zwarenstein & Reeves, 2006). The goal is to help an interprofessional team focus on solving a patient problem rather than seeing the EBP project as the concern of a single discipline, as well as being open to other perspectives and methods for EBP. The orientation and learning programs should expose clinicians to a wide variety of EBP frameworks, methods, and literature that should promote information exchange among disciplines. According to Moyers et al. (2014), addressing problems from only one discipline's perspective does not take into consideration the obstacles to EBP that often exist due to interprofessional relationships and disciplinary biases (p. S23). In their case study, an interprofessional EBP program facilitated participant learning about the value of an interprofessional team in improving work processes and helped the team develop a more holistic view of patient needs.

MENTOR TECHNIQUES AND SUPPORTS

Mentor supports are strategies the program coordinators use to promote the success of the interprofessional EBP program. Program coordinators develop these supports when designing educational materials for the interprofessional EBP program and for development of interprofessional team competencies. The mentor orientation lays the foundation for mentors developing their mentoring techniques partially based on the principles in TeamSTEPPS as outlined in Chapter 4 and the mentoring theory in Chapter 3. The mentor orientation supports mentors working with their teams during the interprofessional program orientation in order to facilitate the team in drafting their team charters, as well as for working with their team throughout the program. Table 6-5 provides examples of supports that program coordinators should include in the mentor and team orientations, and that mentors should role-model as mentor techniques in subsequent team interactions. Other mentor supports to build into the program include strategies that Wallen et al. (2010) and Moyers et al. (2014) identified, which include the following:

- Seminars or intensive workshops on methods for strengthening deliberative and reflective mentoring and for improving team communication

- Interactive lectures and tutorials that include a wide range of approaches from various disciplines to increase knowledge related to the basics of EBP, implementation science, and dissemination strategies

- Scheduled bimonthly meetings for mentors and interprofessional EBP program coordinators for identifying additional learning needs to incorporate as just-in-time learning

	TABLE 6-5
	TeamSTEPPS in an Interprofessional Clinical Scholars Program
TEAMSTEPPS CONCEPTS	**TEAMSTEPPS AND MENTOR TECHNIQUES AND SUPPORTS**
Interprofessional team charter	Educate the team on the importance of using the team charter. Provide instruction for completing the document; ensure the team posts them on the learning platform. The program coordinators should review and provide the mentors and the team with feedback about discussions that improve team transparency.
Briefings before the meetings	Program coordinators and mentors role-model team skills by providing briefings at each educational session and team meetings, and address the required work for teams and the expected goals to accomplish as milestones in the program timeline. Mentors learn to assist the teams in creating agendas that reflect the focus for the work. The program coordinator can review team agendas and provide feedback to mentors about methods to improve clarity regarding team member responsibility.
Debriefings after the meetings	Program coordinators and mentors role-model the use of questions at the end of every meeting teaching teams to ask questions, such as whether the workload is evenly distributed, the team meeting was productive, roles and responsibilities were clearly identified, and all of the concerns were addressed.
Huddles	In between meetings, the program coordinators and the mentors encourage the interprofessional team to use huddles to solve problems that develop. Ongoing mentor and coordinator meetings are a form of a huddle that occurs routinely to identify and plan the next steps and solutions to identified challenges.
Situation monitoring	Program coordinators and mentors role-model keeping the team focused on positive actions and activities, as well as occurrences that are problematic. Mentors help teams to learn to identify mistakes and lapses in actions in a nonjudgmental way and to provide each other with constructive feedback.
Mutual support	Team members learn to anticipate and support their colleagues when they have an understanding of their team member's needs. Mutual support means that members of the team understand each other's responsibilities and workload, offer assistance, and address conflict in a respectful manner. Team mentors are encouraged to routinely ask what support the team needs as a way to role model mutual support.
Call out	A call-out is a strategy used to facilitate critical team communication. The team learns to ask questions when observing mentors engaging in these actions, such as: What deadlines are coming up? What are the next steps? What action will solve the problem? What resources do we need? Who is responsible for this action? When are the assignments due?

- Mentoring tips sent to mentors via a mini-newsletter, blogs, and supportive emails (see book website for "One-Minute Mentoring Updates")

- A celebration party to recognize the work of the EBP mentors and their team members at the end that highlights the learning that occurred (see Chapter 14)

SUMMARY

The orientation programs for mentors and the interprofessional teams are essential for creating an effective interprofessional EBP program. The success of the program is dependent on selecting the most appropriate individuals from both the university and the health care organization to serve as program coordinators. Criteria are helpful for selecting mentors, clinical scholars, faculty, and students. Program coordinators and mentors engage in ongoing planning to address the specific needs of each project, and to solve mentor challenges with well-designed supports. Consistent mentor and program coordinator meetings, as well as a well-established structure for the interprofessional EBP program, help to ensure that participants successfully complete the program.

REFLECTION QUESTIONS

1. How would you structure an interprofessional EBP program differently from a program that includes a single discipline?

2. What are considerations for selecting clinical scholars, students, and faculty for the interprofessional EBP program?

REFERENCES

Albert, N. M., & Siedlecki, S. L. (2008). Developing and implementing a nursing research team in a clinical setting. *Journal of Nursing Administration, 38*(2), 90-96. doi:10.1097/01.nna.0000310714.30721.ca

Austin, T. M., Richter, R. R., & Frese, T. (2009). Using a partnership between academic faculty and a physical therapist liaison to develop a framework for an evidence-based journal club: a discussion. *Physiotherapy Research International, 14*(4), 213-223. doi:10.1002/pri.444

Balakas, K., Sparks, L., Steurer, L., & Bryant, T. (2013). An outcome of evidence-based practice education: Sustained clinical decision-making among bedside nurses. *Journal of Pediatric Nursing, 28* (5), 479-485. doi:10.1016/j.pedn.2012.08.007

Barker, E. R. (2006). Mentoring—a complex relationship. *Journal of the American Academy of Nurse Practitioners, 18*(2), 56-61. doi:10.1111/j.1745-7599.2006.00102.x

Brewer, B. B., Brewer, M. A., & Schultz, A. A. (2009). A collaborative approach to building the capacity for research and evidence-based practice in community hospitals. *Nursing Clinics of North America, 44*(1), 11-25. doi:10.1016/j.cnur.2008.10.003

Brownson, R. C., Colditz, G. A., & Proctor, E. K. (2012). *Dissemination and implementation of research in health: Translating science to Practice.* New York, NY: Oxford University Press.

Centre for the Advancement of Interprofessional Education. (2002). *Interprofessional education: A definition.* Retrieved December 8, 2014, from http://caipe.org.uk/about-us/defining-ipe.

Caldwell, E., Whitehead, M., Fleming, J., & Moes, L. (2008). Evidence-based practice in everyday clinical practice: Strategies for change in a tertiary occupational therapy department. *Australian Occupational Therapy Journal, 55*(2), 79-84. doi:10.1111/j.1440-1630.2007.00669.x

Clinical Scholarship Task Force of Sigma Theta Tau International. (1999). *Clinical scholarship resource paper.* Retrieved December 8, 2014, from http://www.nursingsociety.org/aboutus/PositionPapers/Documents/clinical_scholarship_paper.pdf.

Crist, P., Muñoz, J. P., Hansen, A. M. W., Benson, J., & Provident, I. (2005). The practice-scholar program: An academic partnership to promote the scholarship of "best practices." *Occupational Therapy in Health Care, 19*(1-2), 71-93. doi:10.1300/j003v19n0106

Cullen, L., & Titler, M. G. (2004) Promoting evidence-based practice: An internship for staff nurses. *Worldview on Evidence-Based Nursing, 1*(4), 215-223. doi:10.1111/j.1524-475x.2004.04027.x

D'Amour, D. & Oandasan, I. (2005). Interprofessionality as the field of interprofessional practice and interprofessional education: An emerging concept. *Journal of Interprofessional Care, Supp 1,* 8-20. doi:10.1080/13561820500081604

Dizon, J. M. R., Grimmer-Somers, K. A., & Kumar, S. (2012). Current evidence on evidence-based practice training in allied health: a systematic review of the literature. *International Journal of Evidence-Based Healthcare, 10*(4); 347-360. doi:10.1111/j.1744-1609.2012.00295.x

Dogherty, E. J., Harrison, M. B., Graham, I. D., Vandyk, A. D., & Keeping-Burke, L. (2013). Turning knowledge into action at the point-of-care: The collective experience of nurses facilitating the implementation of evidence-based practice. *Worldviews on Evidence-Based Nursing / Sigma Theta Tau International, Honor Society of Nursing, 10*(3), 129-139. doi:10.1111/wvn.12009

Fineout-Overholt, E., Levin, R. F., & Melnyk, B. M. (2004). Strategies for advancing evidence-based practice in clinical settings. *The Journal of the New York State Nurses' Association, 35*(2), 28-32.

Gawlinski, A. (2008). The power of clinical nursing research: Engage clinicians, improve patients' lives, and forge a professional legacy. *American Journal of Critical Care, 17*(4), 315-327.

Gawlinksi, A., & Miller, P. S. (2011). Advancing nursing research through a mentorship program for staff nurses. *AACN Advanced Critical Care, 22*(3), 190-200. doi:10.1097/nci.0b013e318224786b

Gerrish, K., Nolan, M., McDonnell, A., Tod, A., Kirshbaum, M., & Guillaume, L. (2012). Factors influencing advanced practice nurses' ability to promote evidence-based practice among frontline nurses. *Worldviews on Evidence-Based Nursing / Sigma Theta Tau International, Honor Society of Nursing, 9*(1), 30-39. doi:10.1111/j.1741-6787.2011.00230.x

Gifford, W., Davies, B., Edwards, N., Griffin, P., & Lybanon, V. (2007). Managerial leadership for nurses' use of research evidence: An integrative review of the literature. *Worldviews on Evidence-Based Nursing, 4*(3), 126-145. doi:10.1111/j.1741-6787.2007.00095.x

Graner, T., Sendelbach, S., Boland, L., & Koehn, K. (2011). Evidence based practice fellowships: Changing practice one clinical question at a time. *Nursing Management, 42*(5), 14-17.

Greene, M. T., & Puetzer, M. (2002). The value of mentoring: A strategic approach to retention and recruitment. *Journal of Nursing Care Quality, 17*(1), 63-70. doi:10.1097/00001786-200210000-00008

Harrison, M. B., & Graham, I. D. (2012). Roadmap for a participatory research-practice partnership to implement evidence. *Worldviews on Evidence-Based Nursing / Sigma Theta Tau International, Honor Society of Nursing, 9*(4), 210-220. doi:10.1111/j.1741-6787.2012.00256.x

Interprofessional Education Collaborative Expert Panel. (2011). *Core competencies for interprofessional collaborative practice: Report of an expert panel.* Washington, DC: Interprofessional Education Collaborative.

Jenkins, R. L., Sredl, D., Hsueh, K., & Ding, C. (2007). Evidence-based nursing process (EBNP) consumer culture attribute identity: A message-based persuasion strategy study among nurse executives in the United States of America. *Journal of Medical Sciences-Taipei, 27*(2), 55.

Lundmark, V. A. (2008). Magnet environment for professional nursing practice. In R.G. Hughes, (Ed) Patient Safety and Quality: An Evidence-Based Handbook for Nurses. Rockville, MD: Agency for Healthcare Research and Quality US.

Melnyk, B. M., Fineout-Overholt, E., Feinstein, N. F., Li, H., Small, L., Wilcox, L., & Kraus R. (2004). Nurses' perceived knowledge, beliefs, skills, and needs regarding evidence-based practice: Implications for accelerating the paradigm shift. *Worldviews on Evidence-Based Nursing, 1*(3), 185-193. doi:10.1111/j.1524-475x.2004.04024.x

Melnyk, B. M., Fineout-Overholt, E., Gallagher-Ford, L., & Kaplan, L. (2012). The state of evidence-based practice in US nurses: Critical implications for nurse leaders and educators. *The Journal of Nursing Administration, 42*(9), 410-417. doi:10.1097/nna.0b013e3182664e0a

Moyers, P. A., Finch Guthrie, P. L., Swan, A. R., & Sathe, L. A. (2014). Interprofessional evidence-based clinical scholar program: Learning to work together. *American Journal of Occupational Therapy, 68,* S23–S31. doi:10.5014/ajot.2014.012609

Newhouse, R., Dearholt, S., Poe, S., Pugh, L. C., & White, K. M. (2005). Evidence based practice: A practical approach to implementation. *The Journal of Nursing Administration, 35*(1), 35-40. doi:10.1097/00005110-200501000-00013

Pardue, K. T. (2015). A framework for the design, implementation, and evaluation of interprofessional education. *Nurse Educator, 40*(1), 10-15. doi:10.1097/nne.0000000000000093

Richardson, J., Letts, L., Childs, A., Semogas, D., Stavness, C., Smith, B.J.,…Price, D. (2010). Development of a community scholar program: An interprofessional initiative. *Journal of Physical Therapy Education, 24*(1), 37-43.

Rosswurn, M. A., & Larrabee, J. H. (1999). A model for change to evidence-based practice. *Image: The Journal of Nursing Scholarship, 31*(4), 317-322. doi:10.1111/j.1547-5069.1999.tb00510.x/pdf

Schreiber, J., Downey, P., & Traister, J. (2009). Academic program support for evidence-based practice: A mixed-methods investigation. *Journal of Physical Therapy Education, 23*(1), 36-43.

Schultz, A. (2005). Clinical scholars at the bedside: An EBP mentorship model for today. *Excellence in Nursing Knowledge, 2,* 4-11.

Shediac-Rizkallah, M. C., & Bone, L. R. (1998). Planning for the sustainability of community-based health programs: Conceptual frameworks and future directions for research, practice and policy. *Health Education Research, 13*(1), 87-108.

Sigma Theta Tau International. (1999). Clinical scholarship resource paper. Retrieved December 10, 2014, from http://www.nursingsociety.org/aboutus/PositionPapers/Documents/clinical_scholarship_paper.pdf.

Sredl, D. D., Melnyk, B. M., Hsueh, S., Jenkins, R., Ding, C., & Durham, J. (2011). Health care in crisis! Can nurse executives' beliefs about and implementation of evidence-based practice be key solutions in health care reform? *Teaching and Learning in Nursing, 6*(2), 73; 73-79.

Stetler, C. B., Ritchie, J. A., Rycroft-Malone, J., Schultz, A. A., & Charns, M. P. (2009). Institutionalizing evidence-based practice: an organizational case study using a model of strategic change. *Implementation Science, 4*(1), 78. doi:10.1186/1748-5908-4-78

Strout, T. D., Lancaster, K., & Schultz, A. A. (2009). Development and implementation of an inductive model for evidence-based practice: A grassroots approach for building evidence-based practice capacity in staff nurses. *The Nursing Clinics of North America, 44*(1), 93-102. xi. doi:10.1016/j.cnur.2008.10.007

Titler, M. G., Cullen, L., & Ardery, G. (2002). Evidence-based practice: An administrative perspective. *Reflections on Nursing Leadership / Sigma Theta Tau International, Honor Society of Nursing, 28*(2), 26-27, 46, 45.

Titler, M. G., & Everett, L. Q. (2006). Sustain an infrastructure to support EBP. *Nursing Management, 37*(9), 14-16. doi:10.1097/00006247-200609000-00005

Titler, M. G., Kleiber, C., Steelman, V. J., Rakel, B. A., Budreau, G., Everett, L. Q., … Goode, C. J. (2001). The Iowa model of evidence-based practice to promote quality care. *Critical Care Nursing Clinics of North America, 13*(4), 497-509.

Wallen, G. R., Mitchell, S. A., Melnyk, B., Fineout-Overholt, E., Miller-Davis, C., Yates, J., & Hastings, C. (2010). Implementing evidence-based practice: Effectiveness of a structured multifaceted mentorship programme. *Journal of Advanced Nursing, 66*(12), 2761-2771. doi:10.1111/j.1365-2648.2010.05442.x

Wojciechowski, M. (2009). Forging a groundbreaking clinical-academic research partnership. *PT in Motion, American Physical Therapy Association,* October, 26-32.

Zwarenstein, M., & Reeves, S. (2006). Knowledge translation and interprofessional collaboration: Where the rubber of evidence-based care hits the road of teamwork. *Journal of Continuing Education in the Health Professions, 26,* 46–54.

Supplemental materials for this chapter are available online.
Please refer to the sticker in the front of the book and enter the access code provided.

7

Figuring Out the Problem and Getting Focused

John D. Fleming, EdD, OTR/L

CHAPTER TOPICS

- Understanding the identified practice problem
- Understanding background and foreground questions
- Using evidence to answer background and foreground questions
- Mentor challenges
- Mentor techniques and supports

PERFORMANCE OBJECTIVES

Because of understanding the process for developing projects in an interprofessional evidence-based practice program, team members, mentors, and program coordinators at the conclusion of this chapter will be able to do the following:

1. Describe problem-focused and knowledge-focused triggers and the process for clarifying practice problems.

2. Discuss foreground and background questions as they relate to interprofessional evidence-based practice.

3. Describe answering background and foreground questions as an iterative process.

4. Identify mentor challenges and the corresponding mentor techniques and supports for this beginning phase of the interprofessional evidence-based practice process.

This chapter discusses the first step in the interprofessional evidence-based practice (EBP) process, which is the identification and clarification of the practice problem and the progression to developing the focused EBP question referred to as the *foreground question*. The interprofessional team is ready to start this process after attending an interprofessional EBP program outlined in Chapter 6 about the interprofessional EBP problem and development of interprofessional EBP questions.

The foreground question guides the entire interprofessional EBP project, which makes the steps leading up to determining the foreground question an essential part of EBP. Thus, the interprofessional EBP team starts with understanding the problem so that the foreground question

Moyers, P. A., & Finch-Guthrie, P. L.
Interprofessional Evidence-Based Practice:
A Workbook for Health Professionals (pp 109-122).
© 2016 Taylor and Francis Group.

is the best question to facilitate the project. Practice- and knowledge-focused triggers, along with other strategies, assist with identifying the problem. Answering background questions about the problem helps the interprofessional team to clarify the nature of the practice concern. The process of asking background questions ultimately facilitates the development of the foreground question. This chapter provides definitions of and examples for each type of EBP question, along with a process that interprofessional teams use to work through the formulation of background and foreground EBP questions. This chapter also provides important discussions about mentor challenges that may occur when developing the problem, addressing background questions, and developing the foreground question. Additionally, this chapter highlights considerations for mentoring during this stage of interprofessional EBP. An important team skill to develop during this interprofessional EBP stage is the ability to adjust and revise questions as the interprofessional team discovers themes and clarifies practice issues.

UNDERSTANDING THE IDENTIFIED PRACTICE PROBLEM

Once an interprofessional team forms to address a practice problem that the clinical scholar identified as part of the acceptance process for the interprofessional EBP program (see Chapter 6), the team must obtain evidence from the literature and from other sources that supports changing practice. The interprofessional EBP team generally accumulates published and unpublished evidence from multiple disciplines for the project through searching the available literature and sources of evidence that addresses the identified problem. The interprofessional team should understand that the best and most useful way to identify problems is to examine the needs of patients and factors associated with the care within a health care organization.

Titler et al. (2001), in the Iowa model, identified problem-focused and knowledge-focused triggers as a way to categorize sources for problems that can stimulate the development of EBP questions. Problem-focused triggers stem from patient needs that are unmet or partially met, ineffective health care interventions, and inefficient or unsafe processes or systems. Sources for problem-focused triggers include quality improvement, patient satisfaction, financial, and risk management data, as well as from the practice experience of clinicians and practitioners. Knowledge-focused triggers come from new sources of evidence internal and external to the organization, such as newly published research, changes in national standards, innovative care models, and organizational initiatives in the workplace.

Strategies for regularly identifying problem-focused triggers help clinicians and practitioners develop a spirit of inquiry as part of their regular practice. Specifically, developing a questioning approach is critical for changing practice. Granger (2008) advocated using a strategy and algorithm to investigate clinical questions referred to as *STICK* (Strategies for Investigating Clinical Questions), which serves to promote the clinical reflection necessary for interprofessional EBP practice. Following the idea of "sticky notes," clinicians and practitioners are encouraged to generate and record questions as they come to mind in practice. Categorizing these sticky note questions highlights and identifies recurring themes that lead to identifying practice problems appropriate for interprofessional EBP, especially when professionals from a variety of disciplines share and discuss their sticky notes. Discovering similar practice problems that cross several disciplines necessitates an interprofessional EBP approach to problem solution.

The advantage of the STICK method is that clinicians and practitioners can generate ideas for interprofessional EBP as they work together. Granger (2008) identifies a three-step process in using the method, which includes the following:

1. Placing pads of sticky notes in areas easily accessible to where the interprofessional team works. Use the pads to write down any questions or ideas that come to mind about patient concerns, work processes and procedures, or other questions about patient care.

2. Centralizing storage of the sticky notes helps the interprofessional team to regularly review and respond to problems with further thoughts or refinements.

3. Analyzing the notes for questions that the interprofessional team could answer through an interprofessional EBP process versus questions that might need continuing education/staff development, policy changes, or administrative action (Table 7-1).

Due to the team's focus on patient-centered care, team members from a variety of disciplines are more than likely struggling with similar practice problems. Hearing from multiple disciplines on a team is an advantage over teams consisting of members from the same discipline. Interprofessional teams that welcome a diverse perspective tend to challenge routines that stem from traditions and rituals that inadvertently interfere with practice change. A common problem-focused trigger occurs when the only reason for doing something is that "we have always done it that way."

A dialogue about practice problems also uncovers assumptions and views the interprofessional team may have about another discipline's practice, or the ways specific disciplines work with a group of patients. For example, team members may use similar terminology, but without realizing it, might have different meanings for those seemingly

TABLE 7-1	
WAYS OF ADDRESSING PRACTICE QUESTIONS WITHIN AN ORGANIZATION	
TYPE OF QUESTIONS	**ORGANIZATIONAL RESPONSE**
Questions that call for informing people or providing knowledge	Developing in-services or educational programing (staff development questions)
	Methods of educating may be evidence-based, particularly drawing from implementation science literature, in order to ensure learning results in changes in staff behavior.
Questions that require a change in methods for staff completing day-to-day operations	Creating a policy or procedure (procedural questions)
	Policy questions may be evidence-based, particularly as related to standardizing procedures for interventions, ensuring patient safety, and enhancing process efficiency to reduce costs.
Questions that require administrators of an organization to reach a decision	Making an administrative decision related to mission and vision. (administrative questions)
	Administrative decisions may be evidence-based in that they depend upon financial/productivity data, patient satisfaction, and quality of care indicators
Problems addressing areas of clinical care, areas important to the practice of health care staff, questions that benefit patients, clinical practice, or the organization	EBP questions

familiar terms. The word *function* or *functional* could refer to the operation and health of a particular organ, such as the kidneys, or it could mean a broader set of behaviors related to performing effectively an observable task or activity. The first use of the term might come more readily to those concerned primarily with the physical function of the body; the second is often more familiar to those disciplines concerned with rehabilitation. Teams that do not realize that variations in terminology exist may have trouble communicating and understanding the practice problem.

Talking about concepts, beliefs, and assumptions makes a critical difference in clarifying the interprofessional EBP problem. The interprofessional team uses clarifying questions to understand the practice problem, which includes asking the following:

- What is the basis (e.g., tradition, ritual, research) for this practice?
- Is there a more efficient process?
- Is there a more effective treatment or intervention?
- Is this the best experience possible for patients?
- Is this the most cost-effective way to deliver care?
- What are the ways to reduce any potential harm to the patient?

Another strategy for clarifying the problem is asking "why" five times in a row to get to the root cause of

a practice problem (Lipowski, 2008). For example, a team might ask, "Why does a certain type of patient have longer hospital stays?" If the answer is that the patients are having secondary infections that are prolonging the stay, then the question can become, "Why are patients getting secondary infections?" Answers to this question may include an issue with a specific clinical procedure used in the organization or the level of practitioner or clinician knowledge about preventing infections. Other "why" questions might include: "Why are certain procedures used?" and "Why is staff lacking the knowledge needed for preventing infections?" Answers to the "why" questions can lead the team to fully understand the problem.

Knowledge-focused triggers help to reduce the research-to-practice gap and stimulate innovation. Each member on the interprofessional EBP team needs to stay current within their discipline, as well as needs to understand interprofessional perspectives through reading the professional literature within and outside of one's discipline, and through attending continuing education offerings with other disciplines. When interprofessional team members accept this responsibility, they provide the needed expertise for recognizing knowledge-focused triggers that lead to identifying interprofessional EBP problems. Clinicians and practitioners identify knowledge-focused problems when thinking about innovative ways of providing care. The interprofessional team members ask, "What would happen if we made this change?" For example, the interprofessional team could explore implementing a new way to provide team-based care, using a novel therapeutic approach, and taking an intervention effective with one group of patients and applying the intervention to a new group of patients who may benefit from the intervention. Even though practice- and knowledge-focused triggers come from different sources, both are important for identifying and clarifying interprofessional EBP problems.

Determining the Significance of the Problem for the Organization

The problem, under study, often develops from practice observations, discussions, data, and experiences that an individual or interprofessional team identifies as important; however, the team may have limited knowledge about the perspectives of those outside of the team. Other stakeholders in the organization need to agree that the proposed problem is significant to ensure that the team can obtain the resources they need to study the problem. Bringing others into the team throughout the organization may help determine the interest and importance of the work across the organization. Examining organizational documents, such as mission and vision statements, policy statements, or institutional initiatives, helps the team gauge the interest and potential support from the organization of the team's proposed interprofessional EBP problem. Talking with other practitioners and professionals in the organization also helps with developing consensus and aids the interprofessional team in determining the frequency, pervasiveness, and significance of the problem. The team can also use client or patient satisfaction or stakeholder surveys to determine if other groups are experiencing the problem or would benefit from work on the interprofessional EBP problem.

As discussed in Chapters 2 and 12, achieving "buy-in" from leaders within the health care organization is an important part of successfully addressing an interprofessional EBP problem. Identifying a problem that affects many patients, their professional care providers, and the operations of multiple units or departments of a health care organization is a strong argument for organizational support to launch a project that may improve the situation. The following are some additional questions to ask in the process of determining the significance of the problem:

- What is the most important issue (e.g., change in national standards, poor patient outcomes, or safety)?
- Why is this problem important (e.g., patient satisfaction and improved outcomes)?
- Who is interested in this problem (e.g., the team, the organization, or stakeholders)?
- What do we need to know about this problem before moving forward?

- How can addressing this problem affect the organization and its work?
- What is the feasibility of studying this problem (e.g., resources, time, and practicality)?

Contributions of the Team in Solving the Evidence-Based Practice Problem

The interprofessional EBP competencies include advocating for an interprofessional approach to address patient problems, even when it seems more specific to one discipline. or actively seeking perspectives from other disciplines, even when using primarily a single disciplinary approach for problem solving. A team member may not initially see the connection his or her discipline has with the interprofessional EBP question. However, with some initial review of the literature and reflection regarding the discipline's perspectives related to the question, a team member can develop substantial ways to contribute to the interprofessional EBP process. Some questions each team member should consider about his or her potential contributions include the following:

- What is my profession's scope of practice? How would the profession approach the interprofessional EBP problem?
- What research traditions are common in my discipline? How might these research methods influence the development of the interprofessional EBP question and design of the EBP project?
- Does my profession have any specialized experience working with the population, interventions, or outcome measures considered? How can this expertise contribute to the interprofessional EBP project?
- How does my profession use the terminology considered in the interprofessional EBP project? Does this way of defining the problem have any advantages in development of the interprofessional EBP project?
- What are my personal professional experiences that relate to this project? What contributions can I make from this personal experience?

UNDERSTANDING BACKGROUND AND FOREGROUND QUESTIONS

The heart of any interdisciplinary EBP project is the specific practice problem the team is investigating. Following identification of the problem, the team may decide to generate background questions as part of the process to clarify the problem further. If the problem and the best intervention to

TABLE 7-2

DIFFERENCES AND CHARACTERISTICS OF BACKGROUND AND FOREGROUND QUESTIONS

	BACKGROUND QUESTIONS	FOREGROUND QUESTIONS
CHARACTERISTICS	• Are broad, related to general knowledge (who, what, where, when, how, why?) • When answered, provide a general summary or overview of a topic • When answered, provide the foundation for a complete understanding of the topic • Are written in a general way, such as found in normal conversation or writing	• Are focused, related to specific conditions or situations • Provide answers or research findings related to the specific question • Add detail to basic information; team must have basic foundation for the foreground question to have meaning • Are written in a specific way using a question building technique, such as the PICO technique
TYPES OF SOURCES USED	• General textbooks • Encyclopedias • Medical dictionaries • Narrative reviews, evidence summaries	• Primary sources, such as original research articles in peer reviewed journals • Secondary sources such as systematic reviews
EXAMPLE	• What is type 2 diabetes? • What treatment options are available for type 2 diabetes?	• In adult patients with type 2 diabetes and obesity, is bariatric surgery more effective than standard medical therapy at increasing the probability of remission of diabetes?

address the problem seem evident, the interprofessional team may choose to conduct a focused literature search on specific lines of inquiry. Several researchers (Dearholt & Dang, 2012; Sackett, Rosenburg, Muir Gray, Haynes, & Richardson, 1996; Sackett, Strauss, Richardson, Rosenberg, & Haynes, 2000) describe two types of questions for EBP practice: background and foreground questions.

Background questions are general and broad. Answering these questions generates many subtopics and themes for identifying applicable literature to review. Answering background questions helps the team members educate themselves about factors affecting a practice problem. Background questions may also help the interprofessional team to refine or redefine a problem as the team acquires information and understanding about a problem. The format of background questions includes the traditional question roots of "who, what, where, when, how, and why"; a verb; and then an aspect of a disease, disorder, condition, circumstance, and process or procedure. An example of a background question is, "What are the complications of delirium?" The background question facilitates the interprofessional team to create a context for the project that helps put the problem in perspective for the health care organization and external stakeholders.

Background questions lead to more specific, comparison-based foreground questions that an interprofessional EBP team then uses to conduct specific interprofessional EBP projects in a health care setting. However, it is important to focus on the team's underlying concerns about the problem and to avoid jumping to foreground questions or interprofessional EBP project design before the team understands the problem. Moving to these subsequent interprofessional EBP phases too quickly can limit what the team learns about a problem and may stifle the creative thinking necessary to develop the foreground question. The different perspectives of team members from various disciplines add a deeper understanding of the problem under study, which is vital for developing a foreground question that successfully guides the interprofessional EBP project.

Foreground questions are focused interprofessional EBP questions that use a specific format to look at the effect of a specific intervention. Table 7-2 summarizes the differences between background and foreground questions. Several EBP question frameworks have been developed (Cooke, Smith, & Booth, 2012; Davies, 2011), such as SPICE (setting, population, intervention, comparison, and evaluation), ECLIPSE (expectation, client group, Location, impact, professionals, service), and SPIDER (sample, phenomenon of interest, design, evaluation, research type). The SPIDER approach to foreground question development was created with qualitative research questions in mind (Cooke et al., 2012). The Iowa model, which this text is based on, uses the PICO format to develop a specific EBP question. The letters in the format stand for population/problem, intervention, comparison group, and outcome. The PICO format has also been adapted further to add setting (PICOS) or timeframe (PICOT) to the question (Methley, Campbell, Chew-Graham, McNally, & Cheraghi-Sohi, 2014).

The focus and phrasing of a foreground question allows comparisons between groups, processes, services, or intervention methods that, when answered, supports decision making for changing practice. The PICO format does not necessarily fit every type of foreground question. The interprofessional EBP team may want to answer questions focused on harm, prognosis, diagnosis or an assessment, meaning of an experience, and the economics of health care, which may require altering the format of the identified foreground question (DiCenso, Guyatt, & Ciliska, 2005). For example, the interprofessional team may want to ask an experiential question as part of their evidence-based project, such as, "How do older adults experience the process of transitioning from the hospital to home following an episode of pneumonia?" In this example, one of the other question frameworks may be a better choice.

Interprofessional EBP teams may develop PICO questions to examine the effectiveness of a technique, program, product, or other intervention; whether a behavior, illness, or problem is preventable; or the benefit or usefulness of a particular assessment or evaluation procedure. The PICO question format can also be used to describe a professional behavior or practice and to identify whether the intervention might lessen or eliminate risk (Kloda & Bartlett, 2014). However, the team should recognize that not all foreground questions a team develops are appropriate to move on to an interprofessional EBP project. It is possible that there is a better way to address the question in the organization to get the best results. While Table 7-1 illustrates how to address questions in ways other than the creation of an interprofessional EBP project, note that many of these questions still require evidence as a basis for decision making.

Guidelines for Developing Good PICO Foreground Questions

Development of a strong EBP foreground question is a challenging process and one that often takes the team time and multiple iterations to get the best option. The literature indicates that question development is one of the most difficult parts of the EBP process and one where individual health care practitioners feel that they could use more training in doing (Hastings & Fisher, 2014; Horsley, O'Neill, & Campbell, 2009; Miller & Forest, 2001). Knowledge and understanding about the elements of the PICO question can

help make this part of the interprofessional EBP process less stressful for the team.

The *P* component in the PICO framework stands for *population* or *problem*. Patient or clinical populations are often easier to identify than the specific patient problem because clinicians often see issues in terms of specific patient populations. The patient problem may result from multiple factors, which are not always readily apparent without investigation and reflection. The following questions may help a team develop the *P* component of a question: How would you describe the patient to others (e.g., colleagues and lay persons in the community)? What are the important demographic descriptors of your population group (e.g., age, gender, presence of chronic illness, illness severity, or medical history) that might serve as inclusion and exclusion criteria for the EBP project? How is the problem or situation affecting the lives of an individual or groups of patients (Miller & Forrest, 2001; Sackett et al., 2000)?

The intervention (*I*) component involves the practice change directed to a group of patients or clients and their families, staff, organizational systems, or communities. Interventions for patients and families may include specific procedures or processes, services, diagnostic tests, types of therapeutic procedures, therapeutic protocols or educational programs, the use of medical or therapeutic equipment, or medications. An effective PICO question should match a clear and specific intervention to the population or problem the team wishes to study. The interprofessional team asks the question, what are you going to do with or for this population? In this way, the intervention component of the PICO question is clearly stated. The selected intervention, while potentially useful for many populations, is a relevant intervention for the population or problem in the EBP question. Selecting the intervention or bundle of intervention components can be difficult for an interprofessional team given the variety of expertise concerning interventions specific to a discipline. It is important for the interprofessional team to avoid any turf discussions associated with interventions, especially because there is always overlap in expertise and scope among health care professionals (Barr, 1998; Interprofessional Education Collaborative Expert Panel, 2011). The interprofessional team should view any conversations about interventions as more discovery about what other health professions do within their scope of practice. Remaining patient-centered in the selection of the intervention is important and should reflect the initial work on answering background questions. The intervention should primarily be feasible for the clinical scholar to implement.

The comparison (*C*) component of the PICO question is the main alternative to the intervention that the team chooses for determining the effectiveness of the proposed intervention. The comparison intervention is specific and most often limited to one alternative. Having one specific comparison intervention helps to make searching the literature easier (Sackett et al., 2000). The comparison portion of the PICO question is often optional. In some interprofessional EBP projects, a team may only look at the proposed intervention. An alternative to the selected intervention may not exist or it may be unethical or too difficult to test the new intervention against a control or comparison group. The comparison approach in the question may include the routine standard of care given under normal practice conditions.

The team also identifies the specific outcome (O) component, of a well-defined PICO question. Outcomes are measurable and describe what the interprofessional team plans to accomplish with the new intervention. Outcomes in health care are most useful when they measure a positive change in patient function, the elimination or relief of specific symptoms, an indicator of health or elimination of disease, and enhancement of the experience or quality of life of a patient. The best outcomes indicate *how* a situation or individual lives change due to the intervention and do not measure only outcome improvement (Sackett et al., 2000).

To help create an effective PICO question, the interprofessional team may use a question development tool. There are many such tools available in the literature and through Internet sources. Some tools start with the components of the PICO question but go further to help generate the type of question the project involves, types of literature for which to search, related terms to use in searches, and possible databases to use (see the companion website for this book for a PICO template).

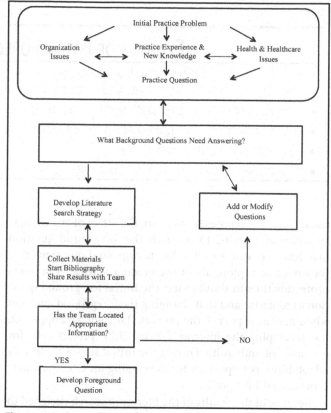

Figure 7-1. Literature search to refine practice questions.

USING EVIDENCE TO ANSWER BACKGROUND AND FOREGROUND QUESTIONS

Information that is more general answers background questions, so textbooks, narrative reviews, and evidence summaries are appropriate literature sources (see Table 7-2). Local data from the organization that were designed to address institution-specific background questions are also helpful to the interprofessional team. Narrative literature reviews are different from systematic reviews and may include evidence-based information, but the interprofessional team should distinguish them from research evidence. Narrative literature reviews generally do not include a description of a systematic search process or explicit criteria for selecting the information included in the review. Narrative literature reviews often include expert opinion as well. However, these narrative reviews do provide a place to start understanding the EBP problem. Evidence summaries that include expert appraisal and synthesis also assist with answering background questions (see Chapter 8). The goal in examining this literature is to identify the elements

needed to construct the foreground question using the PICO format. Information obtained to answer the background question helps determine the patient population most likely to have the problem, as well as helps determine the most common interventions and outcomes. Foreground questions are more complex and require using library databases and other search engines as described in Chapter 8 in order to provide reliable and valid answers.

The literature search process in Figure 7-1 shows the iterative nature of evidence gathering and question development during the initial phases of interprofessional EBP. It is important for teams in this process of question development and obtaining evidence to remain open to new information with the understanding that the background questions for the selected problem might lead the team to revise the problem. The interprofessional team should not treat the initial identification of the problem as immutable, but instead the team should clarify the problem, select a variation of the problem, and add background questions that will help develop understanding as the team progresses. The interprofessional team should also understand that once they clarify the problem and develop a foreground question, the question might need to change as the team starts to search for literature. The team may find information through the literature search that another intervention is superior to the one originally proposed, that the highest risk population is a group other than the one first identified, or that studies

TABLE 7-3
EXAMPLE OF INITIAL FOREGROUND/PICO QUESTION
• Initial PICO: What is the effect of the implementation of a chronic pain management guideline to improve pain management of patients with chronic pain who have opioid tolerance?
• Population: Hospitalized patients with acute and chronic pain with opioid tolerance
• Intervention: Chronic pain management guideline and staff education
• Comparison: Undecided
• Outcome: Improvement in the patient's comfort, reduction of pain, and prevention of opioid tolerance

use different outcomes to measure the effect of the change. In addition, starting to research the foreground question may lead the team to ask other background questions that they need to explore about the practice setting. The interprofessional team should view the initial foreground question as tentative and that changing the foreground question when needed is part of the process. This iterative approach for developing the interprofessional EBP project calls for tolerance of ambiguity. During the initial steps of EBP, this adaptability is important for developing an effective interprofessional EBP project.

Because of the results of the literature search designed to answer the foreground question, there may either be support for changing practice or evidence to support what the health care organization is already doing, thereby making a change unnecessary. Per the Iowa model (Titler et al., 2001), when strong and rich evidence supports a change, the team may propose revising practice to implement recommendations from the literature. In cases of identifying a gap in the literature where the results are ambiguous, the team may need to conduct a research study or a quality improvement project to further investigate a promising intervention.

A Case Example of Using Background/Foreground Questions

One team example of using background and foreground questions at the start of an interprofessional EBP project involved a practice problem the clinical scholar (a staff nurse) in an interprofessional EBP practice program identified. The staff nurse worked in a cardiovascular step-down unit in an acute care hospital where she became concerned about some patients who had high opioid tolerance because of using opioids for managing chronic pain, or who had substance use disorders with alcohol and other illicit substances who also had chronic pain. The nurse believed that adequate evaluation and pain management might not occur because of the patient's high tolerance for opioids. She was thinking that there might be clinicians and practitioners who label these patients as "drug-seeking" rather than as patients with discomfort who are asking for medication because of legitimate acute and chronic pain.

The interdisciplinary team formulated the following background questions:

- What is chronic pain?
- How do the experts define chronic pain?
- What are the causes of chronic pain?
- What are techniques to manage chronic pain in addition to or instead of pharmacology?
- How does chronic pain affect one's lifestyle and quality of life?
- How do practitioners address chronic pain in acute care facilities and for which patient populations?
- How do the experts define opioid tolerance and how does it affect chronic pain?
- How do the experts manage chronic pain in patients with substance abuse disorders?
- What is the incidence of admitting patients with chronic pain and opioid abuse or drug and alcohol use disorders?

In the initial rounds of obtaining evidence to answer these background questions, the interprofessional team found several EBP guidelines (an example of an evidence summary) for persons with chronic pain and substance use disorders. The team then broadened its review to examine all published practice guidelines on the various aspects of the problem and determined how these guidelines might provide more options for pain control when working with patients with chronic pain. Then the team identified an initial foreground question using the PICO format from the information obtained through answering the background questions (Table 7-3).

Following an analysis of the health care organization's patient population, the team determined that there were insufficient numbers of patients with a diagnosis of opioid addiction admitted on a regular basis. Thus, the interprofessional team determined it was not feasible to conduct an interprofessional EBP project on this issue, given the more than likely small sample size compared to the sample size needed to test the effectiveness of an intervention for this population of patients.

TABLE 7-4
EXAMPLE OF A REVISED FOREGROUND/PICO QUESTION
• Revised PICO: What does the implementation of a chronic pain management guideline and staff education do to the knowledge, attitudes, and beliefs of nurses about managing the pain of patients with chronic pain who are hospitalized in an acute care setting? • Population: Nurses working in acute care with patients diagnosed with a disease with chronic pain symptoms • Intervention: Chronic pain management guideline implementation and staff education • Comparison: Attitudes, beliefs, and knowledge of nurses about chronic pain prior to staff education and guideline implementation and then after staff education and guideline implementation • Outcome: Change in nurse's attitude, beliefs, and knowledge of chronic pain

Consequently, the interprofessional team broadened the interprofessional EBP question based on the literature to include other patients with chronic pain rather than limiting the population to those with chronic pain and opioid tolerance. Also, the team identified practice and patient evidence in the institution that nurses primarily focused on acute pain and inconsistently identified whether patients also had chronic pain. In addition, nurses frequently did not document in the electronic health record the specific type of pain. Table 7-4 includes the interprofessional teams' revised foreground PICO question. This question reflects the evidence found about the use of clinical guidelines as a tool to manage knowledge and treatment approaches for chronic pain. Use of clinical guidelines often helps the team incorporate the interprofessional perspectives and concerns related to the question. The revised PICO question identified a way to compare the use of the guideline with a population that was more easily identifiable and accessible to the health care facility in which the team participated and worked. Interprofessional EBP teams use the PICO or other formats for developing foreground questions pertaining to populations and services provided in various health care settings (Table 7-5).

Building a Bibliography of Evidence

No matter the nature of the background and foreground questions, it is important for the team to keep track of the information from the literature and the decisions made for developing the foreground question (see Chapter 8). This search history or trail can help the team select a different question or modify the original foreground question. It is also important for the team to have regular meetings to review the evidence. This regular review helps the team avoid duplication of work effort and check whether the retrieved sources are the most appropriate for the interprofessional EBP problem and question development. Team meetings also help the team more quickly recognize the need to take their interprofessional EBP project in a new direction, especially if the team's interests shift because of the background information found in the literature.

Building a bibliography of the evidence is easier with the evolution of search engines and online databases. It is important to learn how a particular database enables the team to create a search history. Moving back and forth between each initiated search within the same database helps identify key sources as well as refines search terms to make subsequent search processes more effective and focused. Most databases also have mechanisms to print search histories with article abstracts, as well as have the ability to export search results to bibliographic tools, such as RefWorks. These electronic tools remove much of the detailed work of copying or retyping sources in new documents or formats. Table 7-6 lists some of the most common databases that health care professionals use when searching for literature related to interprofessional EBP projects. Databases in the table include publicly available databases and those that are available through a subscription service or institutional source. Access to databases may be limited because of budget constraints, composition of the members in a team, or other issues. Chapter 8 provides some suggestions regarding how to resolve these literature access issues.

A key strategy the interprofessional team uses to identify sources to answer the foreground question is to analyze the information from previous searching when answering the background questions. The goal is to look for trends in the content of articles, to identify important and prolific researchers in the field, and to note key or seminal articles that authors consistently cite. Chapter 8 includes several tools that a team uses for recording and organizing sources found when searching the literature to answer background and foreground questions.

MENTOR CHALLENGES

The interprofessional team must address three key issues in order for effective teamwork and team progress to occur when addressing background questions. First, a team atmosphere supportive of dialogue and communication is necessary. Teams that do not engage in open discourse

TABLE 7-5

EXAMPLES OF CLINICAL PROBLEMS AND PICO QUESTIONS

SETTING/CONCERN	POPULATION (P)	INTERVENTION (I)	COMPARISON (C)	OUTCOME (O)	FINAL QUESTION
Case 1: Independent living elders with concerns about proper nutritional intake/awareness and meal planning (effectiveness question)	Elderly living in an independent living apartment cooking for themselves	Interdisciplinary home program on meal planning and preparation	Stand-alone educational materials about proper nutritional balance and intake	Decreased nutritionally related health problems	For independent living elderly persons, will completion of an interdisciplinary home program for meal planning result in decreased nutritionally related health problems than exposure to educational materials on nutrition and health alone?
Case 2: Concern for teenage pregnancy in teens at risk. Teen population attending programs at a teen resource center in an urban setting (prevention question)	Teenage males and females attending teen resource center programs	Birth control education and information	Educational program on sexual abstinence	Lower pregnancy rates	Will birth control education and information create a lower pregnancy rate for teens at risk compared to an educational program on sexual abstinence?
Case 3: Concern for the health and reengagement of veterans returning to mainstream civilian life (risk question)	Community living veterans with PTSD involved in a community day treatment program	Group cognitive behavioral therapy	Those not getting the group cognitive behavioral theory	Reduced hospital readmissions	How can group therapy provided in community day treatment programs reduce the risk of hospital readmissions in veterans with PTSD?

TABLE 7-6

COMMON SEARCH ENGINES/RESOURCES HEALTH CARE PROFESSIONALS USE FOR EVIDENCE-BASED PRACTICE PROJECTS

SEARCH ENGINES AVAILABLE IN THE PUBLIC DOMAIN

Search Engines	Topic Areas/Disciplines Covered
Cochrane Free Abstracts and Summaries www.cochrane.org/evidence	Free clinical abstracts and summaries through the Cochrane organization about health care issues and treatments
Epocrates https://www.epocrates.com/	Clinical tables information on drugs and diseases, including drug interaction. Also includes patient resources
Evidence Updates from BMJ http://plus.mcmaster.ca/EvidenceUpdates/	From McMaster University, free registration required. Rates articles from over 110 clinical journals
Goggle Scholar	Multidisciplinary
E-Medicine: MedScapes http://emedicine.medscape.com/	Answers to clinical questions by specialty. Free registration.
National Guideline Clearinghouse (NCG) www.guideline.gov	Collection of practice guidelines
Turning Research into Practice (TRIP Database For Evidence-Based Medicine (EBM) www.tripdatabase.com/index.html	Clinical search tool for health practitioners for finding evidence for clinical practice
WebMD www.webmd.com	Medicine, health care, patient information queries

SEARCH ENGINES TYPICALLY AVAILABLE THROUGH CLINICAL OR UNIVERSITY LIBRARIES

Search Engines	Topic Areas/Disciplines Covered
Cochrane Library	Medicine, health care; known for an extensive collection of systematic reviews on Medical subjects
CINAHL: Cumulative Index to Nursing and Allied Health	Nursing, allied health
ERIC: Education Resources Information Center	Education and teaching
MedicinePlus	Medicine
PsycINFO	Psychology, behavioral science, and mental health
PubMed	Biomedical
ScienceDirect	Multidisciplinary
WorldCat	Multidisciplinary, unified catalog of member libraries

often place an emphasis on getting a single answer or going down a particular path too quickly. Consequently, the team risks developing background questions that lack depth, fails to uncover important information to consider, and creates foreground questions that may not address the practice problem effectively.

Secondly, flexibility and acceptance of uncertainty and ambiguity are important for avoiding high levels of anxiety and frustration as the team works toward its final foreground question that guides the design of the interprofessional EBP project. Flexibility fosters a willingness to explore a problem and all its facets before making the actual decision of how to focus the foreground question for the team's EBP project. An attitude of exploration can help the team take the results from addressing background questions to investigate other interesting options. Team members checking with the entire team when they discover options for addressing the EBP problem helps the team maintain an exploratory attitude.

Finally, an understanding that one is unlikely to find the perfect evidence helps prevent constant searching. The team needs to understand that the literature search process is sometimes circular and confusing but evolves given patience and time. As already described earlier in this chapter, addressing the background and foreground questions is iterative and involves a process in which each effort to answer the questions builds on previous efforts. Establishing tolerance and a norm that "nothing is perfect" is also important for the ongoing success and progress of the EBP project. The goals are to define the best foreground question possible and to guide the respective literature search in a way that addresses the specific patient care problem of the health care organization.

Frequent team communication also ensures that individuals develop valid questions and avoid tangential searching of the literature that may not produce a useful outcome. Even with good team communication, organizational factors often create challenges that prevent conducting an interprofessional EBP project in the "ideal" way. The team needs to consult with other members of the organization to learn more about an issue or clarify how the organization operates to better determine what is possible for the interprofessional EBP project.

MENTOR TECHNIQUES AND SUPPORTS

The mentor of a team engaged in developing background and foreground questions must create and support an effective learning team. A valuable concept for effective mentoring is the idea of the mentor as a knowledge broker (Urquhart, Porter, & Grunfeld, 2011). A knowledge broker helps to manage communication among team members and provides opportunities for team members to exchange ideas and become aware of other team member's areas of expertise that may inform the development of background and foreground questions. This knowledge broker role includes the mentor creating structures and methods for sharing the evidence addressing the background questions to avoid duplication of effort, and for creating opportunities to extend work already completed into new areas that need investigating. Effective mentoring at this interprofessional EBP stage also includes encouraging team members to remain persistent and to rethink the problem when searching the literature produces unexpected results.

The mentor does not let the team come too quickly to a foreground question, as being impatient can limit thinking and prevent developing a truly beneficial EBP project for the team and organization. An ongoing interchange between team members that promotes reflection keeps the process moving forward. Approaches that are useful for the mentor to ensure teamwork for developing background and foreground questions include the mentor doing the following:

- Ensuring formal and informal communication through written, electronic, and face-to-face formats that facilitate problem clarification
- Providing meeting time to ensure brainstorming opportunities that facilitate problem identification and development of initial questions
- Actively encouraging members to share their expertise and perspectives that will enhance the evidence-gathering process
- Communicating with the health care organizational leaders and project coordinators as needed to help guide the team in identifying relevant problems and questions
- Balancing the need to keep the team progressing and meeting timelines with the need to conduct a thorough search for information that addresses the background questions
- Providing "just in time" learning to keep the search for evidence progressing
- Providing a structure to regularly summarize the work in order to ask the question, "Is this the direction we want to be going in?" and "How should we change our focus if we need to?"

Being in a Muddy Place

When starting the interprofessional EBP process, the clinical scholar and the interprofessional team members are often excited about the project, wanting to get started. Problem identification and question formulation, while critical to the success of the project, can feel like being stuck in the mud. The mentor may find it challenging to convince the team they are making progress. A mentor technique may include describing the process of asking the right questions as an art that allows creativity. Important mentor techniques to keep the team motivated while exploring background questions as a precursor to developing foreground questions include the following:

- Encouraging the team to regularly share information to answer the background questions
- Supporting members of the team to answer the background questions in which they are most interested
- Creating realistic goals and timelines for answering the background questions
- Keeping the team focused on using the background questions to develop the foreground question

TABLE 7-7	
MENTOR TECHNIQUES AND STRATEGIES	
STRATEGY	**METHODS AND TECHNIQUES**
Finding project resources	• Brainstorming initial ideas and alternative sources as literature search process continues • Creating a common method and location to report resources and results • Team members incorporating their individual resources (human and non-human) that may benefit the project • Educating team members on literature search basics and resources as needed
Addressing team frustrations (e.g., concerns about: the pace of the process, difficulty of developing the foreground question, and getting started on the design and implementation of the project itself)	• Team meetings that include check-ins about the pace of the work and other concerns • Identifying progress with each step and recognizing each team member's accomplishments in meeting these steps • Pointing out how far the team has progressed
Building trust in the process	• Initiating and setting expectations for a regular schedule of meetings and/or reporting opportunities • Encouraging and providing opportunities for every team member to become engaged in the work and report progress at team meetings • Creating agendas and meeting minutes for team meetings
Summarizing progress and identifying next steps	• Using resource managing tools, such as RefWorks • Using search histories and documentation of search forms (see resources in Chapter 8) • Setting deadlines when decisions have to be made

While the mentor should use strategies to make addressing the background and foreground questions as effective as possible, the team may need to realize, based on the state of the science, that the current information may be the best they can find. Encouraging the attitude of "we don't know what we don't know" also creates a learning climate in which the evidence-gathering process represents discovery and exploration (Table 7-7). Senge (2006) described the concept of a learning organization, which is useful for the mentor to incorporate within this stage of interprofessional EBP. Learning organization strategies include the following:

- Nurturing of continuous team learning opportunities
- Promoting inquiry and dialogue through constructively challenging others in the question development process
- Creating means and opportunities to share information in nonthreatening and safe ways

SUMMARY

When starting an interprofessional EBP project, the interprofessional team must first understand the problem that the project addresses. The chapter included a discussion on problem-focused and knowledge-focused triggers that assist a team in identifying significant practice problems. The interprofessional team refines and clarifies the problem through asking background questions and involving stakeholders in determining a relevant focus. The team is able to use strategies such as asking "Why?" five times to get at the root cause of a problem. This early stage of the interprofessional EBP project requires the team to work together to clarify the problem and work together toward developing a foreground question. The mentor encourages the use of mentor strategies that emphasize openness and willingness to revisit and refine the foreground question for the EBP project. Creating team unity and trust at this stage of the interprofessional EBP process pays dividends during the subsequent focused searches of the literature, appraisal of the evidence, and completing the EBP project.

REFLECTION QUESTIONS

1. The chapter provided several questions and considerations an individual EBP team member uses to assess his or her contributions to an EBP project. Review these questions and determine how you can help the team in the process of developing an interprofessional EBP question and searching the literature.

2. Whether you are a mentor or team member on an interprofessional EBP team, what can you do to encourage creativity and flexibility when developing EBP background/foreground questions?

REFERENCES

Barr, H. (1998). Competent to collaborate: Towards a competency-based model for interprofessional education. *Journal of Interprofessional Care, 12*(2), 181-187. doi:10.3109/13561829809014104

Cooke, A., Smith, D., & Booth, A. (2012). Beyond PICO: The SPIDER tool for Qualitative Evidence Synthesis. *Qualitative Health Research, 22*(10), 1435-1433. doi:10.1177/1049732312452938

Davies, K. S. (2011). Formulating the evidence based practice question: A review of the frameworks. *Evidenced Based Library and Information Practice, 6*(2), 75-80.

Dearholt, S. L., & Dang. D. (2012). *Johns Hopkins nursing evidence-based practice: Models and Guidelines* (2nd ed.). Indianapolis, IN: Sigma Theta Tau International.

DiCenso, A., Guyatt, G., & Ciliska, D. (2005). *Evidence-Based Nursing: A guide to clinical practice.* St. Louis, MO: Elsevier Mosby.

Granger, B. B. (2008). Practical steps for evidence based practice: Putting one foot in front of the other. *American Association of Critical Care Nurses Advanced Critical Care, 19*(3), 314-324. doi:10.1097/01.aacn.0000330383.87507.d1

Hastings, C., & Fisher, C. A. (2014). Searching for proof: Creating and using an actionable PICO question. *Nursing Management,* August, 9-12. doi:10.1097/01.numa.0000452006.79838.67

Horsley, T., O'Neill, J., & Campbell, C. (2009). The quality of questions and use of resources in self-directed learning: Personal learning projects in the maintenance of certification. *Journal of Continuing Education in the Health Professions, 29*(2), 91-97. doi:10.1002/chp.20017

Interprofessional Education Collaborative Expert Panel. (2011). Core competencies for interprofessional collaborative practice: Report of an expert panel. Washington, DC: Interprofessional Education Collaborative.

Kloda, L. A., & Bartlett, J. C. (2014). A characterization of clinical questions asked by rehabilitation therapists. *Journal of the Medical Library Association,* April, 65-77. doi: 10.3168/1536-5050.102.2.002

Lipowski, E. E. (2008). Developing great research questions. *American Journal of Health System Pharmacy, 65*(Sept 1), 1667-1670. doi:10.2146/ajhp070276

Methley, A. M., Campbell, S., Chew-Graham, C., McNally, R., & Cheraghi-Sohi, S. (2014). PICO, PICOS, and SPIDER: A comparison study of specificity and sensitivity in three search tools for qualitative systematic reviews. *Bio-Med Central Health Services Research, 14,* 579. doi:10.1186/s12913-014-0579-0.

Miller, S. A., & Forrest, J. L. (2001). Enhancing your practice decision making: PICO, good questions. *Journal of Evidence-Based Dental Practice, 1,* 134-141. doi:10.1067/med2001.118720.

Sackett, D. L., Rosenberg, W. M. C., Muir Gray, J. A., Hayes, R. B., and Richardson, W. S. (1996).Evidence based medicine: What it is and what it isn't. *British Medical Journal, 312,* 71-72. doi:10.1136/bmj.312.7023.71

Sackett, D. L., Strauss, S. E., Richardson, W. S., Rosenberg, W., & Haynes, R. B. (2000). *Evidence based medicine: How to practice and teach EBM* (2nd ed.). Edinburgh, UK: Churchill Livingstone.

Senge, P. M. (2006). *The fifth discipline: The art and practice of a learning organization* (2nd ed.). New York, NY: Doubleday Currency.

Titler, M. G., Kleiber, C., Steelman, V. J., Rakel, B. A., Budreau, G., Eberett, L. Q., ... Goode, C. J. (2001). The Iowa model of evidence-based practice to promote quality care. *Critical Care Nursing Clinics of North America, 13*(4), 497-509.

Urquhart, R., Porter, G. A., & Grunfeld, E. (2011). Reflections on knowledge brokering within a multidisciplinary research team. *Journal of Continuing Education in the Health Professions,* (4), 283-290. doi:/\10.1002/chp.20128

Supplemental materials for this chapter are available online.
Please refer to the sticker in the front of the book and enter the access code provided.

Settling Into the Rhythm of the Interprofessional Evidence-Based Practice Process

John D. Fleming, EdD, OTR/L

CHAPTER TOPICS

- Using a foreground question as the basis of a literature search
- Developing a literature search strategy for addressing a foreground question
- Mentor challenges
- Mentor techniques and mentor supports

PERFORMANCE OBJECTIVES

At the conclusion of this chapter, the interprofessional team members will understand the process of searching the literature and documenting the search and will be able to do the following:

1. Describe a focused, systematic literature search process that addresses a foreground question developed from answering background questions.

2. Use strategies to document the foreground literature search.

3. Identify mentoring challenges in completing a foreground literature search.

4. Use successful mentor techniques and supports to address mentoring challenges arising in the search process.

Gathering appropriate, useful, and credible evidence is critical for addressing the evidence-based practice (EBP) problem. The team initially identifies an interprofessional EBP problem and broad background questions that require investigation. Next, the team reviews evidence (both from the literature and from the practice setting) that helps with understanding the dimensions of the interprofessional EBP problem. The team then develops a foreground question that guides the actual interprofessional EBP project and determines the focus for the literature search. While the mechanics of doing a literature search are the same for answering background and foreground questions, certain search strategies guide the nuances of the search process for foreground questions. This chapter presents the mentor challenges that may occur while the team engages in the search process and describes the mentor techniques and supports for ensuring success with this interprofessional EBP phase.

Moyers, P. A., & Finch-Guthrie, P. L.
Interprofessional Evidence-Based Practice:
A Workbook for Health Professionals (pp 123-136).
© 2016 Taylor and Francis Group.

In the Iowa model (Titler et al., 2001), the literature search process is part of identifying knowledge-focused triggers discussed in Chapter 7 that continues with the step described as assembling relevant research literature (see Chapter 1, Figure 1-2). Collecting literature and appraising the strength and quality of the evidence is necessary for determining whether a practice change has enough evidence for pilot-testing the change. In some cases, implementing a new practice requires the interprofessional EBP team to first conduct a research study to create the needed evidence or the team decides that other non-research evidence can serve as the basis for the recommended change (e.g., case report, expert opinion, scientific principles, and theory). Searching the literature is an essential part of the EBP process.

USING A FOREGROUND QUESTION AS THE BASIS OF A LITERATURE SEARCH

Evidence for answering background questions assists with describing one or more aspects of a problem and possible relationships between factors of the problem. Chapter 7 provided a case example from an interprofessional EBP program of a team developing a foreground question that demonstrated the iterative nature of the process. The interprofessional team in the example used a PICO template to formulate a foreground question from background information (see book website for the template). The team next plans an effective search to answer the foreground question that includes the following:

- Identifying the PICO components (i.e., patient population/problem, intervention, comparison groups, and outcome)

- Identifying search terms stemming from the components in the PICO question

- Developing search strategies for identifying the best databases and sources of evidence, types of evidence that will answer the foreground question, and limits for narrowing the search

- Determining resources, skills, and team education needs to carry out the search

DEVELOPING A LITERATURE SEARCH STRATEGY FOR ADDRESSING A FOREGROUND QUESTION

The goal of searching the literature is to capture relevant evidence through a reproducible search that addresses the foreground question. To ensure an efficient literature search, the interprofessional team develops a written plan to facilitate agreement and overall understanding among team members regarding the steps needed to answer the foreground question. The literature search plan includes addressing access to library resources, as well as determining the education needs of the team for searching the literature. In addition, the plan includes a search strategy that involves identifying key concepts or words in the foreground question; alternate forms of the concepts or word synonyms; databases, search engines, and Internet sources for finding evidence; and limiters or filters for narrowing the search. The interprofessional team learns to use a variety of sources to find relevant evidence in order to address issues of publication bias due to the journals primarily publishing studies with positive results. As part of the plan, the interprofessional team documents the search process and deliberates when to stop the search.

Library Issues and Access in Searching the Literature

Chapter 7 identified a variety of publicly available and institutional sources for conducting a literature search (clinical and university libraries and websites). With Internet availability of free evidence sources and the high cost of library databases, financial support for libraries has decreased, making access to some journals more difficult (Anderson, 2008; Hodge, Manhoff, & Watson, 2013). Many health care organizations with libraries have significantly downsized collections in an attempt to manage costs (Thompson, Toedter, & D'Agostino, 2005). Universities are carefully scrutinizing who has access to their databases and collections (Trail, 2013). Specifically, libraries are making choices regarding subscriptions and, in some cases, charge fees for access to reduce cost to the organization (Balas, 2006; Guarria & Wong, 2011). Thus, part of the interprofessional EBP project budget may need to include funds for conducting the literature search. In addition, the program coordinators need to work with the partnering organizations to address the library needs of the interprofessional EBP program prior to the start of the program. Pooling resources among the interprofessional EBP program sponsors is sometimes possible, thereby enhancing what each organization provides individually.

While the interprofessional team may experience some issues with access to specific journals, a proactive discussion should ensue regarding individual team members' ability to obtain information from various sources. Faculty and students have access to university collections that may include sources other team members may not have within their institution. Team members from various disciplines may have access to journals and websites as part of their membership resources from professional associations that other professions do not have. Clinical members of the team may have access to their facility library or may have

TABLE 8-1

SEARCH TERMS, EVIDENCE, NARROWING THE SEARCH

SEARCH TERMS AND EVIDENCE	CONSIDERATIONS
PICO concepts and keywords	• Patient population • Intervention • Comparison intervention • Patient outcomes
Type of evidence (6S Pyramid of Evidence Resources)	• Are there filtered evidence available (summaries, synopses, syntheses)? • What kind of nonfiltered research evidence will the team include (e.g., type of research methodology, such as quantitative vs. qualitative)? • What kind of expert opinion (e.g., narrative reviews, case reports, clinical articles) evidence is important?

Narrowing the search	• Search may need to go further back in time if there is little information. Some evidence provides historical context for an overall understanding.
	• What limits should narrow the search?
	   ○ Peer-reviewed journals
	   ○ Specific country
	   ○ Language
	   ○ Publication dates
	• Other considerations for narrowing the search (e.g., diagnosis, age, gender, race, length of disease process, type of clinical setting, or other factors)

university access as clinical fieldwork supervisors and preceptors. Creative thinking and sharing among the team regarding library resources before initiating a search is important for developing an effective search strategy as well as for gathering the strongest and most useful evidence.

Developing Skills for Searching the Literature

Health profession educators recommend training for all practicing professionals and health care students in searching the literature because accessing information is an essential competency for practice (Boruff & Thomas, 2011; Wyer et al., 2008). Thus, the interprofessional EBP team as part of planning the literature search ensures team members have familiarity and a comfort level with searching the literature. While many literature databases have common navigation methods, there are differences that are unique to each database. When the team divides the work of searching according to experience and expertise, the search process is more efficient and effective. Pairing inexperienced team members with more experienced members leads to increased comfort in searching.

The sponsoring organizations for the interprofessional EBP program may have librarians to assist team members in using the available printed and electronic resources. In an interprofessional EBP program, the education component about searching for evidence involves hands-on learning with ongoing librarian support during team meeting days. The program coordinators may also want to add library and information management students onto the interprofessional teams and/or academic faculty or student members who have experience in searching. These team members serve as a valuable resource for the team. In addition, there are many tutorials and help guides available online for some of the more common databases. A university partner more than likely has available resources for learning the search process that can support the health care organization if they do not have library services.

Identifying Search Terms

The search strategy starts with identifying essential concepts or key search terms from the elements in the PICO question to identify the population (e.g., patients with orthopedic injuries who also have chronic pain), the intervention (e.g., meditation), comparison (e.g., pain medication), and outcomes (e.g., pain intensity) (Table 8-1). In this example, the search terms resulting from the question include the following:

- Orthopedic injuries
- Chronic pain
- Meditation
- Pain medication
- Pain intensity

The interprofessional team, once they have an initial list of key concepts and words, should expand the list using alternative concepts or synonym words. Examples for alternative terms for pain medication might include pain management, and for pain intensity, an alternative might include pain levels. A good approach is to examine keywords from a target article or search terms described in systematic reviews to obtain ideas for additional terms to use while searching the literature. The team should keep a worksheet for search terms.

When using a database to search, it is important to use predefined or controlled vocabulary for the database. Otherwise the interprofessional team may not find important studies. Generally databases use keywords or search terms to categorize and organize literature in a way that enables individuals conducting a search to find appropriate and relevant evidence. Each database has its own system, which may be similar or very different from other databases. Understanding how each database uses these terms is critical for effective searching. Many databases have a dictionary of terms or a thesaurus in which the searcher can find words the database uses instead of terms the team identified.

Some databases give particular names or labels to their system of keywords. The most well-known of these is the system used in Medical Literature Analysis and Retrieval System Online (MEDLINE), the database of the United States National Library of Medicine, with PubMed providing free access to MEDLINE and links to articles when possible. The organization of the controlled vocabulary or thesaurus in this database includes medical subject headings (MeSH). MEDLINE users may employ keywords in a more general way or may perform a search using MeSH headings. Proper use of MeSH headings in MEDLINE speeds up the search and improves the replication of the search as well. For example, in MEDLINE vocabulary, guided imagery is classified as imagery (psychotherapy). When using this MeSH term, the interprofessional team member would find a greater number of sources compared to when using the general term guided imagery. Therefore, it is important for interprofessional EBP team members to know the search term system of a particular database to produce a replicable search (Facchiano & Snyder, 2012).

Determining Databases and Sources of Evidence

After identifying the search terms, the interprofessional team should determine the databases and sources for the evidence they need to answer the foreground question. The interprofessional team should expect to use more than one database for the search. Matching the question to the database and evidence sources is important because the design of databases and other sources of evidence are different. For example, the Cumulative Index to Nursing and Allied Health Literature (CINAHL) includes literature from nursing and biomedicine, as well as information from alternative and complementary medicine and allied health disciplines (http://health.ebsco.com/products/the-cinahl-database/allied-health-nursing). PubMed, on the other hand, includes literature from the life sciences with a strong focus on biomedical research (http://www.ncbi.nlm.nih.gov/pubmed). Thus, when answering a foreground question regarding effective alternative pain interventions, an interprofessional team would most likely start with CINAHL given the focus on complementary therapy. For abstracts and citations of behavioral and social science research, PsycINFO is an important database (http://www.apa.org/pubs/databases/psycinfo/index.aspx).

When conducting an EBP project, the interprofessional team should also consider starting with filtered sources, using the 6S Pyramid of Evidence Resources (DiCenso, Bayley, & Haynes, 2009; Salmond, 2013; Worster & Haynes, 2012) that provides a hierarchy of evidence for searching the literature. Each part of the 6S Pyramid illustrates a different type of evidence, with filtered sources at the top of the pyramid, followed by unfiltered evidence, and then expert opinion. The authors of filtered sources have appraised the literature, synthesized the information, and identified recommendations for practice. Unfiltered evidence includes primary, original sources and can include randomized controlled trials, cohort studies, case-controlled studies, and case studies. Filtered sources are at the top of the pyramid because busy practitioners have limited time to obtain answers to foreground questions, which involves finding relevant evidence and critically appraising and synthesizing evidence. Starting with filtered sources of evidence provides good information for the strength and quality of the evidence available and assists the team in locating individual studies that they may want to review more closely.

At the top of the 6S Pyramid is the clinical support systems, which include sources of filtered evidence such as those linked to the electronic health record in health care organizations. These evidence systems assist clinicians and practitioners in finding evidence at the point of care specific to problems, treatments, and care for individual patients and clients. The next level of literature in the 6S Pyramid consists of summaries that generally focus on narrow questions or single aspects of care, such as the use of a specific intervention in treating a specific population. Examples of sources of summaries include Dynamed (http://dynamed.ebscohost.com/), Clinical Evidence (http://www.clinicalevidence.com/x/index.html), and Cochrane Summaries (http://summaries.cochrane.org/). A familiar source of summaries is UpToDate (http://www.uptodate.com/home), which many health care institutions connect to their electronic health record. Summaries generally include information from systematic reviews and primary studies that experts critically appraised and synthesized. An important source of summarized information is practice guidelines, which the reader may find on the National Government Clearinghouse website (www.guideline.gov). Well-done summaries note the level and quality of the evidence (see Chapter 9 about leveling and ranking the quality of evidence), which facilitates decision making. Evidence summaries are good sources of evidence to address background and foreground questions.

The next levels of the pyramid include synopses of syntheses and then syntheses. Synopses are generally a one-page article that presents information from systematic reviews and primary studies. This type of evidence usually includes information from high-quality research with the addition of a valuable discussion about the merits of the research. Synopses are often found in EBP journals, such as *Evidence-Based Medicine, Evidence-Based Nursing, Evidence-Based Mental Health*, and *International Journal of Evidence-Based Healthcare*, to name a few.

Syntheses are a form of research (e.g., systematic reviews, meta-analyses, and meta-syntheses) that use a systematic process for reviewing and appraising evidence to answer a predetermined question. These reviews include a comprehensive search protocol to find appropriate published and non-published evidence, criteria for selecting the evidence, and criteria for critically appraising the evidence. The systematic review includes recommendations that stem from the synthesis of the appraised evidence. A meta-analysis is similar to a systematic review but also includes statistical methods to determine the overall effect of an intervention from multiple studies. The Cochrane Database of Systematic Reviews (CDSR) is one source for systematic reviews (http://www.cochrane.org/cochrane-reviews). Syntheses are important sources of high-quality evidence to support answering a foreground question. Often systematic reviews provide the team with an efficient way to launch the literature search as well as give a sense of the scope of the available literature. Further review of the specific published studies in the systematic review assists with understanding the methodology and results important to the interprofessional EBP project.

The interprofessional team may want to use additional databases for obtaining evidence for EBP, such as the databases academic institutions in Australia support, including OTseeker (http://www.otseeker.com/) and the Joanna Briggs Institute (www.joannabriggs.org). OTseeker, which is an open-access database of occupational therapy studies, focuses on abstracts of systematic reviews, randomized controlled trials, and other resources related to occupational therapy interventions. The mission of the Joanna Briggs Institute is to promote the translation, synthesis, and implementation of EBP in health care.

The 6S Pyramid then includes the unfiltered evidence, such as randomized controlled trials, cohort studies, case controlled studies, and other type of primary studies. For some foreground questions, there is not enough research for the creation of filtered evidence, so the interprofessional team will have to access these sources of evidence to answer the foreground question. The type of study in which to search depends on the foreground question (DiCenso, Guyatt, & Ciliska, 2005). For example, the traditional PICO foreground question that is asking about the effectiveness of an intervention calls for finding randomized controlled trials or quasi-experimental studies. For questions of harm, the interprofessional team would search for cohort and/or case-controlled observational studies; for patient experiences, the team would select qualitative studies.

Finally, the last part of the pyramid is expert opinion literature, such as information from textbooks, narrative reviews, and other types of practice articles. These evidence sources are helpful for answering background questions and are not appropriate for foreground questions, unless there is no other type of evidence. When little research is available, the interprofessional team should look for other types of evidence, such as information from published quality improvement reports, consensus statements, patient satisfaction information, case reports, community standards, clinical experience, and input from practice experts and researchers (Dearholt & Dang, 2012) (see Table 8-1).

Using Advanced Search Mechanisms, Special Features, and Other Search Methods

With the amount of literature and search options (see Chapter 7, Table 7-5) available today, a search addressing a foreground question often seems overwhelming. However, an interprofessional EBP project generally involves a more focused search of the literature rather than an exhaustive search. Several systematic search strategies make a literature search more efficient and beneficial (Cronin, Ryan, & Coughlin, 2008; Finfgeld-Connett & Johnson, 2012; Granger, 2008).

Specifically, using advanced search functions helps an interprofessional team narrow the search, such as restricting the search to the type of study (e.g., randomized controlled trial), publication dates, language, journal types or names, author or title, and year of publication used in writing the article. While determination of filters or limits in a focused literature search is important for the cohesiveness and outcome of the results, the team should avoid the temptation to limit the search to only articles accessible as part of the database. This filter or limit will overly simplify the search in a biased way and the team may not access important evidence. While limit features are helpful, the team should also avoid any overuse of the limit features that may prevent finding key evidence (see Table 8-1).

TABLE 8-2	
NESTING AND BOOLEAN OPERATORS: DEFINITIONS OF NESTING AND BOOLEAN OPERATORS FOR LITERATURE SEARCHES	
TOOL	**EXAMPLE**
Boolean operator: OR Using this operator will help find studies that include all of the keywords listed. It will increase the sources for the search.	Chronic pain OR anesthetics (includes studies that address either chronic pain or anesthetics)
Boolean operator: AND Using this will help find studies that include both keywords listed. It will decrease the sources in the search.	Chronic pain AND anesthetics (includes studies that address only chronic pain and anesthetics)
Boolean operator: NOT Using this will exclude studies that contain a specific keyword.	Chronic pain NOT acute pain (excludes studies that mention acute pain as a keyword)
Nesting A way to group terms using parentheses	(guided imagery OR visualization) AND (acute pain) (guided imagery) OR (visualization AND acute pain) • The first grouping would search for studies on acute pain that also included either guided imagery or visualization as keywords. • The second grouping would search for articles on guided imagery that also included both visualization and acute pain as keywords.

Another important strategy is to use Boolean operators, which are conjunctions for combining or excluding studies in order to create a more focused search. Nesting is a technique for ordering combinations of terms to produce a refined search. Table 8-2 provides a description of Boolean operators and nesting. A search structure increasingly available within databases is the faceted search navigation system, which facilitates combining search terms in a quick and easy way. A faceted search system relies on characteristics, or facets, of a topic to help the user define and narrow a search (Fagan, 2010). For example, these methods are available in MEDLINE, PubMed, and CINAHL. In these databases, the user enters a search term as normal, runs the search, and then repeats the process for other keywords. Then, after accessing the search history in CINAHL and MEDLINE and using the advanced search in PubMed, the user selects terms to combine from the search, choosing a Boolean operator (e.g., "and" or "or") to combine the literature searches.

Another way to complement the search process is to use specialized features available in some databases. PubMed, for example, has a clinical queries option that provides results under the three headings of clinical studies, systematic reviews, and medical genetics. CINAHL has evidence-based care sheets that summarize information about a problem and the actions to take to provide care.

Some other strategies to address the foreground question include starting with a seminal or exemplary research study that supports the question and using this study to create a starting point to identify relevant and appropriate articles that relate to the PICO question. "Berry picking" (Bates, 1989) or "Pearl growing" (Schlosser, Wendt, Bhavnani, & Nail-Chiwetalu, 2006) search strategies emphasize reviewing the articles in the reference list of a published study that appear relevant to the PICO question. When deemed appropriate, the interprofessional team obtains the studies in the reference lists and adds them to the search results. In addition, the authors of the selected studies become part of an author search (i.e., the name of the authors are search terms). Through this process, the evidence-based practitioner determines whether the identified authors published current papers on the problem. These techniques for searching the literature are iterative in nature, with one article leading to additional sources, search terms or keywords, and names of researchers for searching by author.

Publication Bias

Publication bias is a challenge that interprofessional EBP practitioners face when conducting any literature search, whether using a focused or exhaustive search approach (Howell & Shields, 2008; Scargle, 2000). Rothstein, Sutton, and Borenstein (2005) defined publication bias as "what occurs whenever the research that appears in the published literature is systematically unrepresentative of the population of completed studies" (p. 1). This bias occurs with all types of published research, quantitative and qualitative. Competition for publishing and finding outlets to publish articles are intense for researchers and scholars. This competition varies by topic or problem under study, discipline, and type of publication. Because of this competition, major journals in many disciplines are selective about the manuscripts they accept for publication. Thus, editors frequently reject studies that have negative, insignificant, or uninteresting results, as well as smaller studies, in favor of studies with large sample sizes. In addition, researchers may also conceal or underreport study findings they believe may lead to potential rejection from the publisher.

In the case of sponsored research, the intent of avoiding the publication of results may occur because of the sponsors and their researchers not wanting to disclose research unsupportive of a specific product, medication, or equipment. Researchers refer to publishing only positive results or incomplete results and withholding results as the "hidden file drawer problem" (Scargle, 2000). This bias has the potential to affect an interprofessional team's decision about implementing a practice change due to the overemphasis on positive findings in the published literature. The proposed practice change may have less benefit or may cause more harm than findings in the published literature indicate.

Some searching strategies that assist in guarding against publication bias include avoiding the use of positive outcomes as search terms (e.g., increased functioning), searching trial registries for completed and ongoing studies, contacting researchers to discuss their work, and searching the databases of regulatory bodies, such as the Food and Drug Administration. While accessing unpublished studies is difficult, the team should keep publication bias in mind and look for other evidence sources to complement the evidence found in electronic database sources. Table 8-3 provides suggestions to expand a search to include other sources of evidence.

Stopping the Search Process

It is often difficult to know when to stop a literature search because it is easy to adopt the attitude that there is definitive evidence still uncovered that will answer the PICO question. There are three considerations for making the decision to stop a search. First, the decision to stop is appropriate if few new citations and the same references reoccur after using all of the combinations of the identified search terms during subsequent searches in other databases. Second, when searching for qualitative research for experiential EBP questions, there is a point of

saturation when finding additional qualitative studies will not necessarily add to the richness and variation of findings (Finfgeld-Connett & Johnson, 2012). The third issue is prematurely stopping the search, which commonly occurs with inexperienced evidence-based practitioners. Lack of skills and ease with conducting a literature search may lead the team to decide erroneously that little evidence is available that answers the foreground question. When the team lacks confidence with searching the literature, the team should contact a librarian for support. When skills are not an issue, the lack of evidence may mean the PICO question is too narrow and requires revision, search filters are overused, or that there is limited evidence to answer the question. When there is little evidence to change practice, the team may need to find another way to address the practice problem, such as conducting research to test the intervention or implementing best practice using a quality improvement approach.

Team members may believe they are spending too much time with the literature search, especially given the time needed to develop a foreground question after doing the background search. Team members may believe they are not making much process in the project overall. In addition, there may be organizational pressures to start implementation, which is the tangible product that health care leaders often value. Strategies to keep the literature search process from being rushed include the following:

- Communicating regularly to team members and organizational stakeholders the progress and rationale for the order and sequencing of team activities in the interprofessional EBP project

- Using a documentation process to maintain the integrity and fidelity of the search

- Having consistent dialogue about search results and evidence for appraisal

Documenting the Literature Search Process and Managing Information

Thorough documentation of the search process is vital to completing an effective search. Documentation of the search process accomplishes the following several purposes:

- Maintains a record of the search to ensure reproducibility

- Enables the team to expand a search or follow up on a theme or keyword

- Provides a record for other team members to prevent duplication

- Assists with decisions and keeping project deadlines

- Provides data for disseminating the project and its results

TABLE 8-3

SOURCES FOR EXPANDING LITERATURE REVIEW SEARCHES

TYPES OF SOURCE AND DESCRIPTION	ADVANTAGES AND DISADVANTAGES OF THE SOURCE	EXAMPLES OF SOURCES
Open access journals or open journals—scholarly journals open to anyone on the Internet without cost or subscription. These are being added and changed all the time. Articles are often peer reviewed and can be specific to a certain discipline.	*Advantages* • Quicker turnaround for publication can make sources more current. • Lower or free cost to access articles • Researchers do not need to be affiliated with any particular institution to access literature. *Disadvantages* • Variations or lack of peer review in some sites may increase concerns about the lower quality of scientific evidence. • Open access sites may not have as high a reputation as some traditional, peer-reviewed, fee-for-service sources. • Quickly changing sources may be difficult for researchers to keep up with and know open access sites that pertain to their EBP question area.	• Nursing Research and Practice: http://www.hindawi.com/journals/nrp/ • The Open Journal of Occupational Therapy: http://scholarworks.wmich.edu/ojot/ • Physiopedia: http://www.physio-pedia.com/Open_Access_Research
Regulatory bodies—agencies that monitor and regulate the use of techniques, procedures, and research for health care	*Advantages* • Contain information on many topics related to general health. • Material up to date reflecting current concerns. • Access to official documents and reports. *Disadvantages* • Can be difficult to search for specific topics. • Information may be more in a newspaper–type article format or a report rather than a research study format.	• http://www.clinicaltrials.com/industry/regulatory_agencies.htm
Registries of controlled trials—includes lists of the design, conduct, and process of clinical trials	*Advantages* • Provides a resource for current clinical trials • Contact information is available for teams to contact the researchers if desired. • Can be useful to see what current initiatives are being pursued in relationship to the EBP topic *Disadvantages* • Trials may be in process or have been stopped, limiting the information that is available. • Results may not be available; teams would need to contact the researchers to gain additional information.	• metaRegister of Controlled Trials: http://www.controlled-trials.com/

(continued)

TABLE 8-3 (CONTINUED)

SOURCES FOR EXPANDING LITERATURE REVIEW SEARCHES

TYPES OF SOURCE AND DESCRIPTION	ADVANTAGES AND DISADVANTAGES OF THE SOURCE	EXAMPLES OF SOURCES
Textbooks	*Advantages* • Can be general or specific; good for overview of a topic and background questions • Goes through a quality review process by the publisher • Can be used with electronic connections • Usually well-referenced; has other sources that can be accessed *Disadvantages* • Can be a long time to publish the evidence; may be outdated • Teams should be careful to use the latest edition of the text • May be hard to share with team members as copies may be limited	• Will vary depending on discipline. There is usually one or two texts that have been in several editions and are considered foundational for the discipline.
Health care blogs	*Advantages* • Can be updated quickly and often, so can be very current • Often talk about topics that are of concern to many at the time of access • Easy to access *Disadvantages* • May contain more personal opinion and anecdotal evidence • Differing levels of quality checking and rigor • May be difficult to know who the sponsoring organization is, risk of bias	• http://www.cision.com/us/2013/10/top-25-healthcare-blogs/
Dissertation abstract depositories—summaries of dissertations and other student scholarly work, done either within a single academic institution or a broader scale	*Advantages* • Some quality checking within the institution and faculty oversight • Often reflect current interests and concerns in health care relating to a discipline • Relatively quick turnaround for publication *Disadvantages* • Complexity and power of projects may be limited due to design or subject size factors • Potential bias brought on by interests and conflicts with faculty review process • May be limited in accessing full information about a study	• Digital Commons Network – Health and Health Science Commons: http://network.bepress.com/medicine-and-health-sciences/ • University of Washington biomedical and health information website: http://www.bhi.washington.edu/vision

(continued)

TABLE 8-3 (CONTINUED)

SOURCES FOR EXPANDING LITERATURE REVIEW SEARCHES

TYPES OF SOURCE AND DESCRIPTION	ADVANTAGES AND DISADVANTAGES OF THE SOURCE	EXAMPLES OF SOURCES
Conference proceedings—description and/or minutes of professional meetings relating to a professional discipline	**Advantages** • Can give a good picture of the current concerns of a discipline • Projects are likely to be current or very recent. **Disadvantages** • The researcher is not sure about any peer-review or other criteria used in selecting the presentations. • Material may only include abstracts instead of detailed results of studies. • Limited access for those outside the attendees or discipline of the conference; may be additional costs for sources	• http://www.proceedings.com/medical-biotechnology-conference-proceedings.html
Health care association documents—white papers, practice guidelines, other official documents	**Advantages** • Specific to a particular health care discipline • Good for a discipline's overall view of an issue or area of practice • Able to trace changes in strategic and policy related changes in a discipline **Disadvantages** • May only be available to members of that association • Old policies and documents may be removed from the site when a revision or new version is made • No consistent search method; have to look at each association to see how things are organized	• American Occupational Therapy Association: http://www.aota.org/ • American Physical Therapy Association: https://www.apta.org/ • American Nurses Association: http://www.nursingworld.org/ • American Medical Association: http://www.ama-assn.org/ama • National Association of Social Workers: https://www.social-workers.org/ • World Health Organization HINARI: www.who.int/hinari/en
State or local historical societies or health care association archives—specific to a particular state, county, local area, or discipline. Many have websites for computerized searching of resources.	**Advantages** • Specific to a particular discipline, locale, or state • Primary documents; able to be seen in the context of the time • May have interlibrary loan or copying options to get a particular resource **Disadvantages** • May only be in a single locale with potentially limited hours for viewing • May have certain requirements or procedures for viewing materials • May have additional costs for printing or loaning resources	• Directory of state historical societies: http://www.stenseth.org/us/statehs.html

TABLE 8-3 (CONTINUED)		
SOURCES FOR EXPANDING LITERATURE REVIEW SEARCHES		
TYPES OF SOURCE AND DESCRIPTION	**ADVANTAGES AND DISADVANTAGES OF THE SOURCE**	**EXAMPLES OF SOURCES**
Newspapers or newsletters—general use as well as discipline-specific newsletters for members	*Advantages* • General sources may be found in many different and publically available places. • May be written for the general public; easier to understand *Disadvantages* • May only be available to members of a discipline or association • May have limited sources for past issues • Those written for the general public may not be detailed or rigorous enough for the team's needs.	• Team members should explore their professional associations to look for special interest groups or association newsletter publications. Membership in a professional association often includes access to special interest groups that publish newsletters at specific times of the year.
Health care social networking tools—specific to a discipline and general use. May have public and discipline-specific/members only forums. Can be grouped around specific professional roles or issues	*Advantages* • Often reflect current issues affecting the discipline • Offer opportunities to talk to professions who have experience or concerns about the topic under study *Disadvantages* • May be limited to the experience of those participating in the forum, anecdotal in nature • Potential bias in evidence	• OT connections: http://otconnections.aota.org/public_forums/f/79/t/300.aspx • Professional list serve forums • Facebook • Twitter

Editors of journals require potential authors to provide enough information about the search process so that others can replicate the search, evaluate the quality of the search process, and determine potential effects of the search process on the quality of the interprofessional EBP project. There are now standards for reporting a search, and many journals use criteria such as the Preferred Reporting Items for Systematic Reviews and Meta-Analyses (PRISMA) (http://www,prisma-statement.org/). The PRISMA guidelines include a 27-item checklist for evaluating a systematic review or meta-analysis. The guideline recommends using a flow chart or algorithm to depict the search and appraisal processes (see Chapter 9, Figure 9-1). Using the PRISMA guideline to construct an algorithm that accurately documents the search/appraisal process ensures that the interprofessional EBP team is producing a quality search.

These efforts to improve standardized reporting are now expanding globally. The Enhancing the Quality of and Transparency of Health Research (EQUATOR) network is a global initiative to improve the quality and transparency

in reporting health research (http://www.equator-network.org/). Several links are available on their website to examine guidelines for published research using many types of research designs, including qualitative research, randomized trials, case reports, diagnostic studies, and quality improvement studies, among others. Teams may take advantage of the guidelines linked there to determine the quality of unfiltered literature sources.

To document a search, the team should include basic information, such as author(s), title, date of publication, and journal or source. The author's contact information is useful for communicating with an author regarding a study or obtaining permission to use study instruments. It is also important to include the retrieval date for the source, the accessed databases or websites, the search terms, the retrieval results with each term and combination of terms, search history, and methods and outcomes for narrowing the search. There are examples listed in Appendix A of several forms for documenting the literature search that are available for use on this book's companion website.

TABLE 8-4	
BIBLIOGRAPHIC TOOLS	
BIBLIOGRAPHIC TOOLS AND LINKS	**WEB ADDRESS**
Bibme	www.bibme.org/
Citation Machine	www.citationmachine.net/
EndNote	http://endnote.com/
Refman	www.refman.com/
RefWorks	www.refworks.com/

The interprofessional team needs a method to manage and centralize the information from the literature search that facilitates sharing documents to ensure effective progress in developing, implementing, and disseminating the EBP project. Online bibliography and citation tools are available to help the interprofessional EBP teams organize, manage, and share search results. However, additional training and consultation with librarians in the health care organization or in the university ensure that the team uses reference management tools effectively. Table 8-4 provides links to some common bibliography and citation management tools. Another useful method is using Google Drive to create shared team folders to store search documents that each team member creates to record his or her search strategy for the EBP project. The team then uses the individual search documents to create a single search documentation form.

MENTORING CHALLENGES

Mentors of an interprofessional team primarily experience three main challenges during the literature search phase of the EBP process. The first challenge is inconsistent documentation and the team's improper management of the search process. Inconsistent documentation and poor management of the search process is a common issue that occurs when multiple members on a team are participating in the search process and are not communicating regularly about the search. Often, problems are due to the lack of skills and knowledge of team members about how to implement the search strategies and documentation process. Mentors may need to assist in training team members on the use of the search documentation forms to ensure that the forms are clear and understandable, create examples of completed forms with sample studies, involve professional librarians in the team learning process, and use library tutorials during the team meetings to review functions of the databases.

Another mentoring issue is advising the team about how to approach what seems like a failed search, which occurs when the team is unable or only finds few sources to answer the foreground question. The mentor works with the interprofessional team to review and modify the search when needed. If the search process is not the issue, the third mentor challenge is helping the interprofessional team determine whether to modify the foreground question. A modified question requires a new search, and if the team does not find additional evidence, the team most likely has identified an unexplored area of practice. The team would need to make decisions about identifying a different problem or solving the current problem with other methods, such as using best practices or community standard.

MENTOR TECHNIQUES AND MENTOR SUPPORTS

The role of the mentor during this phase is often one of a guide who assists the team in following the steps of a systematic search. As a guide, the mentor also ensures team members have the knowledge and support they need to feel confident. The mentor creates a learning environment for using new databases, sources of evidence, and search methods. Table 8-5 provides project coordinators, mentors, and teams with example techniques and supports for completing the literature search process. When the literature search produces inadequate results, the mentor should work with the team to do the following:

- Analyze the search documentation, looking for aspects of the foreground question that the team may not have searched completely, examining search terms and the databases searched

- Based upon the review of the search records, consider expanding the search or using a different search strategy with additional search terms

- Have team members meet with a librarian

- Talk to experts internal and external to the health care organization regarding possible sources of evidence

- Review the foreground/PICO question

Throughout the search process, mentors should stress the importance and usefulness of the search documentation forms to aid team communication and for achieving EBP project deadlines. Documentation, storage of records, and management of the overall plan avoids the rework that occurs from inaccurate or incomplete information, provides a record for determining whether changes or adjustments in the search need to occur, and provides evidence of progress. Accurate and complete search records are essential for dissemination of findings from the project

	TABLE 8-5	

TECHNIQUES AND SUPPORTS		
MEETINGS AND SEARCH APPRAISAL ALGORITHM	**APPLICATION**	
Meeting the project milestone or deadline for the search process	• Developing a communication strategy to share work and notify others of progress • Holding regular meetings with clear agendas to guide team members on upcoming deadlines and expectations • Conducting check-ins with members to see progress and facilitate discussion questions • Using helpful forms, such as those documenting the search process and bibliographic information	
Using a search/appraisal algorithm to assure documentation is available for the dissemination of the EBP project	• Reviewing the search/appraisal algorithm with the team to determine appropriateness and to obtain agreement for its use • Matching search documentation forms to the algorithm as appropriate • Using the algorithm as an organizing structure for team meetings, and for checking progress toward deadlines	

to stakeholders and the larger health care community (see Chapter 15). The team can refer back to these documents when writing an article for publication or preparing professional presentations.

Time management strategies include regular meetings or communication to report on the progress of individual team members in the search. A regular check-in enables the team to make adjustments and changes to the search strategy throughout the process rather than waiting until the search stalls and team members become frustrated. Some useful questions a mentor asks to facilitate a timely search process include the following:

- Documentation of the search: Are the requirements of the form clear? Does the documentation process make sense to team members? Are team members able to find the proper information to fill out the forms completely? Should the team make any changes to the forms to help the team members accomplish assigned work? When should the team review the search documentation?

- Individual team member progress: Is the team member meeting the deadlines the team set for searching? If not, why not? How can the mentor or team members help other members? Are there strategies, suggestions, or specific information the team should share that would help other team members?

- Team progress: Is the team making appropriate progress on the search? How are team results and search experiences affecting the EBP question and overall progress on the project?

SUMMARY

This chapter discussed the process and strategies involved in moving from a search to answer the background question to a more focused search necessary to answer the foreground question. A focused search involves a systematic process that depends on a well-formed foreground question, identifying key concepts and words in the question to serve as search terms, matching the question to specific databases, identifying the type of evidence that will address the question, and narrowing the search. The chapter included a discussion of the 6S Pyramid of Evidence Resources, in which the team starts with filtered evidence. Consideration of library resources, team member skills and resources, and ways to get the most complete sources that minimize or avoid publication bias were discussed. The discussion highlighted the importance of documenting a search process, as well as using bibliography and citation systems to manage information. Mentor challenges include inconsistent documentation and management of the search process, poor time management, and the potential for a failed or inadequate literature search that does not adequately address the foreground question. The primary mentor technique is to serve as a guide to the interprofessional team that focuses on developing and implementing the optimal plan for searching the literature that will address the foreground question.

REFLECTION QUESTIONS

1. Think about your skills, readiness, and resources for conducting literature searches to help the team answer the PICO question. What are your strengths? What are areas that you need further help or mentoring? What kinds of professional contribution and resources can you bring to the search process?

2. Review the links provided in this chapter for resources, databases, and research guidelines. What do you notice about these sources that would help the team create and execute an effective search strategy? How can you share these observations and insights with the rest of the team?

REFERENCES

Anderson, R. (2008). Future-proofing the library: Strategies for acquisitions, cataloging, and collection development. *The serials librarian, 55*(4), 560-567. doi:10.1080/03615260802399908.

Balas, J. L. (2006). Facing budget cuts: Must we rob Peter to pay Paul? Computers in libraries: online treasures. June, pp. 36-38. Retrieved at http://www.infotoday.com.

Bates, M. J. (1989). The design of browsing and berrypicking techniques, for the online search interface. Retrieved at http://pages.gseis.ucla.edu/faculty/bates/berrypicking.html.

Boruff, J. T., & Thomas, A. (2011). Integrating evidence-based practice and information literacy skills in teaching physical and occupational therapy students. *Health Information and Libraries Journal, 28*, 264-272.

Cronin, P., Ryan, F., & Coughlan, M. (2008). Undertaking a literature review: A step-by-step process. *British Journal of Nursing, 17*(1), 38-43.

Dearholt, S. L., & Dang. D. (2012). *Johns Hopkins nursing evidence-based practice: Models and Guidelines.* (2nd ed.). Indianapolis, IN: Sigma Theta Tau International.

DiCenso, A., Bayley, L., & Haynes, R. B. (2009). Accessing preappraised evidence: fine-tuning the 5S model into a 6S model. *ACP Journal, 151*(3), JC3-2-JC3-3.

DiCenso, A., Guyatt, G., & Ciliska, D. (2005). *Evidence-based nursing: A guide to clinical practice.* St. Louis, MO: Elsevier Mosby.

Facchiano, L., & Snyder, C. H. (2012). Evidence-based practice for the busy nurse practitioner: Part two: Searching for the best evidence to clinical inquires. *Journal of the American Academy of Nurse Practitioners, 24*, 640-648.

Fagan, J. C. (2010). Usability studies of faceted browsing: A literature review. *Information Technology and Libraries*, June, 58-66.

Finfgeld-Connett, D., & Johnson, D. (2012). Literature search strategies for conducting knowledge-building and theory-generating qualitative systematic reviews. *Journal of Advanced Nursing, 69*(1), 194-204.

Granger, B. B. (2008). Practical steps for evidence based practice: Putting one foot in front of the other. *American Association of Critical Care Nurses Advanced Critical Care, 19*(3), 314-324.

Guarria, C. I., & Wang, Z. (2011). The economic crisis and its effect on libraries. *New Library World, 112*(5-6), 199-214. doi:10.1108/0307/4801111136248

Hodge, V., Manoff, M., & Watson, G. (2013). Providing access to e-books and e-book collections: struggles and solutions. *The Serials Librarian, 64*, 200-205. doi:10.1080/03615 26X.2013.760411

Howell, R. T., & Shields, A. L. (2008). The file drawer problem in reliability generalization: A strategy to compute a fail-safe N with reliability coefficients. *Educational and Psychological Measurement, 68*(1), 120-128.

Rothstein, H., Sutton, A. J. & Borenstein, M. (2005a). *Publication Bias in Meta-Analysis. Prevention, Assessment and Adjustments.* Chichester, UK: Wiley.

Salmond, S. W. (2013). Finding the evidence to support evidence-based practice. *Orthopedic Nursing, 32*(1), 16-22.

Scargle, J. D. (2000). Publication bias: The "file-drawer" problem in scientific inference. *Journal of Scientific Exploration, 14*(1), 91-106.

Schlosser, R. W., Wendt, O., Bhavani, S., & Nail-Chiwetalu, B. (2006). Use of information-seeking strategies for developing systematic reviews and engaging in evidence-based practice: The application of traditional and comprehensive pearl growing, a review. *International Journal of Language and Communication Disorders*, September-October, 567-582.

Thompson, L. L., Toedter, L. J., D'Agostino, F. J. (2005). Zero-based print journal collection development in a community teaching hospital library: Planning for the future. *Journal of Medical Library Association, 93*(4), 427-430.

Titler, M.G., Kleiber, C., Steelman, V.J., Rakel, B.A. Budreau, G. Eberett, L.Q., Buckwalter, K.C., Tripp-Reimer, T., Goode, C.J. (2001). *The Iowa model of evidence-based practice to promote quality care.* Critical Care Nursing Clinics of North America, 13(4), 497-509.

Trail, M. A. (2013). Evolving with the faculty to face library budget cuts. *The Serials Librarian, 65*, 213-220.

Worster, A., & Haynes, R. B. (2012). How do I find a point-of-care answer to my clinical question? *Canadian Journal of Emergency Medicine, 14*(1), 31-35.

Wyer, P. C., Naqvi, Z., Dayan, P. S., Celentano, J. J., Eskin, B., & Graham, M. J. (2009). Do workshops in evidence-based practice equip participants to identify and answer questions requiring consideration of clinical research? A diagnostic skill assessment. *Advances in Health Sciences Education, 14*, 515-533.

Supplemental materials for this chapter are available online.
Please refer to the sticker in the front of the book and enter the access code provided.

9

Transitioning Into Interprofessional Evidence-Based Practitioners

VaLinda I. Pearson, PhD, RN, CRRN and Patricia L. Finch-Guthrie, PhD, RN

CHAPTER TOPICS

- What is a critical appraisal?
- Screening for relevancy
- Appraising the evidence
- Synthesizing results into practice recommendations
- Mentor challenges
- Mentor techniques and supports

PERFORMANCE OBJECTIVES

By the end of the chapter, the mentors and team members will be able to do the following:

1. Screen studies to fit with the PICO question using the title and an abstract review.

2. Appraise a research study determining the level and quality of the evidence, documenting the appraisal results.

3. Synthesize the evidence and make recommendation for changing practice.

4. Identify and manage team issues and mentor challenges.

When the interprofessional team has collected potentially relevant studies from multiple disciplines through searching the literature (Chapter 8), the next part of the interprofessional evidence-based practice (EBP) process is to differentiate useful studies from studies that are not helpful in answering the PICO question. The results from the grounded theory study on mentoring (Chapter 3) indicate that clinicians new to interprofessional EBP start to feel they are evidence-based practitioners as they engage in the intense learning associated with appraising and synthesizing evidence. The purpose of this chapter is to assist the interprofessional team in learning how to select, appraise, and synthesize the literature.

In the Iowa model (Titler et al., 2001), appraisal of evidence is a significant step in determining if there is sufficient evidence to move forward to pilot a practice

Moyers, P. A., & Finch-Guthrie, P. L.
*Interprofessional Evidence-Based Practice:
A Workbook for Health Professionals* (pp 137-151).
© 2016 Taylor and Francis Group.

change (see Chapter 1, Figure 1-2). The decision regarding sufficient evidence requires an evaluation of the strength and quality of the available evidence. If the evidence is insufficient, then the interprofessional team may decide to conduct research to supplement the evidence identified in the search process. However, the Iowa model (Titler et al.) also maintains that other types of evidence, such as case reports and expert opinions, may provide enough evidence to support some forms of practice change.

WHAT IS A CRITICAL APPRAISAL?

According to D'Auria (2007), critical appraisal is a "careful and systematic examination of the research evidence" (p. 343); however, non-research evidence also needs appraising. Goals for examining evidence include judging the quality and credibility of reported findings and deciding whether to use the evidence to make practice recommendations implemented in an EBP project (Chapters 10 through 12). The interprofessional team members need a systematic method and a variety of tools to assist them in carefully determining the strength and quality of the evidence to make good decisions and ensure the reliability and validity of the appraisal process. Most peer-reviewed research has had some critical appraisal for internal and external validity through the publishing process; however, the consumer of research must conduct his or her own appraisal in relationship to the practice context and the EBP question driving a practice change.

Interprofessional Appraisal

Program coordinators should offer a variety of appraisal tools to the mentors and teams as part of the toolkit for the interprofessional EBP program, thus saving the team's time in searching for the best appraisal tools (see Table 9-1 for a summary of three evidence hierarchies). Program coordinators should also carefully select an appraisal approach as the main method guiding the evidence leveling and quality appraisal process as a place for teams to start or further develop their knowledge and skills. Having all teams in the interprofessional EBP program use the same leveling system has some advantages, including a common language about EBP, which is important when multiple disciplines work together. The program coordinators provide education for the interprofessional teams on the program's selected appraisal processes and methods.

Not every interprofessional EBP program should use the same appraisal process. Program coordinators might consider the Johns Hopkins appraisal system (Dearholt & Dang, 2012). This system addresses two general types of evidence: research and non-research evidence. The hierarchy for the research evidence includes three levels designated I through III, and for the non-research evidence, the appraisal approach designates two levels: IV and V. Level I

is the highest level of evidence (see Table 9-1). When selecting the basic appraisal method for the interprofessional teams to use, the program coordinators should do the following when possible:

- Accommodate the practice scope of disciplines involved in the program
- Match participant knowledge, skill, and expertise in the interprofessional EBP program
- Afford ease of use
- Focus on the types of EBP questions appropriate to the program (e.g., intervention)
- Use available predeveloped educational materials and supports regarding appraisal

Evidence hierarchies for leveling evidence as part of the appraisal process vary based on disciplines and professional organizations, which contributes to each interprofessional team possibly having to make unique decisions about their appraisal processes that do not incorporate the main appraisal approach of the program. The program coordinators encourage teams to make decisions about appraisal approaches using an interprofessional EBP process where the disciplines involved, the type of PICO question, and the variety of evidence require the team to select the most appropriate approach given the nature of the EBP project. Organizations of health professionals, such as the American Association of Critical Care Nurses, American Medical Association, or the American Occupational Therapy Association have hierarchies for leveling evidence depending on the type of evidence. Organizations, such as Johns Hopkins University and Hospital, have specific guidelines for leveling and appraising evidence as well (Dearholt & Dang, 2012).

Team members from multiple disciplines, in deciding how to appraise relevant studies, have to engage in careful deliberation, negotiation, collaboration, and knowledge exchange in order to recognize the team members' differences in expertise, experience, culture, values, and traditions. The value of an interprofessional appraisal process comes with various interpretations and perspectives that advance understanding of the evidence. The interprofessional EBP team should address the following questions before settling with one or more appraisal tools:

- What kind of PICO question has the interprofessional team developed (e.g., is it an intervention question)?
- What types of evidence has the interprofessional team found (e.g., randomized controlled trials [RCTs], systematic reviews, practice guidelines, qualitative studies, and quality improvement)?
- How does each discipline on the interprofessional team normally appraise these kinds of evidence, what is the comfort level with each possible appraisal tool, and which tools seem to fit the interprofessional EBP project best?

TABLE 9-1

SUMMARY OF LEVELING SCHEMA FOR EVIDENCE-BASED PRACTICE

SOURCE	BASIC LEVELS	QUALITY
CEBM Levels of Evidence Working Group. "The Oxford Levels of Evidence 2. Oxford Centre for Evidence-Based Medicine. http://www.cebm.net/index.aspx?o=5653 (for Intervention Studies)	*Level 1* • Systematic review of RCTs *Level 2* • RCT or observational study with dramatic effect *Level 3* • Nonrandomized cohort study with follow-up *Level 4* • Case series, case control *Level 5* • Mechanism-based reasoning (involves an inferential chain linking the intervention with a clinical outcome)	Level may be graded down on the basis of study quality, imprecision, indirectness (study PICO does not match questions PICO) because of inconsistency between studies or because the absolute effect size is very small; Level may be graded up if there is a large or very large effect size.
Dearholt, S. L., & Dang, D. (2012). *Johns Hopkins Nursing Evidence-Based Practice: Model and Guidelines* (2nd ed.). Indianapolis, IN: Sigma Theta Tau International.	*Level I* • RCT • Systematic review of RCTs, with or without meta-analysis *Level II* • Quasi-experimental study • Systematic review of a combination of RCTs and quasi-experimental, or quasi-experimental alone, with or without meta-analysis *Level III* • Nonexperimental study • Systematic review of combination of RCTs, quasi-experimental and nonexperimental, or nonexperimental studies only, with or without meta-analysis • Qualitative study or systematic review, with or without meta-synthesis *Level IV* • Opinion of respected authorities, nationally recognized expert committees/consensus panels based on scientific evidence (e.g., practice guidelines) *Level V* • Based on experimental and non-research evidence • Literature reviews • Quality improvement • Case reports	*Research Levels I Through III* High, Good, Low Generalizability, sample size, control, conclusions, recommendations based on literature review *Research Level IV* High, Good, Low Sponsorship, documentation of search, number of well-designed studies, criteria-based evaluation of strength and quality, national experience evident, developed within the past 5 years *Level V* High, Good, Low Expertise evident Definitive conclusions Scientific rationale Thought leaders

(continued)

TABLE 9-1 (CONTINUED)

SUMMARY OF LEVELING SCHEMA FOR EVIDENCE-BASED PRACTICE

SOURCE	BASIC LEVELS	QUALITY
Fineout-Overholt, E., Melnyk, B. M., Schulz, A. (2005). Transforming health care from the inside out: Advancing evidence-based practice in the 21st Century. *Journal of Professional Nursing, 21,* 335–344.	*Evidence Pyramid for Answering Questions About Effectiveness of Interventions (top to bottom)* • Systematic review or meta-analysis of RCTs • Evidence-based clinical practice guidelines based on RCTs • RCT • Controlled trials without randomization and case control and cohort studies • Systematic reviews of descriptive and qualitative studies • Descriptive and qualitative studies • Opinions of authorities and reports of expert committees *Evidence Pyramid for Answering Questions About Meaning (top to bottom)* • Systematic reviews of descriptive and qualitative studies • Descriptive and qualitative studies • Opinions of authorities and reports of expert committees • Evidence-based clinical practice guidelines based on RCTs • Controlled trials without randomization and case control and cohort studies • Systematic review or meta-analysis of RCTs • RCT	(1) Are the results of the study or systematic review valid? (i.e., as close to the truth as possible); (2) What are the results? (i.e., are they meaningful and reliable—if applied, I can get the same results); and (3) Are the findings clinically relevant to my patients?

• How does the context of the recommendation for practice change influence the appraisal approach selected?

Characteristics of Appraisal Systems and Tools

In most evidence hierarchies, there are between five and seven levels of evidence (Dearholt & Dang, 2012; Ho, Peterson, & Masoudi, 2008; Krainovitch-Miller, Haber, & Jacobs, 2009; Peterson et al., 2014). EBP experts tend to agree that the smaller the number used to identify an appraisal level (for example, level I), the greater the strength of the evidence. RCTs often receive a higher ranking when compared to quasi-experimental designs because they provide strong evidence for determining the existence of a cause-and-effect relationship between the independent (i.e., intervention) and dependent (i.e., outcome) study variables. Most EBP experts agree that level I typically involves a synthesis of many RCTs in a meta-analysis or in a systematic review.

In contrast, some appraisal leveling systems differ with the placement of clinical guidelines within a hierarchy. For example, in the Johns Hopkins hierarchy (Dearholt & Dang, 2012), clinical guidelines are part of non-research evidence with a level of IV. Other hierarchies treat clinical guidelines similar to systematic reviews and classify guidelines developed from RCTs as level I evidence, and guidelines developed from expert opinion as lower-level evidence (Fineout-Overholt, Melnyk, & Schulz, 2005). In addition, evidence hierarchies from medicine include a greater emphasis on observational studies in ranking evidence (see Table 9-1).

One problem with evidence hierarchies is that the original developers designed the structures primarily to answer questions about interventions regarding the demonstrated efficacy under controlled research conditions. For instance, initial RCTs were drug trials with rigid inclusion and exclusion criteria for selected subjects, and with detailed, specific guidelines or protocols for the drug treatment administered to subjects (Atkins, 2007). While this high degree of control manages the effect of potential confounding variables, the rigor incorporated in the RCT also raises questions about applying results to practice. The question RCTs answer is whether an intervention has merit or potential to improve outcomes. These types of studies do not answer the EBP question regarding whether the intervention will work in everyday life. While RCTs have substantial internal validity, external validity is often insufficient to determine applicability and relevance of the intervention to other populations and to conditions that occur under circumstances different from the context of the study.

In addition, patients generally have multiple health problems, are often dissimilar to subjects in RCTs, and have lives that may not allow for adherence to detailed intervention protocols. As Atkins (2007) noted, the outcomes measured in the RCT may include the costs and benefits of greatest importance to researchers. These costs and benefits may not be those that are most important to patients. The inclusion of patient values is one of the definitional components of EBP and, because other research methods are better at uncovering patient values, it is necessary to obtain patient perspectives from other types of evidence.

In general, EBP questions are not answerable with RCT studies alone. Most EBP questions also require evidence from clinical experience, expert wisdom and patient values (Ilott, 2012), as well as from implementation and dissemination research. Without evidence regarding the best implementation approach for an identified intervention, a greater number of negative results may occur in the applied setting in comparison to the results of the RCT. Comparative effectiveness research is important to include in the appraisal process because these studies attempt to answer real-world questions, such as which interventions are most effective, which patients will benefit the most, the conditions necessary for the intervention to work, and the cost of multiple approaches (Glasgow & Steiner, 2012). These studies compare interventions with alternative treatments or current practice to examine the benefits and harms associated with a practice change, rather than comparing outcomes with subjects who do not receive any intervention or receive a placebo (i.e., control group). Comparing groups who receive an intervention to those who do not receive an intervention provides only information that the intervention has an effect, but RCTs typically do not inform clinicians whether the intervention is better than current treatments. Without that information, the interprofessional team may still struggle with whether the proposed change is truly beneficial and cost-effective.

Unfortunately, many authors and practitioners have also applied appraisal hierarchies designed to rank evidence for efficacy to other types of EBP questions (e.g., harm, diagnosis, prognosis, and experience). The interprofessional team should note that when appraising studies for other types of PICO questions as discussed in Chapter 7, other leveling systems provide better guidance. For example, Fineout-Overholt et al. (2005) identified a system for meaningful questions (see Table 9-1). Meta-syntheses of qualitative studies and individual qualitative studies are at the top of the hierarchy, with RCTs at the lower levels of evidence. Critical appraisals that assist teams in effective decision making regarding the next steps in the interprofessional EBP process (i.e., sufficient or insufficient evidence for trialing a practice change) require the interprofessional team to discuss the nature of the EBP question, the wide range of evidence required to answer the question, as well as evidence that guides implementing a practice change. The Oxford Center for Evidence-Based Medicine (CEBM) has an evidence hierarchy for other types of EBP questions that may assist with appraising evidence (www.cebm.net/oxford-centre-evidence-based-medicine-levels-evidence-march-2009/).

Compared to hierarchies for leveling evidence, the strategies for assessing the quality of the evidence are less clear. Often, the leveling system includes a separate set of evaluative questions for quality (see Table 9-1). Other hierarchies have quality criteria built into the levels, such as the hierarchy from CEBM. For example, one of the levels in the CEBM evidence hierarchy includes evidence from an individual RCT with narrow confidence intervals (see Chapter 14). The appraiser would rate this type of evidence as level 2b. The evidence is level 2 because it includes only a single RCT. The quality of the evidence is "b" because the narrow confidence interval may make the evidence less generalizable to other situations. In order for the evidence to be level 1, the evidence would need to be a systematic review of several RCTs and not a single RCT. Evidence that is "a" level quality meets criteria for generalizability, larger sample size, and large effect size.

Often, clinicians and practitioners have difficulty in leveling and determining quality in one appraisal step. Separating the leveling process from determining quality is often easier. Quality ratings are separate from the leveling hierarchy in the Johns Hopkins system (Dearholt & Dang, 2012). Once the reviewer has leveled the study, they assign the evidence a quality rating after answering a set of questions. In the Johns Hopkins approach, both types of evidence (i.e., research and non-research) use a quality rating ranging from A to C, with A representing high quality, B good, and C low-quality evidence (see Table 9-1).

According to Whiffin and Hasselder (2013), appraisal forms are either research design-led or are generic in that they are applicable to a variety of evidence types. Design-led forms include questions specific to a particular type of study—qualitative or quantitative. An example of a set of design-led appraisal forms are those found on the Critical Appraisal Skills Programme (CASP) website (www.casp-uk.net), which includes tools for RCTs, cohort studies, qualitative studies, and systematic reviews. An advantage of these appraisal tools is that CASP has a Creative Commons license, which allows anyone to use the appraisal tools without copyright infringement, as long as the user is not using the tools for commercial purposes. Appraisal tools also exist for reviewing data collection instruments or screening tools, practice guidelines and expert consensus documents, and quality improvement studies.

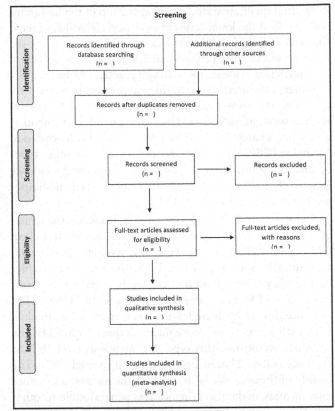

Figure 9-1. PRISMA 2009 flow diagram. (Reprinted from The PRISMA Statement distributed under the terms of the Creative Commons Attribution License, which permits unrestricted use, distribution, and reproduction in any medium. Moher, Liberati, Tetzlaff, & Altman, the PRISMA Group (2009). Copyright: © 2009 Moher et al. This is an open-access article distributed under the terms of the Creative Commons Attribution License, which permits unrestricted use, distribution, and reproduction in any medium, provided the original author and source are credited. http://www.prisma-statement.org/PRISMAStatement. aspx.)

SCREENING FOR RELEVANCY

As the interprofessional team is obtaining evidence from the literature search, the team tracks all the evidence they selected for appraisal and the evidence the team decided not to use for the EBP project. Documenting the decisions involve using an algorithm (Figure 9-1) in which the evidence lost to each step in the search and appraisal processes is important for making the process transparent. This documentation process ensures transparency to stakeholders who support the project and to future readers of the published project who want to evaluate the quality and applicability of the EBP project to their institutions.

The interprofessional team first identifies the total number of records in the literature search process initially identified from selected databases and other sources. The next step is to remove duplicate records, calculating the number of sources remaining. The interprofessional team screens the remaining records for relevancy to the EBP question

to reduce further the number of records for appraisal. For example, a study focusing on fall prevention for community-dwelling older adults is not relevant for fall prevention in long-term care. In this situation, the interprofessional team would eliminate the community falls study from further appraisal.

An efficient method to determine relevancy for answering the PICO question includes reviewing both the title and the abstract. For the most part, the title and abstract should give a clear idea of the nature of the study, especially when authors provide a structured abstract that includes a description of the study background, purpose/research questions, methods, results, and conclusions. If the abstract indicates the study is consistent with the PICO question, then the study is appropriate for a full appraisal of the strength and quality of the evidence. If the abstract still does not fully delineate the information needed to determine fit with the PICO question, then reading the entire study is necessary. If the evidence does not fit the PICO question or the patient population, then the team should save the evidence in an electronic file or in RefWorks and should add the information to the algorithm to document elimination of the study.

Experts vary in their opinions about how to screen abstracts of published research studies to determine fit with a PICO question or practice concern, as well as the number of questions to consider for relevancy. Based on a literature review, some authors use five to seven questions to review an abstract (Alderson, 2012; Assadi, Zarghi, Shamloo, & Nikooiyan, 2012; Young & Solomon, 2009). However, the primary determination is dependent on whether the study aligns with the PICO question. The interprofessional team should take time to practice screening using the following abstract and PICO question created specifically for this book, which represents a fictitious quantitative research study. The practice PICO question is, "Is there a difference in resting heart rate and systolic blood pressure in older women who exercise compared to those who do not exercise?"

The aim of this study is to investigate whether health outcomes improve for older, minority women with regular exercise. Forty-five African American women between 60 to 70 years of age participated in the study. The researchers randomly assigned the study participants to either a control or an intervention group. Women in the control group received instructions to follow their usual exercise practices for 4 months. Women in the intervention group walked at a comfortable pace for 30 minutes three times a week for 16 weeks. Women in both groups recorded their resting pulse rate and blood pressure using an automatic blood pressure cuff three times per week. Each participant completed a standardized exercise and lifestyle questionnaire at the start and the conclusion of the study, along with weighing at the beginning and at the end of the study. On average at the end of the study, a six-point difference in systolic blood pressure existed for women in the intervention compared to the control group, with no difference in resting pulse rate between groups. Women in the intervention group had an average weight loss of 10 pounds, whereas the control group did not experience weight loss.

The team discusses whether the abstract depicts a study that is a good fit for the PICO question. Team members may differ in their decision regarding the relevance to the PICO question given the study's single focus on one study population (i.e., African American women). In addition, the abstract does not identify statistical analyses necessary to determine a significant difference in blood pressure and weight, nor does the abstract determine the magnitude of the effect of the intervention on the health outcomes (see Chapter 14). The information in the abstract does seem to match the basic elements of the PICO question, but the full study needs appraisal as to the strength and quality of the evidence. Based on the abstract, the study may assist the team when combined with other studies in understanding outcomes for different populations of older women. The PICO question was not specific regarding the population except for the age of the women. The team may find that the abstract does not answer all of the questions regarding the study. Having unanswered questions does not mean that the interprofessional team should discard the study. It does mean that team members need to pay close attention to those unanswered questions when reading the complete study for the full appraisal.

APPRAISING THE EVIDENCE

The second step of the process is to appraise the screened evidence in a systematic fashion and to use the selected appraisal tool to record the comments of team members. While the team may decide to eliminate evidence from consideration based on a brief review of the title and abstract, the team should not identify evidence as supportive of making a practice change when reviewing only the abstract. The team appraises all of the screened evidence that seems to answer the PICO question, as well as evidence where it is unclear whether the study addresses the question.

According to Alderson (2012), there are three basic assessments for appraisal of research:

1. Quality of the study design (Does the study have the right design given the purpose?)

2. Quality of results (Does the study address both statistical and clinical significance if quantitative? Does the qualitative study demonstrate thickness of description?)

3. Applicability or external validity of the results (Do results support changing practice?)

Metzler and Metz (2010) indicated that appraisers should carefully consider applicability of study findings to the practice context. Determining whether to change practice is challenging when few if any similarities exist between the organization described in the study and the organization wanting to implement a similar intervention in terms of context of the practice situation and conditions (e.g., acute vs long-term care). Values, mission, purpose, and philosophy of care vary across health care organizations (e.g., short lengths of stay in acute care vs in long-term care where the facility is the home of the resident), thereby affecting the translation of interventions. Therefore, the interprofessional team needs to detail the differences in the practice context before using study results to support the EBP project.

Leveling Evidence

Determining the strength of a research study is dependent on the study design (e.g., RCT, quasi-experimental, cohort and case-control, correlational, and qualitative). The interprofessional EBP team identifies the study design or type of evidence to assign an evidence level according to the appropriate evidence hierarchy adopted for the appraisal process. The most credible and most respected type of research in health care for testing the efficacy of an intervention is the RCT. RCTs have three essential elements that include randomization of subjects to a control or intervention group, manipulation of the independent variable (at least one group receives the intervention and the others do not), and control of extraneous variables with potential to affect the dependent variable. A well-done RCT has a sample size designed to detect a significant difference between the intervention group(s) and control group(s). The primary question is, does the intervention have a significant effect on the dependent variable in the treatment group when compared to the outcomes of the control group? This difference in outcomes between the two groups indicates the intervention has potential to improve practice within the organization.

A typical evidence hierarchy ranks systematic reviews and meta-analyses as level I because these kinds of evidence include a standardized process for appraising multiple, independent studies to draw conclusions and make recommendations for practice. Meta-analyses, unlike systematic reviews, use statistical methods to combine results from studies to examine the effectiveness of interventions. Systematic reviews and meta-analyses are stronger when including only RCTs compared to reviews that also include quasi-experimental or other studies with nonexperimental designs (e.g., correlational, cohort, case-control, and qualitative). When conducting a critical appraisal of systematic reviews and meta-analyses, publication bias is a significant consideration because the validity of this type of evidence is reliant on a comprehensive literature search of both published and unpublished research (see Chapter 8).

Because negative findings or smaller studies are often not published (i.e., the "hidden file drawer"), the interprofessional EBP team may reach an incorrect decision about the actual effectiveness of an intervention if the meta-analysis only includes published findings. While meta-analyses are strong evidence for changing practice, they still need careful appraisal. There are different methods that authors of meta-analyses use to reduce or test for the potential effect of publication bias on their analysis, such as the failsafe-N statistic and the trim-and-fill method (Rothstein, 2008; Rothstein, Sutton, & Borenstein, 2005; Song, Hooper, & Loke, 2013). A funnel plot, another publication bias method, visually examines the relationship between sample size and the estimated effect size of the intervention in each study within the meta-analysis. Skewed or incomplete funnels may indicate publication bias or that there is a systematic difference between studies with small and large samples (Noordzij, Hooft, Dekker, Zoccali, & Jager, 2009; Song et al., 2013). Consequently, when using meta-analyses as evidence for a practice change, the team needs to examine the comprehensive nature of the literature search, comparing numbers of published and unpublished studies included in the analysis, and the researcher's use of statistical methodology to assess for publication bias (Rothstein et al., 2005).

Clinical guidelines also provide strong evidence and are most helpful when authors clearly describe the classification schemes they use to appraise the evidence supporting the guideline. In addition, well-done guidelines use pre-established criteria to indicate the strength of each practice recommendation. For example, the label "A" may indicate that a specific recommendation stems from level I evidence.

Quasi-experimental studies are a less rigorous type of experimental study that generally lacks the control that RCTs have as part of their design. These studies do not have equivalent comparison groups because of the inability to randomize subjects to groups. These studies use convenient (i.e., non-probability samples) or repeated measures with the same group of subjects. For example, a researcher may test the effect of a weight loss program by measuring the weight for a group of subjects before the start of a program, after 3 months, and at the end of the program. Quasi-experimental research evidence is usually at a lower level on the evidence hierarchy compared to RCTs. However, these studies are closer to a real life situation and provide support for changing practice, especially when synthesized with RCTs demonstrating efficacy.

Observational studies (e.g., cohort and case-control) studies are important studies comparing differences between naturally occurring groups. The cohort study is most often prospective, in which one group of subjects has exposure to a specific factor or variable of importance and the other group does not. A researcher follows the two groups to determine differences in specific outcomes. For example, a researcher may follow a group of older patients attending an exercise program specifically designed for older adults and compare them to another similar group of older adults attending a program that includes younger adults to determine differences in exercise adherence. These studies are more pragmatic than RCTs and are helpful in examining real-world effectiveness and answering the question, "Will this intervention work in everyday life?" Cohort studies when combined with RCTs provide good evidence for implementing a practice change.

Case-control studies are retrospective, in which the researcher uses existing records to compare a group with a known outcome ("case") to a group who did not develop the outcome in order to determine differences in specific factors potentially leading to the outcome. For example, a researcher might compare hospitalized adults who developed a hospital-acquired infection with a similar group of patients who did not develop the infection. The purpose of the case-control study is to determine factors potentially associated with the occurrence of the infection. Observational studies lack the control of RCTs (i.e., the researcher does not randomize subjects to groups or manipulate the intervention). Case-control studies are specifically important for assessing risk and harm, which is not often possible to do in RCTs because of the rare occurrence of harm. These studies are essential to review when an intervention has potential for creating harm as well as benefit.

Descriptive and correlational studies provide some evidence for a practice change, but because they do not determine a cause-and-effect relationship between an intervention and an outcome, they provide lower-level evidence for changing practice. They are most helpful in providing answers to background questions for an EBP project. Descriptive studies provide information that describes behavior, a population, a concept, a condition, or circumstance. For example, a descriptive study might describe older adults who engage in exercise programs, which is useful for targeting an intervention to the right population. These studies use quantitative or qualitative methods of data collection. Correlational studies are quantitative and examine the relationship or association between variables. As an example, a researcher may use correlational methods to examine potential relationships between activity level of adults and their employment status.

Qualitative studies have a variety of designs, such as grounded theory, case study, phenomenology, ethnography, and historical to name a few. These studies are important sources of evidence because of their focus on the experiences of individuals within a real life context. The intent of qualitative studies is to discover new insights or ways to understand a phenomenon. Because these studies do not test interventions, they are usually lower in the hierarchy of evidence for those types of EBP questions. However, from the point of view of a clinician or practitioner who is concerned whether an intervention is acceptable to a patient

TABLE 9-2	
RESEARCH DESIGN AND CRITICAL APPRAISAL FORMS	
DESIGN	**APPRAISAL FORMS**
Meta-Analysis/ Systematic Reviews	Systematic Review Appraisal Sheet. Centre for Evidence Based Medicine. University of Oxford: www.cebm.net/critical-appraisal/ AMSTAR, the validated systematic review measurement tool: http://amstar.ca/Amstar_Checklist.php CASP. CASP Systematic Review Checklist: www.casp-uk.net/#!casp-tools-checklists/c18f8
Key Quality Factors	• Focused question • Documented search strategy • Inclusion/exclusion criteria for studies • Flow diagram of eliminated studies • Appraisal of study level and quality • Overview of studies included • Conclusion based on results • Identification of review limitations • Appropriate studies combined and summary statistic if meta-analysis
Randomized Controlled Trials	Therapy/RCT Critical Appraisal Sheet. Centre for Evidence Based Medicine. University of Oxford: www.cebm.net/critical-appraisal/Critical Appraisal Skills Programme. CASP Randomized Clinical Trial Checklist: http://www.casp-uk.net/#!casp-tools-checklists/c18f8
Key Quality Factors	• Purpose clearly presented • Sample size sufficient • Control of subject selection bias • Use of a control group/all groups treated equally except intervention • Randomization • Few withdrawal and dropouts • Instruments reliable and valid • Data collection described • Results presented clearly • Study limitations identified • Conclusions based on results

(continued)

population, the results from a qualitative study may significantly affect the design of an interprofessional EBP project.

Appraising the Quality of Evidence

Determining the quality of evidence is dependent on the validity of the study methods and the rigor researchers use to implement the study. Quality standards for each type of study are at the basis of a critical appraisal. Because an interprofessional team is appraising studies with different designs, the members of the team need to consider critical aspects specific to each study design (Table 9-2). Criteria important for one type of design are not necessarily applicable when appraising the quality of other study designs. For example, sample size is critical for quantitative studies, but small sample sizes are relevant for qualitative studies in which participants represent the examined experience. Randomization is important for experimental studies but

TABLE 9-2 (CONTINUED)

RESEARCH DESIGN AND CRITICAL APPRAISAL FORMS

DESIGN	APPRAISAL FORMS
Research (General)	Effective Public Health Practice Project. (EPHPP) Quality Assessment Tool for Quantitative Studies: www.ephpp.ca/tools.html The TREND Statement. Centre for Disease Control and Prevention (CDC): www.cdc.gov/trend-statement/docs/AJPH_Mar2004_Trendstatement.pdf
Key Quality Factors	• Selection bias • Study design • Confounders (differences in groups prior to intervention) • Blinding • Data collection methods • Withdrawals and dropouts • Intervention integrity • Analyses
Case Control	CASP. CASP Case Control Checklist: www.casp-uk.net/#!casp-tools-checklists/c18f8
Key Quality Factors	• Clearly focused problem • Case control method appropriate for problem • Recruitment acceptable • Selection bias for controls controlled • Exposure measured accurately • Taken account of confounding factors • Precision of risk estimate
Cohort Study	CASP. CASP Cohort Study Checklist: www.casp-uk.net/#!casp-tools-checklists/c18f8
Key Quality Factors	• Clearly focused issue • Cohort recruitment acceptable • Exposure measured accurately • Outcome accurately measured • Identified confounding factors • Follow-up of participants complete and long enough • Precision of results
Qualitative	CASP. CASP Qualitative Checklist: www.casp-uk.net/#!casp-tools-checklists/c18f8
Key Quality Factors	• Study aims clear • Qualitative methodology appropriate • Research design appropriate for study aims • Recruitment strategy • Data collection • Relationship between researcher and participant • Ethical issues addressed • Data analysis sufficiently rigorous • Clear statement of findings

(continued)

TABLE 9-2 (CONTINUED)

RESEARCH DESIGN AND CRITICAL APPRAISAL FORMS

DESIGN	APPRAISAL FORMS
Practice Guidelines	Appraisal of Guidelines Research & Evaluation: www.agreetrust.org/
Key Quality Factors	<ul><li>Scope and purpose</li><li>Stakeholder involvement</li><li>Rigor of development</li><li>Clarity of presentation</li><li>Applicability</li><li>Editorial independence</li><li>External review</li></ul>

is not appropriate for a cohort study comparing naturally occurring groups. The important issue for a cohort study is the similarity of the comparison groups and the researcher's process for matching groups on important subject characteristics. A criterion of quality for RCTs and quasi-experimental studies is a clear description of the interventions or treatments, as well as the control condition.

Non-research evidence, which includes expert and consensus panels and practice guidelines, has criteria for quality (see Table 9-2). The quality of consensus statements and clinical guidelines depends on the reputation of the expert and the expert's connections to professional or governmental organizations. The reason reputation is essential is that these sources of evidence depend on opinion for developing practice recommendations and interpreting available evidence. If the credentials and experience of identified experts are unknown, team members should take time to investigate qualifications of the expert through an author search of a database or contacting the professional organization publishing the consensus document. Practice guidelines require updating within 5 years, and the best guidelines have an external review process to ensure their validity and applicability.

Just because a publisher accepts a study for publication in a journal does not guarantee high quality. Unfortunately, poor-quality research does get published; however, as journals adopt standard guidelines for specific studies, such as the CONSORT Statement (www.consort-statement.org) for RCTs, the PRISMA Statement (www.prisma-statement.org) for systematic reviews, and the STROBE Statement (www.strobe-statement.org) for cohort studies, there will be greater consistency in quality of published evidence. However, an interprofessional EBP team should be aware that guidelines outline the minimum standard for transparent reporting.

Identifying and Scrutinizing Studies With Questionable Results

Researchers may overstate or inflate their study results and understate the study limitations (Montori et al., 2004). The interprofessional team should scrutinize and understand the study limitations when appraising each study, especially those studies that support the interprofessional EBP project. Strategies for remaining objective include the following:

- Refraining from reading the discussion section of the study until appraising the results in order for the team to make an independent determination of whether results support the interprofessional EBP project

- Being wary of studies in which researchers had insignificant results for addressing the primary research questions but identified findings of minor importance in subgroup comparisons

- Questioning studies with reported results that do not answer the research question(s) and are inconsistent with the study aims

- Assessing the transparency of the researchers reflected in the discussion of study limitations and their potential effect on study results

  ○ Identify threats for quantitative studies to internal validity, such as a small sample size and the attrition of participants throughout the study

  ○ Identify issues with trustworthiness for qualitative studies (e.g., credibility, transferability, dependability, and confirmability [Lincoln & Guba, 1985])

  ○ Examine potential conflicts of interest, as well as the organizations that provided financial support for the research to determine bias in favor of the funder

TABLE 9-3

LEVELS AND STRENGTH SYNTHESIS

STUDY QUALITY (HIGH, GOOD, LOW)

Level	Appraisal 1	Appraisal 2	Appraisal 3
Level I	High		
Level II			Good
Level III		Good	
Level IV—No studies of this level appraised			
Level V—No studies of this level appraised			

TABLE 9-4

SYNTHESIS OF THE OUTCOMES OF APPRAISED STUDIES

OUTCOMES	APPRAISAL 1 LEVEL I, A	APPRAISAL 2 LEVEL II, B	APPRAISAL 3 LEVEL III, B
Outcome 1: Improved quality of life in the experimental group	Met	Not evaluated	Met
Outcome 2: Decreased blood pressure in the experimental group	No change	Met	Not evaluated
Outcome 3: Increased duration of ambulation in the experimental group	No change	Met	Not evaluated

SYNTHESIZING RESULTS INTO PRACTICE RECOMMENDATIONS

The next step of the interprofessional EBP process is to summarize and synthesize evidence that supports the interprofessional team in making practice recommendations. Synthesis means combining evidence from multiple sources into a logical discussion (Aveyard, 2010; Whiffin & Hasselder, 2013). The team needs to summarize and synthesize results from appraised studies in a structured, succinct, and understandable way through the creation of a variety of summary charts to categorize results. For example, synthesis tables might summarize the levels of evidence and quality ratings, outcomes, and the essential elements of the intervention tested across studies (see Tables 9-3, 9-4, and 9-5 as examples).

Once the team has synthesized the evidence, the team makes recommendations for changing practice. Recommendations are easier to make with strong, high-quality evidence compared to evidence that is weak and of low quality. In some circumstances, the best recommendation may include continuing with the same practice.

Important questions answered when synthesizing evidence include the following: (a) is the intervention efficacious (answered through RCTs and meta-analysis of RCTs), (b) is the intervention effective (answered through outcome registries and comparative effectiveness research), and (c) what are the benefit-harm considerations of the intervention (answered through cohort, case-controlled, comparative effectiveness research, and qualitative research) (Atkins, 2007; Glasgow & Steiner, 2012)? Other considerations when making recommendations include the feasibility, the cost and the required resources for the change, the fit of the change with the organizational culture, and patient and staff acceptance of the intervention. Following a decision to change practice, the next step is to design the actual interprofessional EBP project and plan for implementation as outlined in Chapters 10, 11, and 12.

MENTOR CHALLENGES

Members of an interprofessional team may make unwarranted assumptions about the EBP educational preparation of team members without understanding the differences in

TABLE 9-5

SYNTHESIS OF INTERVENTIONS RELATED TO SPECIFIC STUDY OUTCOMES

	APPRAISAL 1 LEVEL I, A	APPRAISAL 2 LEVEL II, B	APPRAISAL 3 LEVEL III, B
Outcome 1: Improved Quality of Life in the Experimental Group			
Intervention 1: Support group	All experimental group participates ranked support group participation as improving their quality of life ($p < 0.05$)	This outcome not included in the study	95% of experimental group participants rated support group participation as very effective in improving their quality of life
Intervention 2	Data on results of intervention 2	Data on results of intervention 2	Data on results of intervention 2
Outcome 2: Decreased Blood Pressure in the Experimental Group			
Intervention 1: Structured meditation practice	Before and after readings of blood pressure showed no significant change	Before and after blood pressure readings decreased an average of 6 points ($p < 0.05$) for all experimental group participants	This outcome not evaluated in the study
Intervention 2	Data on results of intervention 2	Data on results of intervention 2	Data on results of intervention 2
Outcome 3: Increased Duration of Ambulation in the Experimental Group			
Intervention 1: Timed ambulation activity	No change in duration of ambulation before and after intervention	Distance ambulated and length of ambulation time tolerated increased by an average of 100 feet and 10 minutes ($p<0.05$) for all experimental group participants	This outcome not evaluated in the study
Intervention 2	Data on results of intervention 2	Data on results of intervention 2	Data on results of intervention 2

education background. A variety of disciplines has various levels of EBP education included in their entry-level curricula, often with more emphasis in advanced professional programs. In addition, the interprofessional team has practitioners with a wide range of years of clinical practice. The practicing clinician may have little experience with conducting an organized review of the literature and appraising articles, in addition to having little time to develop the appraisal skill set required (Clark, Burkett, & Stanko-Lopp, 2009; Salbach, Jablal, Korner-Bitensky, Rappolt, & Davis, 2007). No matter the educational level that health care professionals attain, there is at least one generation of clinicians whose undergraduate or graduate curricula provided little education about EBP or the process of critical appraisal of the research literature (Currow & Agar, 2012).

A major team issue is to ensure team members are comfortable and not intimidated when appraising a variety of research designs and analysis methods. Learning to appraise different types of evidence requires coaching and time. The team member leading the appraisal process should have skills in conducting appraisals. McCurtin and Roddam (2012) found that experience in applying search strategies, using databases, and conducting critical appraisals are skill sets more commonly found among recent graduates and beginning practitioners than among more experienced speech and language practitioners. Zidarov, Thomas, and Poissant (2013) reported that experienced physical therapists identified that they had a lack of skills in conducting literature searches and critical appraisals (p. 1572). Therefore, the team might need coaching to have the practitioner or clinician who most recently completed his or her professional education, a faculty member, or a student who completed a research/EBP course lead this interprofessional EBP task. Team members should practice their appraisal skills even when team members have some expertise in appraisal in order to achieve consistency.

TABLE 9-6	
APPRAISAL SUCCESS STRATEGIES	
STRATEGY	**CONSIDERATIONS**
Anticipate the need for experts to guide the appraisal process.	• Are the experts within the team? Outside of the team? • What expertise is needed for the appraisal? Statistical analysis? Methodological analysis? Content analysis?
Develop a plan for how to organize and store the appraisal results.	• Will you store results electronically? In paper format? Who will have access to the results? Who can update the appraisal results? Are you organizing results by author, by topic, or by person who completed the appraisal?
Establish clear expectations for all members of the team in conducting the appraisal in terms of numbers of studies to review, and the deadline for completion.	• Review the One Minute Mentor Update on team member roles and responsibility • Set deadlines and keep them • Keep to a meeting schedule
Anticipate conflict during the appraisal process, such as disagreements about the quality of studies, quantity of studies to review, relevance of a study to the EBP project, meeting deadlines, and meeting expectations.	• Review the One Minute Mentor Update on Interprofessional Communication • Review and apply suggestions from Chapters 4 and 5

MENTOR TECHNIQUES AND SUPPORTS

The program coordinators need to work with mentors who are inexperienced with appraisal and research designs. Having mentors practice appraisal within the mentor meetings provides reassurance or validation that mentors are ready to work with their teams on this EBP task. Program coordinators should encourage mentors who have expertise to help those mentors who might need more development in their skills. Program coordinators should check in with mentors to see if they would like a research expert to attend one of the interprofessional EBP team meetings, particularly when the team is grappling with a complicated study or a study with a design unfamiliar to the team. Program coordinators should offer to review any of the appraisals about which the team has questions. Program coordinators should consider having joint check-in meetings of all the teams centered on discussing difficult appraisals as a way of learning and sharing how teams have managed these tougher appraisals. Table 9-6 outlines strategies to improve the appraisal process.

SUMMARY

This chapter focused on the process of appraising evidence collected for the team's interprofessional EBP project. There was an opportunity to review an abstract for determination of the relevancy of the study to the PICO question. The chapter addressed the barriers that may happen during the appraisal process and provided suggestions for overcoming those barriers. The chapter primarily focused on developing sound appraisal skills, including ways to organize the evidence in a manner that supports progress with this phase of the interprofessional EBP process. There are samples of synthesis tools included in this chapter.

REFLECTION QUESTIONS

1. Think about a practice change that may improve patient outcomes and identify the various types of evidence needed to recommend implementing the practice change.

2. Identify a type of evidence with which you are unfamiliar and read background information that clarifies the appropriate use of that type of evidence.

REFERENCES

Alderson, D. (2012). How to critically appraise a research paper. *Surgery, 30*(9), 477-480.doi:10.1016/j.mpsur.2012.06.002

Assadi, R., Zarghi, N., Shamloo, A., & Nikooiyan, Y. (2012). Evidence-based abstracts: What research summaries should contain to support evidence-based medicine. *International Journal of Evidence-Based Healthcare, 10,*154-158.

Atkins, D. (2007). Creating and synthesizing evidence with decision makers in mind: Integrating evidence from clinical trials and other study designs. *Medical Care, 10*(Suppl 2), S16-S22. doi:10.1097/mlr.0b013e3180616c3f

Aveyard, H. (2010). *Doing a literature review in health and social care: A practical guide* (2nd ed.). Maidenhead, UK: Open University Press.

Clark, E., Burkett, K., & Stanko-Lopp, D. (2009). Let Evidence Guide Every New Decision (LEGEND): An evidence evaluation system for point-of-care clinicians and guideline development teams. *Journal of Evaluation in Clinical Practice, 15*,1054-1060.doi:10.1111/j.1365-2753.2009.01314.x

Currow, D., & Agar, M. (2012). Evidence-based practice—Where does the buck stop? *Journal of Pharmacy Practice & Research, 42*, 91-93. doi:10.1002/j.2055-2335.2012.tb00140.x

D'Auria, J. P. (2007). Using an evidence-based approach to critical appraisal. *Journal of Pediatric Health Care, 21*(5), 343-346. doi:10.1016/j.pedhc.2007.06.002

Dearholt, S. L. & Dang, D. (2012). *Johns Hopkins nursing evidence-based practice: Model and guidelines* (2nd ed.). Indianapolis, IN: Sigma Theta Tau International.

Facchiano, L. & Snyder, C. (2012). Evidence-based practice for the busy nurse practitioner: Part three: Critical appraisal process. *Journal of the American Academy of Nurse Practitioners, 24*, 704-715. doi:10.1111/j.1745-7599.2012.00752.x

Fineout-Overholt, E., Melnyk, B. M., & Schultz, A. (2005). Transforming healthcare form the inside out: Advancing evidence-based practice in the 21st century. *Journal of Professional Nursing, 21*(6), 335-344. doi:10.1016/j.profnurs.2005.10.005

Glasgow, R. E., & Steiner, J. F. (2012). Comparative effectiveness research to accelerate translation: Recommendations for an emerging field of science. In R. C. Brownson, G. A. Colditz, & E. K. Proctor (Eds.), *Dissemination and implementation research in health: Translating science to practice.* New York, NY: Oxford University Press, 72-93.doi:10.1093/acprof:oso/9780199751877.003.0004

Ho, P. M., Peterson, P. N., & Masoudi, F. A. (2008). Evaluating the evidence: Is there a rigid hierarchy? *Circulation, 118*, 1675-1684. doi:10.1161/circulationaha.107.721357

Ilott, I. (2012). Evidence-based practice: A critical appraisal. *Occupational Therapy International, 19*, 1-6. doi:10.1002/oti.1322

Krainovich-Miller, B., Haber, J., & Jacobs, S. (2009). Evidence-based practice challenge: Teaching critical appraisal of systematic reviews and clinical practice guidelines to graduate students. *Journal of Nursing Education, 48*(4), 186-195. doi:10.3928/01484834-20090401-07

Lincoln, Y. S., & Guba, E. G. (1985). *Naturalistic Inquiry.* Beverly Hills, CA: Sage.

McCurtin, A., & Roddam, H. (2012). Evidence-based practice: SLTs under siege or opportunity for growth? The use and nature of research evidence in the profession. *International Journal of Language and Communication Disorders, 47*, 11-26. doi:10.1111/j.1460-6984.2011.00074.x

Metzler, M., & Metz, G. (2010). Translating knowledge to practice: An occupational therapy perspective. *Australian Occupational Therapy Journal, 57*, 373-379. doi:10.1111/j.1440-1630.2010.00873.x

Montori, V. M., Jaeschke, R., Schünemann, H. J., Bhandari, M., Brozek, J. I., Devereaux, P. J., & Guyatt, G. H. (2004). User's guide to detecting misleading claims in clinical research reports. *British Medical Journal (Clinical Research Edition), 329*(6), 1093-1096.doi:10.1136/bmj.329.7474.1093

Noordzij, M., Hooft, L., Dekker, F. W., Zoccali, C., & Jager, K. J. (2009). Systematic reviews and meta-analyses: When they are useful and when to be careful. *Kidney International, 78*, 1130-1136. doi:10.1038/ki.2009.339

Peterson, M., Barnason, S., Donnelly, B., Hill, K., Miley, H., Riggs, L, & Whiteman, K. (2014). Choosing the best evidence to guide clinical practice: Application of AACN Levels of Evidence. *Critical Care Nurse, 34*(2), 58-68. doi:10.4037/ccn2014411

Rothstein, H. R. (2008). Publication bias as a threat to the validity of meta-analytic results. *Journal of Experimental Criminology, 4*, 61-81. doi:10.1007/s11292-007-9046-9

Rothstein, H., Sutton, A. J., & Borenstein, M. (2005). *Publication bias in meta-analysis. Prevention, assessment and adjustments.* Chichester, UK: Wiley.doi: 10.1002/0470870168

Salbach, N., Jablal, S., Korner-Bitensky, N., Rappolt, S., & Davis, D. (2007). Practitioner and organizational barriers to evidence-based practice of physical therapists for people with stroke. *Physical Therapy, 87*, 1284-1303. doi:10.2522/ptj.20070040

Song, F., Hooper, L., & Loke, Y. K., (2013). Publication bias: what is it? How do we measure it? How do we avoid it? *Open Access Journal of Clinical Trials, 5*, 71-81. doi:10.2147/oajct.s34419

Titler, M. G., Kleiber, C., Steelman, V. J., Rakel, B. A. Budreau, G. Eberett, L. Q., … Goode, C. J. (2001). *The Iowa model of evidence-based practice to promote quality care.* Critical Care Nursing Clinics of North America, 13(4), 497-509.

Whiffin, C. J., & Hasselder, A. (2013). Making the link between critical appraisal, thinking and analysis. *British Journal of Nursing, 22*(14), 831-835. doi:10.12968/bjon.2013.22.14.831

Young, J. M., & Solomon, M. J. (2009). How to critically appraise an article. *Nature Clinical Practice: Gastroenterology and Hepatology, 6*(2), 82-91. doi:10.1038/ncpgasthep1331

Zidorov, D., Thomas, A., & Poissant, L. (2013). Knowledge translation in physical therapy: From theory to practice. *Disability and Rehabilitation, 35*, 1571-1577. doi:10.3109/09638288.2012.748841

Supplemental materials for this chapter are available online.
Please refer to the sticker in the front of the book and enter the access code provided.

Section III

- Preparation for an Interprofessional Evidence-Based Practice Program

  Section I

- Immersion Into the Evidence

  Section II

- Completion and Dissemination of the Interprofessional Evidence-Based Project

  Section III

Chapter 10	Designing the Interprofessional Evidence-Based Practice Project	What kind of project design should the interprofessional team use to study the practice change?
Chapter 11	Linking the Design to the Ethics of Evidence-Based Practice and Grant Funding	What are the ethical and grant funding issues that might occur in an evidence-based practice project?
Chapter 12	Planning and Implementing the Interprofessional Evidence-Based Practice Project	What implementation science principles guide the interprofessional team in managing their evidence-based practice project?
Chapter 13	Evaluating and Analyzing the Interprofessional Evidence-Based Practice Project	How does the interprofessional team analyze and interpret their results and arrive at recommendations for changing practice?
Chapter 14	Wrapping Up the Interprofessional Evidence-Based Practice Project	How does the interprofessional team make sure all evidence-based project tasks are completed on time and within budget?
Chapter 15	Disseminating the Interprofessional Evidence-Based Practice Project	How does the interprofessional team disseminate the results of the evidence-based practice project?

10

Designing the Interprofessional Evidence-Based Practice Project

David D. Chapman, PhD, PT/L and Vicky J. Larson, PhD, RN, CNE

CHAPTER TOPICS

- Designing the evidence-based practice project
- Research designs
- Non-research designs
- Selecting relevant outcome measures
- Determining the sample
- Data collection and analysis plan
- Mentor challenges
- Mentor techniques and supports

PERFORMANCE OBJECTIVES

At the conclusion of this chapter, the engaged reader will be able to state and explain the following:

1. Considerations guiding the team's decision making in regard to the design of the interprofessional evidence-based practice project.

2. Factors that the team considers when selecting relevant outcome measures for the interprofessional evidence-based practice project.

At this point, the team has already completed many significant steps toward completing the interprofessional evidence-based practice (EBP) project. The team has identified essential partners, succeeded in developing good team communication, selected the specific problem the team wanted to address, and spent considerable time refining the PICO question. Relevant research and related literature has been reviewed, critiqued, and synthesized (Everett & Titler, 2006) (see Chapter 9). Based on this foundation, the team is at the major decision point described in the Iowa model (Titler et al., 2001) to determine whether there is sufficient evidence collected from the literature to pilot

Moyers, P. A., & Finch-Guthrie, P. L.
Interprofessional Evidence-Based Practice:
A Workbook for Health Professionals (pp 155-165).
© 2016 Taylor and Francis Group.

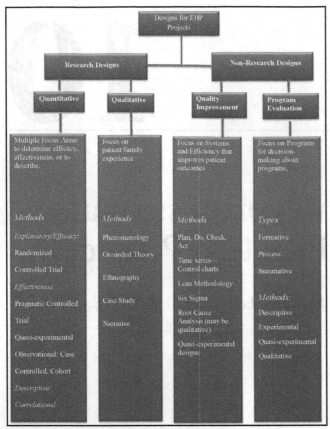

Figure 10-1. Designs for EBP projects.

methods, while non-research methodologies include QI and program evaluation. Note that QI and program evaluation may use both quantitative and qualitative designs, but are not considered research due to the purposes and goals of these methods. The goal of QI is to understand issues of efficiency and effectiveness of process and systems within the health care system, while the goal of program evaluation is to make decisions about a program. In fact, program evaluation might be more appropriate if occurring in the last steps of the Iowa model (Titler et al., 2001) where the determination to adapt the change in practice has been made and the organization seeks to scale implementation and assess the outcomes of the widespread practice change. However, QI methods are used either at the pilot of a practice change or during this last stage in the Iowa model (Titler et al.) sequence. Exemplar PICO questions are presented in Table 10-1 along with the research designs the interprofessional EBP team may use to answer the sample PICO questions.

Figure 10-2 highlights the various design components of the EBP practice project. The team should begin with the PICO question (see Chapter 7), located at the center of Figure 10-2, as it will guide the team's design process. For instance, the purpose of the EBP project could be to implement a well-supported intervention to determine its local effect on patient outcomes, design a QI project, or conduct an effectiveness study to explore an intervention further. Figure 10-2 is referred to throughout this chapter as the design components for an EBP project are discussed, including choosing a project design, selecting relevant outcome measures, determining the sample, and developing a data collection and analysis plan. However, two EBP project design components, funding and dissemination, are described in Chapters 11 and 15, respectively.

an interprofessional EBP practice change. If there is not sufficient literature, the question is whether the interprofessional team should design a research study to collect additional data that may be needed, or whether there are other types of data, such as case reports or expert opinion to guide the development of a EBP practice change pilot (see Chapter 1, Figure 1-2).

Once the interprofessional team makes a decision either to go forward with a pilot of a practice change or to conduct research, the interprofessional team is ready to design an EBP project that ultimately results in effective and sustainable change that supports the quality improvement (QI) goals of the health care organization. To help the team plan an appropriate and manageable interprofessional EBP project, this chapter provides an overview of several types of designs for the team to consider.

DESIGNING THE EVIDENCE-BASED PRACTICE PROJECT

For simplicity, Figure 10-1 categorizes EBP project designs broadly into research and non-research. Research methodologies include quantitative, qualitative, and mixed

RESEARCH DESIGNS

The research designs, according to Figures 10-1 and 10-2, include several quantitative approaches including studies determining efficacy of the intervention when using a randomized controlled trial (RCT) or determining the effectiveness of the intervention with a pragmatic controlled trial or an observational design. Descriptive or correlational designs might be helpful when the interprofessional team has specific questions about the percent of the population that improves as the result of the intervention, particularly noting whether key outcomes are correlated with population characteristics. Qualitative research, including ethnography, phenomenology, grounded theory, or a narrative study, is appropriate for addressing a meaning-related PICO question that the evidence has not clearly answered. A case study method is helpful when examining questions related to a process or how something occurred.

TABLE 10-1

EXEMPLAR PICO QUESTIONS WITH RESEARCH DESIGNS AND OUTCOME MEASURES

EXAMPLE PICO QUESTIONS	POSSIBLE DESIGNS	POSSIBLE OUTCOME MEASURES
What is the difference in daily pain ratings recorded in a pain diary for older adults living in the community with arthritis who participate in daily exercise compared to those who are sedentary?	• Experimental • True experiments • Quasi-experimental • Cross-sectional study • Cohort study	• Visual Analogue (Gallagher, Liebman, & Bijur, 2001) • Pain intensity scales (Hjermstad et al., 2011)
What is the difference in body mass index (BMI) for adolescents in 7th grade at the end of the academic year who are attending a school with a school-based obesity prevention program throughout the year compared to those who attend a school that does not have a prevention program?	• Nonexperimental • Cohort Study • Cross-sectional study	• Body Mass Index (BMI) http://www.nhlbi.nih.gov/health/educational/lose_wt/BMI/bmicalc.htm
What are the factors (number of concussions, years playing football, football position, age when starting to play football.) that predict the development of cognitive impairment?	• Nonexperimental • Correlational • Regression	• Automated Neuropsychological Assessment Metrics (Cernich, Reeves, Sun, & Bleiberg, 2007)
What is the lived experience for caregivers caring for a family member receiving hemodialysis in an outpatient clinic?	• Nonexperimental • Qualitative: interpretive or descriptive phenomenology	• Interviews • Focus groups • Observations

Quantitative Designs

There are several types of quantitative research designs including RCTs, pragmatic clinical trials (PCTs), quasi-experimental studies, and observational and descriptive studies that may be used to achieve the goal of the EBP project (Meyer, Wheeler, Weibberger, Chen, & Carpenter, 2014). Irrespective of the type of quantitative approach the team chooses to implement, the results will be organized as numbers (e.g., frequency counts, means, and standard deviations) (see Chapter 13). In selecting a quantitative design, the team may consider implementing an experimental approach, such as a RCT, which is the current gold standard for assessing the efficacy of a given intervention. These types of studies are challenging to complete in an applied practice setting because RCTs require that participants meeting the inclusion criteria be randomly assigned to a given intervention technique in order to determine whether a treatment works (Meyer et al., 2014). While these studies have strong internal validity, they have less external validity. Typically, RCTs involve homogeneous groups of participants who tend to have fewer comorbidities than would be found in the general patient population (Gartlehner, Hansen, Bissman, Lohr, & Carey, 2006), which

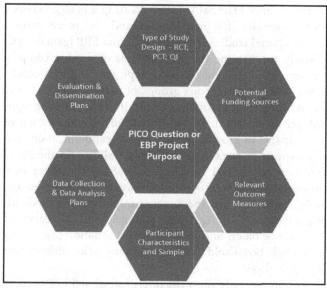

Figure 10-2. Elements of the EBP project design.

makes generalizing the treatment to a larger population difficult. In addition, RCTs tend to test more simplistic interventions, such as a single medication against a control group whose participants do not receive the medication.

Figure 10-3. Overview of RCTs and PCTs.

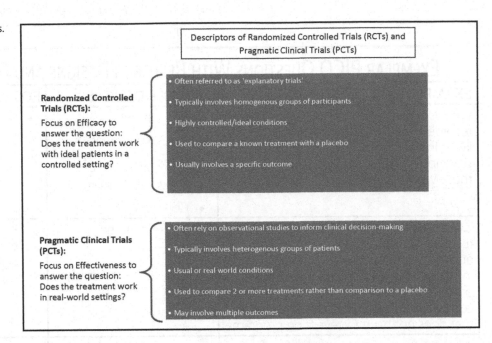

These types of studies have also been described as explanatory trials because they seek to assess the treatment effect under ideal and often highly controlled conditions (Gartlehner et al., 2006).

Observational studies, such as cohort and case-control designs, while having stronger external validity because of their study of populations under natural conditions, have less internal validity, making it hard to determine cause and effect relationships. PCTs or real-world trials provide a design that has significant internal validity while also having higher external validity, creating a bridge between experimentally designed studies and the more natural observational studies. Within a PCT, the EBP team designs a study to examine the effectiveness of a more complex treatment or intervention under typical or everyday conditions with heterogeneous groups of participants that may be subdivided into smaller clinically relevant subgroups (Meyer et al., 2014). PCTs still include randomization of participants to groups or use a cluster randomization process, which ensures greater internal validity. In the PICO question mentioned in Chapter 9 about the effect of a 30-minute walking program on pulse rate, blood pressure, weight, and lifestyle, the analysis might include subdividing participants by age (e.g., younger than 75 years and 75 years or older) and by their living situation (e.g., living in a single household dwelling or living in an independent living facility).

Pragmatic trials allow the interprofessional EBP team to examine potential practice differences across settings and across providers, comparing interventions with alternative interventions versus using the traditional control group of no intervention. When the pragmatic trial indicates the effectiveness of an intervention that is also supported with evidence from the appraisal process indicating its efficacy,

the interprofessional team is able to make recommendations for a permanent change in practice, an important step in the Iowa model (Titler et al., 2001). Figure 10-3 summarizes the characteristics of RCTs and PCTs.

The interprofessional EBP team would benefit from examining the Pragmatic-Explanatory Continuum Indicator Summary (PRECIS) model as a guide for designing a pragmatic trial (Thorpe, Zwarenstein, & Oxman, 2009; Zwarenstein, Treweek, Gagnier, & CONSORT Group, 2008) when the aim is to determine effectiveness and generalize to a broader population. The CONSORT Work Group on Pragmatic Trials originally developed the PRECIS model as an approach that investigators use to evaluate the relative clinical applicability of a given project in comparison to a project that aims to determine a specific cause or mechanism for an observed effect (Elder & Munk, 2014). The PRECIS model outlines 10 dimensions of a study to assess, including the relative flexibility of the experimental intervention, practitioner research expertise, eligibility criteria of the participants, and practitioner adherence. According to Elder and Munk (2014) and Gaglio, Phillips, Heurtin-Roberts, Sanchez, and Glasgow, (2014), team members rate their decisions regarding participant eligibility from low (1) to high (5), with a highly pragmatic study design receiving a 5. If the team planned to enroll participants who have the condition of interest regardless of their comorbidities, previous levels of compliance with a specific treatment, and the participant's potential responsiveness to treatment, the team would rate their design as a 5, indicating one criterion for a pragmatic design is met.

Another quantitative research design that might be used in an EBP project is a quasi-experimental design. The key difference between experimental or quasi-experimental techniques is how participants are assigned to groups. In the experimental approach, the investigator randomly assigns participants to any group within the study design. In quasi-experimental studies, the researcher assigns participants conveniently to the control or treatment condition (e.g., as they are admitted to a care unit) or the design does not have a control group but includes multiple measurements of the same participants (e.g., pre- and post-test, or delayed post-test). The interprofessional team might choose a quasi-experimental design when randomization is not possible or is not ethically desirable. Shapira, Barak, and Gal (2007) conducted a quasi-experimental study that examined older adult's well-being after they received Internet training. In this study, the goal was to provide Internet training to all of the elders who wanted the education, so randomization was not possible.

Observational designs were described in Chapter 9 as involving case-control and cohort designs, where for both designs a comparison group is carefully matched with a naturally occurring group that underwent the experience of interest. Both groups are then followed either retrospectively (i.e., in case-control studies) or prospectively (i.e., in cohort studies) in order to determine differences between the two groups on factors of interest. Descriptive research methods may be more familiar to the team where collecting data is for helping the team describe or assess current levels of performance (e.g., once the physician makes a referral for a patient to receive speech and language therapy, how many days does it take a patient to begin this service?). The interprofessional team may decide to determine the relative strength of the relationship between two or more variables using a correlational research method (e.g., what is the relationship between gender and levels of pain experienced following total hip replacement surgery?). Notice these observational and descriptive designs do not manipulate an independent variable as is true of experimental or quasi-experimental research designs. Only experimental designs determine whether an intervention strategy leads to a particular patient response or creates a difference in outcomes between two groups or more.

Qualitative Research

Within the qualitative approach, there are three distinct traditions (Brown, 2012). One method is phenomenology, which the team may use to understand the "lived experience" of individuals. For example, if the team members were working to understand better the lived experience of person(s) with a certain diagnosis or condition, this would be an appropriate methodology to employ. However, if the team were concerned about meeting the needs of individuals from a unique cultural background, then it would be more appropriate to use ethnographic techniques, in which the norms, values, social rules, and roles of people who come from a particular culture become the focus (Brown, 2012). Alternatively, if the purpose of the EBP project is to

develop a "tentative, coherent explanation" (p. 42) about how health care is being delivered in the organization, then the team may want to use grounded theory research (Brown, 2012).

All three qualitative approaches may require the team to complete observations of the persons in which the team is interested, to review documents and artifacts, and to conduct interviews that consist of open-ended questions. From the observation notes, documents, and interview transcripts, the team works inductively to develop codes representing key categories. How these categories are interrelated is the discovery that occurs as part of the process of identifying themes. The team then interprets these themes in relationship to the PICO question of the EBP project. Jacobson et al. (2008) used qualitative methodology to understand the patients' perceptions of total knee replacement surgery.

Mixed Methods

Another research approach the team may consider in designing the EBP project is a combination of qualitative and quantitative methods. This combination is often referred to as a *mixed-methods approach*. The team collects qualitative data via observations and interviews and quantitative data through various measurement strategies, such as surveys and self-assessment measures of knowledge, attitudes, and skills. Mixed-methods research is surprisingly complex and requires enough time and an understanding of the variety of ways to mix the qualitative with the quantitative data in order to produce a coherent study from start to finish (Creswell & Plano Clark, 2011). Mix-method designs do not involve a casual combination of the different forms of data but instead involve such strategies as merging, connecting, and embedding data.

Merging or convergent designs occurs when the researcher reports quantitative statistical results and then provides qualitative quotes or themes that support or refute the quantitative results (Sandelowski, Voils, & Knafl, 2009). In order to enable comparison with the quantitative data set, another way to merge the data occurs when the qualitative data set is transformed through the counting of the occurrence of themes. Creswell and Plano Clark (2011) described the process of connecting data or explanatory mixed methods as occurring when the analysis of one data set informs subsequent design and data collection for a second phase of the study. Perhaps the results of a quantitative survey guides development of the qualitative interview questions used subsequently. The embedding type of designs happens when the analysis of a data set of secondary importance is included within the analysis of the primary set of data. Asking qualitative questions as participants concurrently engage in an experimental trial to determine how they would describe their experience of the intervention is an example of embedding.

NON-RESEARCH DESIGNS

Non-research designs include QI and program evaluation. Each has a focus distinctive from research and from each other. The aim of QI is the systematic evaluation of performance (e.g., increasing efficiency) and quality (e.g., reducing medical errors), and the methods to improve both. The goal of QI or performance improvement is to remove waste in the system in order to decrease costs and increase value. The purpose of program evaluation, in contrast, is to determine whether the program achieved its pre-identified patient goals or outcomes and program effectiveness goals, such as costs.

Quality Improvement Designs

A commonly used method in health care organizations and systems is QI. QI typically involves systematic efforts aimed at improving the health care services provided to select patient populations (U.S. Department of Health and Human Services, 2011). QI methods have been described as the "unceasing efforts" of each individual involved in the health care system to implement new or different modes of service delivery to improve patient outcomes (Batalden & Davidoff, 2007).

It is common for the team to have questions about the differences between QI projects and research studies. The mentor and team members should keep in mind that QI projects usually involve collecting data from small samples. In addition, QI often involves multiple changes in protocols or interventions as the team continues to learn about and refine their work to improve patient outcomes and services. The focus of QI is on local application of efforts rather than trying to collect data or information generalized from a given sample to a general population (Varkey, Reller, & Resar, 2007).

In contrast, research studies usually collect data from larger samples of participants, rely on relatively strict protocols that do not change or vary during the study, and focus more on collecting data that can be generalized from the local situation to a more global setting. There are instances, however, when a QI project may also be considered research. This occurs if the QI project involves comparing a new intervention with an established practice or procedure, individual patients serving as participants, randomly assigning treatments and patients to the study conditions, and exposing participants to risks that they would normally not experience if they were not involved with the QI project (Varkey et al., 2007).

Typically, QI projects rely on plan, do, study, act (PDSA) cycles, Six Sigma, and Lean methodology as the team works to improve patient outcomes, the competence of staff, and the efficiency and safety of the service delivery system (Batalden & Davidoff, 2007; Varkey et al., 2007). The PDSA approach is the most common method used in QI projects (Varkey et al.). This approach involves four repetitive steps that are implemented on a small scale, such as at the unit level, before being applied throughout an entire department or organization. The four PDSA steps include the following (Varkey et al.):

1. Plan: Objectives are developed, potential outcomes are identified, and an implementation plan is developed.

2. Do: The plan is implemented.

3. Study: The team summarizes what was learned or observed from the initial trial.

4. Act: The outcomes of the first application trial are used to inform the team regarding what changes should be incorporated into future trials.

Six Sigma began in the mid-1980s and involves five key steps (Varkey et al., 2007). These include the following:

1. Define: The team works to identify the customer's needs, the scope of the project, project goals, criteria of success, team member selection and roles, and time deadlines.

2. Measurement: The team develops and implements their data collection plan in order to determine how errors are currently being made as services are provided.

3. Analysis: The team focuses on outcomes that deviate from the expected level of performance and why those deviations occurred.

4. Improve: The team develops and implements strategies that are designed to improve the expected outcome, (i.e., reduce the observed deviations from the expected levels of performance).

5. Control: The team develops and implements new policies, guidelines, and tactics aimed at minimizing the deviations from the expected outcome in the future.

Consider the application of the Six Sigma approach to a hospital unit treating patients who have had total hip or knee replacement surgeries. These surgical procedures are well-planned, involving multiple steps (e.g., preoperative skin preparation and antibiotic administration, initiation of therapy services, and timing of pain medications) that can be studied and potentially improved through the Six Sigma approach. For example, the number of minutes or hours that elapse between when the patient arrives in the room following the procedure and the beginning of physical therapy is studied in order to decrease the time lapse between the two events. Likewise, QI targets the timing of when pain medications are administered relative to therapy sessions so that the patient's pain is well-controlled during therapy.

Lean methodology is a third approach that QI teams commonly use to improve patient outcomes and service delivery models (Varkey et al., 2007). The Lean approach focuses on removing or eliminating non–value-added services or activities. Any type of activity that does not add value for the patient or customer is considered waste within the Lean methodology. QI teams that use this technique focus on reducing the following:

- Over- or under-production (e.g., low staff productivity and staff overtime)

- Wasted inventory of supplies

- Errors in performance (e.g., lags in pain medications being dispensed or incomplete documentation)

- Wasted motion (e.g., inefficient ergonomic work stations)

- Patient or customer wait times

- Policies and procedures that increase waste (e.g. using paper output when electronic records are available)

- Transportation time waste (e.g., the time waste that occurs when transporting patients from their room to the rehabilitation area in comparison to the time waste that occurs when therapists see the patient in the hospital room)

Program Evaluation

Program evaluation methods are appropriate if a practice change includes implementation of various programs or modifications of existing programs, such as a patient education program, a competency program for staff, or a prevention program for population health problems. Program evaluation typically involves several types of evaluation. For instance, formative evaluation occurring before the program informs program development, process evaluation occurring while the program is running examines program implementation, and summative evaluation occurring when the program has been completed assesses the short- and long-term changes of participant performance, health status, or behavior change (Berkowitz et al., 2008).

For programs to be effective, they must lead to real reductions in risk or improvements in health or performance (Goldsmith & Harris, 2013). Measurable change to one or more of the assessment metrics used in the summative program evaluation results only when the program fully engages enough participants. Engagement in the program is more than mere attendance. Finally, improvements must be sustainable long term to derive an important difference. Programs are not effective if change lasts for only several days or months once the participant has completed the program (Goldsmith & Harris).

Program evaluation designs depend on the purpose, whether formative, process, or summative. All program evaluation methods may use a mix of qualitative and quantitative methods, such as a market survey (quantitative) and focus groups (qualitative) as data collection tools

for a formative evaluation to develop a program. Process program evaluations typically determine fidelity of the program in terms of whether the participants actively engage (e.g., course evaluations, attendance records, number of program activities completed, and participation level during program activities) and learn throughout the program (pre- and post-knowledge testing or competency demonstrations). Summative evaluations may involve qualitative interviews and quantitative self-assessment surveys, and observation of skill demonstrations at multiple points after completion of the program (e.g., at the program end, and at 3- and 6-month follow-up). The results of the process and summative program evaluations are compared to the program goals and objectives to interpret program success.

In terms of training programs, the model of program evaluation Kirkpatrick and Kirkpatrick (2006) developed is helpful. This model consists of four levels: reaction (e.g., participant satisfaction or how the learner plans to act), learning (e.g., changes in cognitive, psychomotor, or affective domains), behavior (e.g., participants using or applying what they learned in practice), and results (e.g., impact of the learning on the organization).

SELECTING RELEVANT OUTCOME MEASURES

Most EBP project designs require the interprofessional team to select relevant outcome measures for the project (see Figure 10-2). The interprofessional team previously defined conceptually the outcome in the PICO question, which becomes the basis for operationalizing the outcome. Review Table 10-1 for possible outcome measures for each of the exemplar PICO questions. If the team decides to define pain as whatever the patient says it is, for example, then the team would consider a measure of the patient's subjective experience of pain. Selecting relevant outcome measures may be the most important step the team completes to develop a successful EBP project. In general, outcome measures focus on measuring the following: (a) *health care processes* (e.g., provider productivity or how a patient experiences his or her care); (b) *patient-reported outcome measures* (PROMs) that address specific questions (e.g., did the health care service improve the patient's health and sense of well-being?); and (c) *population health measures* that assess the effectiveness of selected interventions on population health traits (e.g., the incidence of hypertension within a given patient population) (Hostetter & Klein, 2012). The Agency for Healthcare Research and Quality (2014) described similar purposes of outcome measures, such as measuring the quality of the patient care provided, assessing caregiver accountability, supplying the data needed to answer a particular patient care-related research question, or measuring a combination of these purposes.

A productive starting point for identifying an outcome measure is to work with the stakeholders in the organization to determine whether the health care organization is already using measures that would address the outcome (McGlynn, 1997). For example, the Joint Commission on Hospital Accreditation requires acute care organizations to collect core measures around heart failure, stroke, and acute myocardial infarction (The Joint Commission, n.d.). In addition, many organizations collect information on patient satisfaction. Specifically, the Hospital Consumer Assessment of Healthcare Providers (HCAHPS, n.d.) is a standardized survey for determining patient perceptions of the quality of care benchmarked to national scores. This survey is available in multiple languages through the Centers for Medicare and Medicaid Services (www.CMS.gov). Many organizations also have patient registries, which they use to evaluate both process and outcomes of patient care. If the PICO question involves a rehabilitation problem, the team may want to measure staff productivity, patient gains on the Functional Independence Measure (FIM) (Uniform Data System for Medical Rehabilitation, n.d.) and patient responses to the 36-Item Short-Form Health Survey Version 2.0 (SF-36v2) (Ware, Snow, Kosinski, & Gandek, 1993; Ware, Kosinski, & Dewey, 2000; Ware & Kosinski, 2001). Staff productivity provides the efficiency and cost data of an individual provider or of a team, such as a rehabilitation team. Data from the FIM assesses the caregiver's effectiveness in facilitating the patient gains in daily functional performance, such as in activities of daily living. Patient perceptions regarding an intervention's effectiveness in improving overall health status, functional status, and health-related quality of life are measured with the SF-36v2.

Even though the health care organization may collect multiple measures of health care effectiveness, it may not be feasible or productive for the team to use the data from all of those measures. Moreover, the EBP interprofessional team may determine one or more of their chosen outcome measures may not be important or financially relevant to the health care organization. Thus, the team will have to choose wisely regarding which outcome measures to include in the interprofessional EBP project. Stakeholder feedback about the possible outcome measure is often warranted given that staff in the health care organization may be using a new outcome measure of which the team is currently unaware.

Once the team has identified a potential outcome measure, the team will need to assess the relative quality of each measure the team wants to implement as part of the interprofessional EBP project (Agency for Healthcare Quality and Research, 2014). The team should answer the following four broad questions to assess the quality of each outcome measure:

1. Is the measure important or *relevant* to the various stakeholders within the health care organization?

2. Is the measure *scientifically sound* (e.g., is it valid, reliable, and sensitive to the proposed practice change)?

3. Is it feasible to collect and analyze the data on the phenomenon that the outcome measure is intended to assess?

4. Does the outcome measure capture the impact of the practice change on patient care?

In addition to the considerations described, the team should think about how important the outcome measure is to the health and well-being of the patients. The interprofessional team needs to decide whether the practice change has potential to improve the outcome the team is evaluating. The team also needs to evaluate whether the measure under consideration is strategically as well as financially important to the stakeholders (Agency for Healthcare Research and Quality, 2014). It is possible that the team will not be able to improve the performance on a given outcome measure if the resources needed to influence that measure are beyond the control of the health care organization. For example, if a separate organization owns and operates the ambulance service for an acute care organization, it may not be possible to improve the transport times for patients who may be having a cerebrovascular accident. Thus, it may not be prudent to pursue an interprofessional EBP project designed to reduce the transport times of these patients unless a strong and collaborative partnership exists between the two organizations.

The team should consider whether the outcome measure is clinically logical, significant, and applicable to the patients in the facility. In addition to validity and reliability, the team should also determine whether the staff members view the outcome measure as helpful in clinical decision making. As a result, the team needs to determine whether the outcome measure is relevant to the key stakeholders that the team identified early in the design phase of the interprofessional EBP project (Agency for Healthcare Research and Quality, 2014). The reader should examine information on the National Quality Measures Clearinghouse (www.qualitymeasures.ahrq.gov/) and on the National Quality Forum (www.qualityforum.org) about potential measures appropriate for an interprofessional EBP project.

The interprofessional EBP team verifies that they have the abilities and resources needed to answer their PICO question as well as to achieve the goal of the EBP project within the prescribed time. The team determines whether they have the knowledge and skills needed to analyze the data they plan to collect during the EBP project. This is a good reminder that it is often wise to consult with statisticians and research methodologists early in the design phase of the EBP project. This additional step, although time-consuming and potentially costly, allows the team to move forward with confidence knowing that they have an appropriately designed EBP project as well as possess the skills and resources needed to fully analyze the data collected during the implementation of the EBP project (see Chapter 13).

The team should also verify that the outcome measures they have selected would accurately measure the results of the practice change. For example, to assess a change in practice regarding how patient pain is treated, the team may need to collect valid and reliable pain ratings from their patients prior to beginning the new intervention as well as at the end of the of the EBP project. In this straightforward example, if the team does not collect baseline pain ratings before they begin their practice change, it is difficult, if not impossible, to fully assess the effectiveness of the EBP practice change.

DETERMINING THE SAMPLE

An important step in designing an interprofessional EBP project is to determine the sample that represents the population identified in the PICO question and the literature synthesis (see Figure 10-2). There are different methods for sampling such as randomization, convenient, or purposeful that the team selects based on the PICO question and the methodology. For example, purposeful samples are appropriate for qualitative methods because the goal is to understand the experience of the participants. Randomized samples are appropriate for interprofessional EBP projects with an experimental design. When randomization is not possible, the team may need to use a convenient sample. The team should consider the following about the sample:

- Inclusion and exclusion criteria for the sample
- Size of the sample (larger samples tend to be more representative of a given population [Domholdt, 2000]; it is wise to plan for a small amount of participant attrition)
- The relative strength of the interventions (e.g., stronger interventions usually lead to using a smaller sample size)
- The number of variables measured and manipulated
- The analysis approach

DATA COLLECTION AND ANALYSIS PLAN

In order to design an achievable interprofessional EBP project, the team needs to develop data collection strategies and data analysis approaches (see Figure 10-2). The mentor ensures that the team members have the skills and expertise needed to collect and analyze the data. For determining the details of the data analysis portion of the design, the team solicits and secures the advice of a statistician. Statisticians

point out potential limitations to the project design, which is helpful to the team in making changes to the design when possible in order to reduce the effect of these limitations on the interpretation of the outcomes. Note that the team should include the costs associated with using a statistician in the budget for the interprofessional EBP project. To verify the feasibility of the data collection and analysis, the team should consider the following questions:

- How long will it take the team to collect the data? (Remember, the length of time to complete an EBP project typically depends on the length of the program.)
- Will the team collect *retrospective data* from electronic health records, medical databases, or financial records? Or will the team collect *prospective data* as a result of implementing a new intervention strategy or cost-saving approach?
- What are the financial costs associated with collecting data?
- Does the team have the people and technological resources to collect and analyze the data?
- How does the sample size for the data collection affect the project resources?

MENTOR CHALLENGES

The design phase of the interprofessional EBP project is detailed, time-consuming, and requires that team members employ skills related to design, outcome measure selection, and data analysis. The mentor needs to facilitate self-assessment of each team members' knowledge and skills in these three main areas so that the team may strategize ways to obtain the additional support needed. The mentor must confront the unrealistic expectations of team members that the team does not need outside help with the design and the required statistical analysis, especially when team members possess a basic level of these skills. The team must be prepared to handle frustration of team members who may be working near the limits of their expertise, while simultaneously holding team members accountable for timely completion of each task within the design process (e.g., selecting relevant outcome measures).

MENTOR TECHNIQUES AND SUPPORTS

Mentors use mentor techniques to ensure the team not only meet on a consistent basis, but that the team members schedule extra meetings to design the project in order to avoid spending too many weeks on this EBP phase. The mentor provides realistic and positive feedback to each team member, hears the concerns of the team, and assigns each person to work on tasks that are well-matched to his or her strengths, such as having the students conduct a literature search on specific outcome measures.

Mentor supports that are especially important to consider during the design phase of the EBP project include having a program coordinator who can mentor or instruct the mentor and team members regarding the tasks that may be new to the team and the mentor. For example, having a program coordinator assist the team with evaluating the pros and cons of potential outcome measures can be critical to team success. It may be productive for the team to receive education or training about different research designs (e.g., observational studies, and cross-sectional versus longitudinal designs that may be used to help the team answer their PICO question). In addition, program coordinators should secure outside experts as needed for feedback about the design and the planned statistical analysis.

SUMMARY

The purpose of the design phase is to create a manageable interprofessional EBP project for practice change based on the appraisal and synthesis of the literature. Design requires knowledge of research and non-research approaches that appropriately match the purpose of the EBP project and the PICO question. In addition, the interprofessional EBP team selects relevant outcome measures that are important strategically and financially to the organization. The leader of this design phase of the project assists the team in developing an interprofessional EBP project that is manageable and that leads to a sustainable, effective practice change for the health care organization. As the team completes the design phase of the work, the team will be well-prepared to obtain institutional review board approval if needed and to develop a successful funding proposal.

REFLECTION QUESTIONS

1. What factors should the interprofessional EBP team consider as they select a project design?

2. How will the interprofessional EBP team verify the feasibility of the data collection and analysis plan?

REFERENCES

Agency for Healthcare Research and Quality. (2014) *Tutorials on quality measures.* Retrieved from www.qualitymeasures.ahrq.gov/tutorial/varieties.aspx

Batalden, P. B., & Davidoff, F. (2007). What is "quality improvement" and how can it transform healthcare? *Quality Safe Healthcare, 16*(1) 2-3. http://dx.doi.org/10.1136/qshc.2006.022046.

Berkowitz, J., Huhman, M., Heitzler, C., Potter, L., Nolin, M. J., & Banspach, S. (2008). Overview of formative, process, and outcome evaluation methods used in the VERB Campaign. *American Journal of Preventive Medicine, 34*, S222–S22. doi:10.1016/j.amepre.2008.03.008

Brown, S. J. (2012). *Evidence-based nursing: The research-practice connection* (2nd ed.). Sudbury, MA: Jones and Bartlett Learning.

Cernich, A., Reeves, D., Sun, W., & Bleiberg, J. (2007). Automated neuropsychological assessment metrics sports medicine battery. *Archives of Clinical Medicine, 22* (Supplement 1), S101-114. doi: 10.1016/j.acn.2006.10.008

Creswell, J. W., & Plano Clark, V. L. (2011). *Designing and conducting mixed methods research.* Los Angeles, CA: Sage.

Domholdt, E. (2000). *Physical therapy research: Principles and applications* (2nd ed.). Philadelphia, PA: WB Saunders.

Elder, W. G., & Munk, N. (2014). Using the pragmatic-explanatory continuum indicator summary (PRECIS) model in clinical research: Application to refine a practice-based research network (PBRN) study. *Journal of the American Board of Family Medicine, 27*(6), 846-854.

Everett, L. Q., & Titler, M. G. (2006). Making EBP part of clinical practice: The Iowa model. In R.F. Levin & H.R. Feldman (Eds.), *Teaching evidence-based practice in nursing* (pp. 295-324). New York, NY: Springer Publishing Company.

Gaglio, B., Phillips, S. M., Heurtin-Roberts, S., Sanchez, M. A., & Glasgow, R. E. (2014). How pragmatic is it? Lessons learned using PRECIS and RE-AIM for determining pragmatic characteristics of research. *Implementation Science, 9*(1),1-11. doi:10.1186/s13012-014-0096-x

Gallagher, E. J., Liebman, M., & Bijur, P. E. (2001). Prospective validation of clinically important changes in pain severity measured on a visual analog scale. *Annals of Emergency Medicine, 38*, 633-638. doi:10.1067/mem.2001.118863

Gartlehner, G., Hansen, R., Bissman, D., Lohr, K., & Carey, T. (2006). *Criteria for distinguishing effectiveness from efficacy trials in systematic reviews. Technical Review 12.* Rockville, MD: Agency of Healthcare and Research Quality.

Goldsmith, R., & Harris, S. (2013). Thinking inside the box: The health cube paradigm for health and wellness program evaluation and design. *Population Health Management, 16*, 291-295.doi: 10.1089/pop.2012.0103

Hjermstad, M. J., Fayers, P. M., Haugen, D. F., Caraceni, A., Hanks, G. W., Loge, J. H.,... Kaasa, S. (2011). Studies comparing numerical rating scales, verbal rating scales, and visual analogue scales for assessment of pain intensity in adults: A systematic literature review. *Journal of Pain and Symptom Management, 41*, 1073-1093. doi:10.1016/j.jpainsymman.2010.08.016

Hospital Consumer Assessment of Healthcare Providers and Systems (HCAHPS). (n.d.). Survey instruments. Retrieved from http://hcahpsonline.org/surveyinstrument.aspx., June 30, 2015.

Hostetter, M., & Klein, S. (2012). Quality matters: The commonwealth fund. Retrieved from www.commonwealthfund.org/publications/newsletters/quality-matters/2012/october-november/in-focus

Jacobson, A. F., Muerscough, R. P., Delambo, D., Fleming, E., Huddleston, A. M., Bright, N., & Varley, J. D. (2008). Patients' perspectives on total knee replacement. *American Journal of Nursing, 108*(5), 54-63. doi:10.1097/01.naj.0000318000.62786.fb

Kirkpatrick, D. L., & Kirkpatrick, J. D. (2006). *Evaluating training programs: The four levels* (3rd ed.). San Francisco, CA: Berrett-Koehler.

McGlynn, E. A. (1997). Six challenges in measuring the quality of health care, *Health Affairs, 16*(3), 7-21. doi:10.1377/hlthaff.16.3.7

Meyer, A. M., Wheeler, S. B., Weibberger, M., Chen, R. C., & Carpenter, W. R. (2014). An overview of methods for comparative effectiveness research. *Seminars in Radiation Oncology, 24*(1), 5-13. doi:10.1016/j.semradonc.2013.09.002

Sandelowski, M., Voils, C. I., & Knafl, G. (2009). On quantitizing. *Journal of Mixed Methods Research, 3*(3), 208-222. doi:10.1177/1558689809334210

Shapira, N., Barak, A., & Gal, I. (2007). Promoting older adults' well-being through Internet training and use. *Aging & Mental Health, 11*(5), 477-484.

The Joint Commission. (n.d.). *Specifications manual for National Hospital Inpatient Quality Measures.* Retrieved from www.jointcommission.org/specifications_manual_for_national_hospital_inpatient_quality_measures.aspx, June 30, 2015.

Thorpe, K. E., Zwarenstein, M., & Oxman, A. D. (2009). A pragmatic-explanatory continuum indicator summary (PRECIS): A tool to help trial designers. *Journal of Clinical Epidemiology, 62*(5), 464-475. doi:10.1016/j.jclinepi.2008.12.011

Titler, M. G., Kleiber, C. Steelman, V. J., Rakel, B. A., Budreau, G., Everett, L. Q., & Goode, C. J. (2001). The Iowa model of evidence-based practice to promote quality care. *Critical Care Nursing Clinics of North America, 13*(4), 497-509.

Uniform Data System for Medical Rehabilitation. (n.d.). Retrieved from www.udsmr.org/WebModules/FIM/Fim_About.aspx, August 8, 2015.

U.S. Department of Health and Human Services Health Resources and Services Administration. (2011, April). Quality Improvement. http://www.hrsa.gov/quality/toolbox/508pdfs/qualityimprovement.pdf.

Varkey, P., Reller, M. K., & Resar, R. K. (2007). Basics of quality improvement in healthcare. *Mayo Clinic Proceedings, 82*(6):735-739. doi:10.1016/s0025-6196(11)61194-4

Ware, J. E., Snow, K. K., Kosinski, M., & Gandek, B. (1993). *SF-36® health survey manual and interpretation guide.* Boston, MA: New England Medical Center, The Health Institute.

Ware, J. E., Kosinski, M. & Dewey, J. E. (2000). *How to score version two of the SF-36 health survey.* Lincoln, RI: QualityMetric, Incorporated.

Ware, J. E., & Kosinski, M. (2001). *SF-36 Physical and mental health summary scales: A manual for users of version 1, second edition.* Lincoln, RI: QualityMetric Incorporated.

Zwarenstein, M., Treweek, S., & Gagnier, J. J., CONSORT Group; Pragmatic Trials in Healthcare Group. (2008). Improving the reporting of pragmatic trials: An extension of the CONSORT statement. *British Medical Journal, 337,* a2390. doi:10.1136/bmj.a2390

Supplemental materials for this chapter are available online.
Please refer to the sticker in the front of the book and enter the access code provided.

11

Linking the Design to the Ethics of Evidence-Based Practice and Grant Funding

*David D. Chapman, PhD, PT/L; Vicky J. Larson, PhD, RN, CNE; and
Patricia L. Finch-Guthrie, PhD, RN*

CHAPTER TOPICS

- Ethical considerations for designing an evidence-based practice project
- Linking the project design with institutional review board approval
- Funding the interprofessional evidence-based practice project
- Mentor challenges
- Mentor techniques and mentor supports

PERFORMANCE OBJECTIVES

At the conclusion of this chapter, the engaged reader will be able to do the following:

1. Design a practice change project that considers the ethical protection of human subjects.

2. Determine whether institutional review board approval is needed for non-research projects.

3. Understand how to submit the evidence-based practice project to the institutional review board.

4. Prepare a successful external funding application to support the interprofessional evidence-based practice project.

Following the design phase of an interprofessional evidence-based practice (EBP) project, team members are excited to initiate their project. During the design process, the team addresses any ethical concerns relevant to protecting human subjects and subsequently makes necessary changes within the design to safeguard the rights of the participants. An important ethical issue involves the interprofessional team making sure the project is well-designed. Limited internal validity within a project creates results that are not reliable, thereby causing undue risk for participants and a waste of limited resources (Emanuel, Wendler, & Grady, 2000). The federal statutes for conducting research (United States Department of Health and Human Services [USDHHS], 2009, Title 45 Code for Federal Regulations [CFR] 46) create a common understanding in which all disciplines are responsible to protect the rights of human subjects. However, ethical standards for implementing non-research–based EBP (e.g., quality improvement and

Moyers, P. A., & Finch-Guthrie, P. L.
*Interprofessional Evidence-Based Practice:
A Workbook for Health Professionals* (pp 167-181).
© 2016 Taylor and Francis Group.

program evaluation) is currently lacking (Carter et al., 2011; Gondolf, 2000; Kumar, Grimmer-Somers, & Hughes, 2010; Loi & McDermott, 2010). In addition, many institutions do not have formal processes for reviewing the quality of non-research EBP change projects, which makes it more important that an interprofessional team carefully considers potential ethical issues when using non-research methods (Platteborze et al., 2010).

The ethics of conducting EBP also include having the financial support necessary to implement the project and disseminate the findings, as well as ensuring appropriate management of finite resources (Emanuel et al., 2000). The interprofessional team works with the EBP program coordinators to assure funding is available within the operational budget of the health care organization. Applying for grant funding is another strategy the interprofessional team may use to support a project and cover costs associated with new equipment and instruments, education of staff and the interprofessional team, and collecting and analyzing data. The purpose of this chapter is to provide a discussion about the ethical considerations inherent in the design of an EBP project, as well as the process for obtaining external funding to support a well-designed EBP project. Later in this chapter, two exemplars of interprofessional EBP projects illustrate unique human subjects issues associated with the project design.

ETHICAL CONSIDERATIONS FOR DESIGNING AN EVIDENCE-BASED PRACTICE PROJECT

Because ethical considerations link with the design of an EBP project, it is important to review the Iowa EBP model (Titler et al., 2001). According to the Iowa EBP model (see Chapter 1, Figure 1-2), the interprofessional EBP team, based on their appraisal and synthesis of the literature, may decide to design a pilot of a practice change or a research study. When there is substantial evidence supporting a proposed practice change (Chapter 9), an interprofessional EBP team will most likely conduct a pilot of a practice change. Conducting additional research to determine the efficacy of an intervention when strong evidence exists is inappropriate (Emanuel et al., 2000). Instead, reducing the gap between research and practice is the primary focus for EBP.

In situations where the literature provides limited evidence for supporting an intervention or change in practice, the interprofessional team may need to conduct a research study to strengthen the existing evidence. However, the interprofessional team may still decide to conduct a practice change pilot even with limited evidence, based on the type of evidence available, level of risk, patient safety, availability of alternative interventions, benefits, costs, patient

preferences and values, and staff acceptability. Thus, in the context of limited evidence, determining the next step in the EBP process is less clear. Understanding the ethical considerations is a significant requirement for the team in order to guide their selection of the most appropriate project design.

Identifying and evaluating potential ethical issues associated with an EBP project occurs throughout the design phase of a project and is not specific to projects using a research design. However, the literature primarily focuses on the ethical concerns for conducting clinical research (Emanuel et al., 2000; Hardicre, 2014; Neff, 2008; Seale & Barnard, 1999). Because the primary objective of research is to create generalizable knowledge and not to provide patient care, knowledge generation creates potential to exploit human subjects when testing a proposed intervention that exposes participants to possible harm. Thus, ethical requirements are essential for ensuring respectful treatment of participants and avoiding inadvertent mistreatment or undue risk.

Elucidating ethical considerations are the responsibility of the interprofessional team, mentors, program coordinators, and sponsors of the interprofessional EBP program. To identify ethical issues, no matter the design of the project, the interprofessional EBP team should answer the following important questions that stem from the ethical principles outlined in the Nuremberg Code (1947), Declaration of Helsinki (2008), Belmont Report (1979), and the Common Rule (USDHHS, 2009, 45 CFR 46):

- Is there societal value or good associated with the project?

- Does the project build on what is already known about the problem?

- Do the benefits of the project outweigh the risk of harm, is the well-being of the participant a primary concern, and are vulnerable participants protected?

- Has proper preparation occurred for ensuring privacy and confidentiality of personal information?

- Does the project require independent review?

- Are subject selection processes fair?

- Are the project design, measurement, and analysis processes transparent and rigorous (scientific validity) as well as respectful of the individual?

- Does the interprofessional team have the capacity to conduct the EBP project?

- Is the interprofessional team willing to terminate a project when results indicate unnecessary harm, injury, or death is occurring because of the intervention?

Another potentially useful framework for assisting the interprofessional team in developing a well-designed EBP project includes the six dimensions of quality outlined in the Institute of Medicine (2001) *Crossing the Quality Chasm* report. The interprofessional team can review their project in relationship to the quality aims that care is safe, effective, efficient, timely, patient centered, and equitable. Additional ethical considerations not previously addressed that apply to program evaluations include ensuring that a program is need-based, well-suited to users, offering choices to participants, involving the users, and empowering staff and participants (Bruce & Paxton, 2002).

LINKING THE PROJECT DESIGN WITH INSTITUTIONAL REVIEW BOARD APPROVAL

Because an interprofessional EBP team has many interests when engaging in EBP (e.g., improving patient outcomes, conducting an EBP project efficiently, obtaining grants, limiting project costs, and engaging in professional scholarship), an independent review of a project prevents competing agendas from inappropriately affecting the team's design decisions. In addition, an interprofessional team often becomes immersed in a project and may not identify important ethical concerns. For research studies, an institutional review board (IRB) provides an independent review and is a committee with at least five members with various backgrounds (e.g., scientists, non-scientists, and ethicists) that serve to protect the rights, welfare, and dignity of individuals who participate in research studies (USDHHS, 2009, 45 CFR, 46.107).

The IRB approves research studies prior to their implementation and ensures that research studies meet standard guidelines for human subject protection, organizational policies and procedures, and codes for professional conduct, as well as meet any applicable laws. Human subjects protection however is a shared responsibility among IRBs, researchers, clinicians, students, faculty, advisors, and organizations. IRBs do provide valuable guidance to interprofessional EBP teams regarding the safe and ethical implementation of the team's project.

Specifically, an IRB focuses on the privacy of research participants and ensures participants are able to maintain their autonomy and dignity throughout the research process and that each participant fully understands what is required and the time needed to complete the study before agreeing to participate. Most importantly, the IRB considers multiple types of participant risks potentially present in a research study that include not only physical or emotional risk, but also financial and employment risk, criminal/civil liability, stigmatization, insurability, and embarrassment (USDHHS, 2009, 45 CFR, 46).

According to federal regulations, there is no requirement that institutions engaged in human subject research have an IRB (USDHHS, 2009, 45 CFR, 46.107). Instead, an institution or organization may have an external IRB review and approve study applications. The interprofessional EBP team needs to identify how the health care organization meets the federal requirements for research with human subjects, as well identify individuals who chair, are members, and support the functions of the IRB. The interprofessional EBP team should access these individuals when needing support for preparing for an IRB review.

However, it is not always clear when to seek IRB approval for a pilot of a practice change. Depending on the intent of a practice change pilot, the interprofessional team may use a variety of project designs (e.g., quality improvement, pragmatic clinical trial, quasi-experimental) (Chapter 10), some of which are research methods. While a pilot of a practice change always requires ethical treatment of patients and maintaining patient confidentiality, a practice change pilot with a quality improvement (QI) design (i.e., a non-research method) may or may not require IRB approval. Knowing when to obtain IRB approval is important because misclassifying research projects as QI may not only violate federal regulations, but has potential to expose patients to unnecessary risk. On the other hand, classifying QI projects as research adds to the work of the interprofessional EBP team and the IRB (Platteborze, 2010). IRB approval for a QI type of EBP project depends on the nature of the QI methods, the intent of the project, and the specific IRB requirements of the health care organization and the university (Lynn et al., 2007).

To determine whether a project with a QI design needs IRB approval, it is important to first define QI, which is the "systematic, data-guided activities designed to bring about immediate improvements in health care delivery in particular settings" (Lynn et al., 2007, p. 666). Quality improvement is essential for continuous improvement of patient care and is an intrinsic part of health care delivery. The intent of QI is much different from a research study, which is about generalizing the results to the larger population of patients. Quality improvement focuses on improving the process of care within an organization with methods, such as plan, do, study, act (PDSA), in order to make system changes.

According to federal guidelines for conducting research, IRB approval is required when an EBP project involves collecting data through intervention or interaction with individuals, and when data about or from human subjects is identifiable (USDHHS, 2009, 45 CFR, 46.102). However, this definition may lead many to interpret that a wide range of EBP projects constitute human subject research and require IRB approval. For example, QI generally involves the collection of data from the health records of individual patients, and often involves observations following the implementation of a practice change to determine whether care improved.

The difference between QI and research becomes more complicated when health care professionals publish QI activities. Some experts argue that the act of publication involves generalizing results beyond an institution (Neff, 2008). Some organizations require an IRB review for QI studies when the plan includes publishing results, which may simply involve the chair reviewing the study to ensure confidentiality of data management and reporting. In addition, health care organizations often require an IRB review when seeking external funding to support an EBP project, regardless of how the team conceptualized the EBP project (e.g., QI project, research study, or practice change pilot). Conflicts of interest may exist when accepting external funding (e.g., a product company), which requires careful evaluation and possibly an independent review to elucidate potential effects on the implementation and outcomes of the project.

With advancement of QI using comparative effectiveness methods, the distinction between research and QI is more difficult to distinguish even for experts. Consequently, careful consideration of ethical issues associated with QI projects become even more critical (Lynn et al., 2007; Newhouse, Pettit, Poe, & Rocco, 2006). For example, Lindenauer, Benjamin, Naglieri-Prescod, Fitzgerald, and Pekow (2002) in a study exploring congruence between experts for determining the need for IRB approval for six different scenarios found agreement ranged from 44% to 96%. The author's conclusion was that the role of IRBs in approving QI projects needed greater clarity.

Interprofessional EBP team members should consider the following guiding questions to determine whether a pilot of a practice change requires IRB approval (Cacchione, 2011; Lynn et al., 2007; Ogrinc, Nelson, Adams, & O'Hara, 2013; Platteborze, 2010):

- Will all patients receive the intervention within the standard of patient care? If the answer is no (e.g., the project includes randomizing an intervention to a control and an intervention group), then the EBP team should have the IRB review the project.

- Are risks to participants greater than those normally associated with providing patient care (minimal risk)? If the EBP team answers yes, then IRB involvement is necessary.

- Is the intent of the project *primarily* to generate generalizable knowledge? If the EBP team answers yes, then the IRB should review the project.

- Does the project intend to evaluate the use of medications or medical devices? If the EBP team answers yes, then the IRB should review the project.

- Does this project involve vulnerable populations, (e.g., children, or people with a disability)? If the EBP team answers yes to this question, then the intent, risk, and design of the project needs greater scrutiny.

The interprofessional EBP team should use the organization's research policies and obtain consultation from the IRB to determine whether IRB approval is necessary. Using factors identified in the literature, Table 11-1 provides additional questions that the interprofessional team should consider (Millum & Grady, 2013; Newhouse et al., 2006; Ogrinc et al., 2013) when determining whether an EBP project requires IRB approval.

Securing Institutional Review Board Approval

The team should inquire about the IRB application and approval processes early in the design phase of a project because the time for an IRB review ranges from several weeks to several months depending on the type of review required, the process, the workload of the IRB, and whether multiple IRBs are involved (Petersen, Simpson, SoRelle, Urech, & Chitwood, 2012). With involvement of faculty and students on the interprofessional EBP team, the IRB of the university will also need to approve the study. However, the program coordinators may obtain collaborative agreements between IRBs regarding the primary IRB on record for the project.

Table 11-2 provides a list of common topics the interprofessional team needs to address in an IRB application. As one of the first steps in completing an IRB application, the interprofessional team identifies the level of risk for human subjects and the type of review (i.e., exempt, expedited, or full IRB review) that best fits the study. However, the IRB makes the final decision regarding the type of review required based on their own independent assessment. According to the federal rules and regulations (USDHHS, 2009, 45 CFR, 46.107b), studies meeting the *exempt review criteria* involve minimal risk, which means the potential for and degree of harm is no greater than what subjects encounter in daily life or with routine physical or psychological assessments (Table 11-3). An *expedited study,* which requires two IRB members to review, involves no more than minimal risk, includes appropriate consent procedures, does not rely on intentional deception as part of participant permission and/or data collection procedures, and does not involve sensitive populations or topics (USDHHS, 2009, 45 CFR, 46.110) (see Table 11-3).

Any study not meeting the exempt or expedited criteria, requires a full IRB review. These are generally studies that place participants at greater than minimal risk and those involving a protected class of participants. Vulnerable populations include a variety of groups, such as fetuses, children, prisoners, pregnant women, mentally disabled or cognitively impaired persons, terminally ill patients, older adults, students, and employees; survey research that involves AIDS information either with the general public or with vulnerable populations; and economically

TABLE 11-1

CLARIFYING QUESTIONS REGARDING QUALITY IMPROVEMENT PROJECTS VERSUS INSTITUTIONAL REVIEW BOARD REVIEWS

PROJECT ELEMENT	DESIGN: PILOT OF A PRACTICE CHANGE USING QUALITY IMPROVEMENT	DESIGN: RESEARCH WITH HUMAN SUBJECTS
Purpose	• Is the purpose of the project to improve performance of the standard of care within the health care organization? • Do you plan to publish? The purpose becomes less clear with publishing. Will you publish lessons learned or the effectiveness of an outcome?	• Is the purpose of the project to fill a "gap" in the existing literature and/or test a specific hypothesis(es) in order to generate new knowledge? • Publishing is an expectation.
Study methods	• Will staff deliver the change in practice as part of their care within the typical patient-care relationship? • Will the data collected be unidentifiable? • Will the project's interventions change over time based on feedback obtained during the project (Plan, Do, Study, Act)? • Is it rapid cycle change? • Will the project include assessing how service(s) are provided? • Is a large enough sample used to demonstrate change? • Will statistical tools assist with evaluating differences in the system or how services are provided (e.g., control charts)?	• Will the project include collecting identifiable private information outside of the typical clinician patient relationship? • Will the project study medications and devices? • Will the project rely on a specific protocol that defines the intervention, who will administer the intervention and/or the interaction(s) with participants? • Is the sample carefully determined using power analysis? • Will the project make comparisons between groups to test the project hypothesis(es)? • Will the project rely primarily on statistical analysis to compare differences between groups or to verify the relationship(s) between variables?
Proposed outcomes	• Will the project result in direct benefit(s) to the participants? • Will the health care organization benefit from improved services and care processes?	• Will the project directly benefit each participant or the institution? • If the answer to this question is no or uncertain then will the project benefit society by developing new or advance current knowledge about a problem?
Levels of risk	• What type of risk exists? Are the risks similar to those that normally occur with receiving care? Minimal risk is most often related to data management and confidentiality. • Risk is often greater if the continued care is not changed.	• Are there risks with the intervention or change in practice that are greater than those in receiving normal care? • Are risks more than those associated with data management and confidentiality?

or educationally disadvantaged persons (USDHHS, 2009, 45 CFR, 46.111b).

When an IRB reviews a study that includes patient health information, they determine whether the interprofessional EBP team is complying with the Health Insurance Portability and Accountability Act (HIPAA) that protects patient privacy (www.hhs.gov/ocr/privacy/hipaa/administrative/privacyrule/). The IRB is looking to see whether the researcher is obtaining permission to access the clinical record in the informed consent. In addition,

TABLE 11-2

ELEMENTS OF AN INSTITUTIONAL REVIEW BOARD APPLICATION

IRB ELEMENT	DESCRIPTION
Anticipated level of review	Indication of the required level of review: exempt, expedited, or full review.
Summary of the research project	The summary should include the following: • The purpose of the project • A brief review of the literature or background for the project • The methods to complete the project • The research questions
Expectations of the participants	An explanation of what the participants will be expected to do as they participate in this project
Estimated time commitment of the participants	A good faith estimate of how much time will be required for a participant to complete his or her participation in the project
Description of the participants	The description should include a statement of the following: • Total number of participants • Number of males and females • Specific inclusion and/or exclusion criteria, including the recruitment of special and/or vulnerable populations, like pregnant women, children, or people with disabilities
Risks and benefits	Discussion of the relative risks and benefits that each participant can reasonably expect to experience and/or receive as they participate in the project (relative benefits should outweigh relative risks)
Participant recruitment plan	This should include the following: • Description of subject recruitment • Hard copies of any written materials, advertisement flyers, and/or emails for recruiting participants • Hard copy of a phone script to recruit participants by telephone • A description of any incentives for subject participation that are minimal to avoid coercion (e.g., $10.00 gift card).
Informed consent document	Informed consent document that includes an explanation of the purpose of the project, procedures, expectations, time frames, risks and benefits, alternatives when applicable, and process for withdrawing from the study, a place for each participant to sign acknowledging the study. If accessing protected information from the electronic record, must include a discussion about rights identified in the Health Insurance Portability and Accountability Act (HIPPA).
Data management plan	This plan should include the following: • The data storage plan • Who will have access to the data • How long will the data be available to the researchers • When will the data be destroyed • The plan for protecting the confidentiality of the data

TABLE 11-3

FEDERAL GUIDELINES FOR EXEMPT AND EXPEDITED RESEARCH

EXEMPT	EXPEDITED
• Research in educational settings that focus on typical educational practices, instructional strategies, curricula, classroom management	• Studies of medications or medical devices that are ready for marketing, are not new, and are used as intended
• Research that includes collecting unidentifiable results from educational tests, surveys, interviews, or observation of public behaviors	• Collection of blood samples using finger, heel, or venipuncture. Venipuncture can be used within specific guidelines for adults (see 45 CFR 46).
• Surveys, interviews, observations of public behaviors of elected or appointed public officials and those running for office. Confidentiality of personal information is still required.	• Collection of biological, noninvasive specimens, such as nail clippings
• Research including publicly available data from documents, records, pathological specimens or diagnostic specimens when the identity of subjects is protected	• Collection of noninvasive data routinely employed in clinical practice. X-rays, microwaves, and general anesthesia are excluded from this category.
• Research and demonstration projects that examine public benefit programs	• Data collected from documents, records, or specimens that are collected as part of care
• Consumer studies, tasting food meeting the Food and Drug Administration standard	• Collection of data from voice, video, digital, or image recordings for research purposes
	• Information about individual or group characteristics or behaviors from surveys, interviews, oral histories, focus groups that explore perceptions, motivation, cultural beliefs, cognition, communication

the study should include a plan for accessing only a limited set of data specific to the study, de-identifying collected data, protecting the health information, destroying the identifiers as soon as possible, and assuring that the health information is not reused or disclosed to anyone unless the law dictates. The Health Insurance Portability and Accountability Act describes health information that is potentially identifiable as demographic data related to an individual's physical or mental health (i.e., past, present, or future) and their health care, as well as information about financial payment of services. Types of information include a patient's name, age, address, birthdate, Social Security number, telephone number, address, Internet protocol address/numbers, medical record number, dates of services, and full-face images. Some IRBs require an additional consent form specific to the use of health information and others recommend adding it to the study informed consent.

Research Roles and Education of the Interprofessional Team

As the EBP team works to complete the IRB application process, they also need to clarify the role of individual team members in carrying out and managing the study protocol. The interprofessional team needs to designate one or more team members as the principal investigator (PI)

and co-investigators. According to the federal regulations for research, investigators are responsible for ensuring the protection of subject rights and welfare and for the quality of the study (USDHHS, 2009, 45 CFR 46).

The expectation is that the investigator will carry out the approved protocol that includes obtaining and documenting subject consent, obtaining prior approval from the IRB of any protocol changes, completing IRB-required progress reports and requesting continuing review as needed, reporting any unanticipated subject risks and noncompliance, and keeping records for at least 3 years following completion of the study. The PI generally serves as the "supervisor" of the project and functions as the primary contact with and for the IRB. As such, this individual(s) should have the skills, experience, and expertise needed to guide the team through the IRB process and the completion of the EBP project.

In addition, each team member, depending on the health care institution requirements and the individual's role in the project need to complete certain educational activities prior to being involved with the EBP project. For instance, most organizations involved with human subjects research require that each team member complete training about the responsible conduct of research, data management, and security (including data storage and who will have access to the team's data). An excellent and cost-effective source of this type of education is the CITI program housed at the University of Miami (www.citiprogram.org/). Other sources of training include the Office of Human Research Protection (OHRP) that offers training videos and webinars for protecting human subjects, and the National Institutes of Health (NIH) also has a training module for investigators (https://phrp.nihtraining.com/users/login.php).

Exemplars of Evidence-Based Practice Projects and Ethical Considerations

Interprofessional EBP teams design their projects to answer a PICO question developed based on an appraisal and synthesis of the literature. Two exemplars of interprofessional EBP projects (Tables 11-4 and 11-5) are presented to illustrate the link between the design of the project and the IRB related issues. In both cases, limited research evidence existed to support the proposed intervention; however, the interprofessional teams chose different designs (i.e., pilot of a practice change vs a research study). Their choices illustrate various ethical considerations related to the design of the EBP project.

The interprofessional team for the study described in the first exemplar (see Table 11-4) worked through several essential decisions developing their EBP project. The focus of the study was to change chest tube management strategies that would facilitate early patient ambulation after open-heart surgery. The goal of the EBP project was to change from the traditional practice of placing chest tubes to wall suction (a fixed device that limits patient movement) until chest tube removal to a practice of using water seal with a chest tube drainage collection system (a mobile device) on the first postoperative day (Benz & Sendelbach, 2014). In particular, they found evidence for putting chest tubes to water seal for patients who underwent pulmonary-related surgery (Cerfolio, Bass, & Katholi, 2001; Coughlin, Emmerton-Coughlin, & Malthaner, 2012), but not for patients undergoing open-heart surgery. However, a pilot of a practice change using a quasi-experimental approach (i.e., before and after design) was chosen because of the health care organization's successful use of water seal with pulmonary surgical patients. The cardiac surgeon offered leadership support for changing practice as the interprofessional team outlined. The cardiac surgeons viewed the study as a quality improvement study and not as a project for determining the intervention's efficacy.

Table 11-4 illustrates that the study has elements from both quality improvement and a research approach, which blurred the distinction between the two methods. Thus, the interprofessional team consulted with the IRB chair to determine whether IRB approval was necessary. The IRB chair determined it was a QI study and believed the study presented minimal risk because the approach being proposed was currently in use within the institution for pulmonary surgical patients. For the pulmonary surgical patients, water seal had demonstrated evidence of preventing chest tube complications. In addition, the IRB was satisfied with the QI design because the cardiac surgeons were involved in the QI study and believed it was an improvement to current practice. In addition, the surgeons identified the use of wall suction following open-heart surgery was based more on tradition than evidence and was most likely a function of where the surgeons were trained (Cerfolio et al., 2001). The risk was deemed no greater than the risk that currently exists when providing open-heart surgery.

Data collection strictly involved a chart audit in which the study protocol met the HIPAA regulations. The protocol involved limiting the chart audit data to chest tube outcomes and the patient demographics of gender, age, type of surgery, number of chest tubes, and the dates for chest tube removal. In addition, the data were de-identified, which prevented a link between the study data and the medical record number and the patient name. Other safeguards included collecting data only for those patients who signed the hospital admission consent that gave permission for using electronic health information in research or quality improvement. Additionally, only the staff nurse working at the health care institution who was on the interprofessional team extracted the data from the patient's electronic medical record. The project was funded through an internal hospital foundation grant rather than an external funding agent.

The second case was conducted to add to the limited evidence in the literature about the effectiveness of using aromatherapy as an adjunct to pain management for trauma patients (Moyers, Finch Guthrie, Swan, & Anderson Sathe, 2014). This EBP team primarily found evidence for using aromatherapy for addressing symptoms of anxiety rather than for pain management in patients with significant injuries. Because there is a relationship between anxiety and pain and because essential oils were being used for pain management in many clinical situations in the community, the team decided to conduct a research study to extend the literature and apply this intervention to patients with pain recovering from traumatic injuries. While this proposed intervention was novel for managing pain in this population of patients at this clinical site, the health care organization was using aromatherapy to improve care for other populations in acute care and as a result supported the study.

The primary ethical consideration for this EBP project was the use of a placebo as a comparison intervention for aromatherapy. The interprofessional EBP team used an explanatory, randomized controlled design to determine whether the aromatherapy intervention was efficacious. The gold standard according to the United States Food and Drug Administration (2014) for testing new medications is with placebo comparisons (U.S. Food and Drug

TABLE 11-4		

PILOT OF A PRACTICE CHANGE EXEMPLAR: BLURRING BETWEEN QUALITY IMPROVEMENT AND RESEARCH DESIGNS

Issue: Is the EBP project quality improvement or research requiring IRB review?

Study Title: Place Atrium to Waterseal (PAWS): A quality improvement project to assess wall suction versus water seal in chest tubes after open-heart surgery

Evidence-Based Practice Question: For adult patients undergoing open heart surgery (OHS) is there a difference in complications associated with chest tubes, measured output, and dwell time when chest tubes remain connected to wall suction until discontinued (usual care) versus placing chest tubes to water seal the morning following surgery?

STUDY ELEMENT	HOW THE EBP PROJECT MET QUALITY IMPROVEMENT REQUIREMENTS	HOW THE EBP PROJECT MET RESEARCH REQUIREMENTS
Purpose	Goal: Adopt a practice for facilitating early ambulation. Placing chest tubes to water seal has potential for creating greater freedom of movement for patients.	Compare two chest tube management processes for postoperative OHS patients, including the traditional approach of placing chest tubes to wall suction versus placing chest tubes to water seal the first postoperative day.
Evidence from the literature	Evidence did not exist for using water seal in OHS patients	Use of water seal in pulmonary surgical patients is effective.
Study methods sample	At least 30 post-OHS patients before and 30 patients after change, used QI sampling guidelines	No power analysis
Design	Before and after implementation of the new practice	1. The first group of patients in the study before changing practice received wall suction until their chest tubes were discontinued. 2. The second group of patients after changing practice to using water seal received water seal on the first postoperative day until their chest tubes were discontinued
Implementation	The change of chest tube placement to water seal was part of the delivery of care to all open heart surgery patients following baseline data collection	Protocol used to define the intervention and the process
Data collection	The study did not include collecting data about care processes, but included chart reviews	OHS patient outcomes: chest tube dwell time, output, and complications
Analysis	The study did not include traditional QI analysis methods like control charts	Statistical analysis to determine differences between pre- and post-groups
Benefits	Potential to decrease dwell time for chest tubes, promoting early ambulation	Creation of new knowledge, water seal previously used in pulmonary surgery patients and not OHS patients
Funding	Internal foundation funding	No external funding
Dissemination	Publication was not restricted to internal dissemination	Plan for publication

TABLE 11-5		
RESEARCH STUDY SECOND EXEMPLAR		
Issue: Ethical Use of a Placebo in a Control Group		
Study Title: Use of aromatherapy in managing pain for patients on the trauma specialty care unit		
Evidence-Based Practice Question: For adult patients on the trauma specialty unit, what is the effect of using aromatherapy as an adjuvant treatment for pain management on pain intensity, anxiety, and patient satisfaction compared to those patients receiving a placebo in addition to their pain management plan?		
UNETHICAL USES OF A PLACEBO	**ETHICAL USES OF PLACEBO**	**EBP PRACTICE CHANGE RESEARCH PROTOCOL**
As a sham pain management treatment as part of the care plan outside of a research study Often used when complaints of pain were not felt by caregivers as true physical pain	Use of a proven therapeutic treatment for pain when caring for patients reporting pain	Placebo was not used as a clinical treatment in the protocol as a replacement for therapeutic pain management in the patient's care
Controls in a study receive placebos in place of known alternative treatments	Control group should not receive a placebo when known alternative treatments for comparison exist	Both the control and the treatment group received provider ordered pain medications as needed for pain. Aromatherapy and the placebo was in addition to their current prescribed treatment
Patient is unaware of receiving a placebo	Patient has complete information about the use of the placebo	Use of the placebo was described in the consent. The patient had a right to withdraw from the study.
Lack of safeguards for patients receiving a placebo in a study	Well-developed research protocol for randomization and management of the intervention and control conditions	Investigator blinded to random assignment—predetermined Those administering the aromatherapy and the placebo were not caring for the patient or determining when to administer the provider ordered pain medications.

Administration, CFR 21, 314.126). In addition, previous aromatherapy studies included the use of a placebo, such as the use of water vapor or other inert essential oils (Han, Hur, Buckle, Choi, & Lee, 2006; Ni et al., 2013) in response to criticism in the literature that aromatherapy was not being tested with rigorous research methods similar to testing new medications (Ernst, 2000). However, while there is support for the use of placebos in research, a number of ethical issues exist concerning protecting participants when using placebos as a comparison treatment. Table 11-5 is an exemplar of the aromatherapy study that compares ethical and unethical uses of placebos with the aromatherapy study protocol involving a placebo.

The interprofessional team first distinguished their project as different from the ethical controversy for using placebos as a sham pain treatment in the clinical care of patients. The deceptive use of a placebo to treat a patient's pain in clinical practice is unethical (Arnstein, Broglio, Wubrman, & Kean, 2011). At one time, clinicians used placebos when they believed a patient's pain complaint was not physically based, or when they did not believe the patient's account of his or her discomfort. Research use of placebos also has ethical issues when known alternative medications exist that are available for comparison. Millum and Grady (2013) indicated that international guidelines permit the use of placebos in clinical trials when the science indicates their use under four circumstances: (1) when there is no proven alternative, (2) when withholding treatment is associated with minimal risk, (3) when there are methodological reasons to include a placebo and the use does not create undue harm to the participant, and (4) when the intent of the study is to create treatment options for the population from which the participants are recruited for the study (p. 510).

The interprofessional team designed the study to prevent undue harm, with the patient receiving the aromatherapy or the placebo in addition to their provider-ordered pain management (see Table 11-5). The interprofessional team chose a placebo-controlled trial design because it was not

TABLE 11-6

POTENTIAL FUNDING SOURCES

FUNDING SOURCE	TYPE OF FUNDING PROVIDED
SPIN	40,000+ funding opportunities in all disciplines
SPIN SMART	Sign up for email alerts for new funding opportunities
Grants.gov	Single portal access for all federal grant opportunities
Foundation Center	Search private U.S. Foundations
FedBizOpps	Search federal government contract opportunities
Fellowship Listing	Search links to fellowship opportunities
The State's Office of Grants Management	Search state grant opportunities
US Department of Health and Human Services	Search health research, education, and program funds
Association of Healthcare Research and Quality	Search health care improvement research funds
Health Resources and Services Administration	Search health care education funds
National Institutes of Health	Search health research, biomedical workforce education and investigator career development funds

clear whether aromatherapy provides added pain relief or whether the caregiver providing additional presence was the added intervention. To prevent participant deception, the consent clearly outlined that participants had potential to receive a placebo instead of the aromatherapy. The IRB reviewed and approved the study.

Both of the EBP exemplars illustrate that interprofessional EBP teams may make different decisions regarding the design of a project when only limited evidence is available to the team. The exemplars also highlight the ethical considerations an interprofessional team considers related to the design of an EBP project. In addition, the exemplars reveal that not every interprofessional EBP project will need IRB approval; however, the exemplars show the importance of working with the health care organization's IRB to ensure that the rights and safety of all participants are protected throughout the study process.

FUNDING THE INTERPROFESSIONAL EVIDENCE-BASED PRACTICE PROJECT

Multiple sources may be appropriate for funding the interprofessional EBP project, including the operating budgets of the health care organization, internal grants of the university or health care organization, as well as external funding from professional associations, foundations, and government. This chapter focuses on funding from external sources, which all have unique expectations, requirements, and deadlines for securing financial support for the project. A critical first step is to find a funding source whose mission and goals align closely with the interprofessional EBP

project. Contacting the program officer of the grant agency is helpful to verify fit with the funding source and to obtain information needed to refine the grant proposal (Blanco & Lee, 2012). Table 11-6 provides a list of potential funding sources.

All funders require the team to write a competitive proposal that is well-referenced throughout to substantiate the interprofessional team's choices in the design of the EBP project (Inouye & Fiellin, 2005). Table 11-7 highlights the basic steps in writing a funding proposal for an EBP project. Writing a grant proposal for an EBP project is slightly different from writing one for a traditional research or a program evaluation project (Proctor, Powell, Baumann, Hamilton, & Santens, 2012). Grant proposals for implementation projects have to focus on why the interprofessional EBP project needs to be completed in light of the gaps in care or quality. The interprofessional team establishes significance of the EBP project when including literature about the extent of the gaps in practice and the costs to the patient and the health care system in terms of the expense engendered when care is not effective. The interprofessional team should describe the innovation or practice change the interprofessional team plans to evaluate and should highlight the way in which policy trends are beginning to identify the need for this innovation.

Next, the interprofessional team clearly and briefly describes evidence of the efficacy or potential effectiveness of the practice change. In some cases, there is not strong support from the literature for the practice change due to the literature search discovering studies primarily conducted at the lower levels of strength and quality (see Chapter 9). In this situation, according to the Iowa model (Titler et al., 2001), the accumulation of lower levels of

TABLE 11-7

SUCCESSFUL GRANT WRITING FOR IMPLEMENTATION EVIDENCE-BASED PRACTICE PROJECTS

	GRANT WRITING TIP	MAIN IDEA
1	Identify funding agencies and resources	Internal funding of university or health care organization; professional organizations; foundations; government
2	Know the funding agency and verify fit	Understand mission and goals; examine profile of previous grant recipients; does the EBP project meet their goals? Talk to program officer.
3	Follow the grant directions	Note instructions; make a checklist; note required order, format, and length; include required attachments (curriculum vitae, letters of support)
4	Write clearly	Avoid jargon; use headings if permitted; use bullets; include key diagrams/charts; proofread
5	Make a case for the need of the EBP project. What is the care or quality gap? Can you substantiate this care or quality gap? Does the EBP project align with policy trends?	EBP project addresses timely and relevant question (1) Why is your project important? (2) Did you make the case for the EBP project's need? (3) Did you state the purpose? (4) Did the aims of the EBP project address the purpose? (5) Does the team have a track record to accomplish the aims/goals? (6) Have you described the organizational support for the EBP project?
6	Describe the proposed evidence-based treatment and its evidence.	Cite appropriate evidence to demonstrate the potential effectiveness for the program, treatment, or set of services.
7	Describe conceptual model or theoretical justification of treatment or intervention	The conceptual model should inform the design of the EBP project and its variables.
8	Design appropriate methodology	Describe methodology, evaluation methods, participants, sample selection and size, IRB process, measurable outcomes and type of data, instruments and tools, methods of data analysis to answer PICO question. Is there a measurement plan for each construct? Is the data analysis plan clear how relationships between constructs are tested?
9	Plan a feasible EBP project with timeline	Consider the grant period; Allow extra time within grant period; Factor in time to obtain IRB approval; Outline implementation strategies and justification. Describe contingency plans. Demonstrate capacity of the health care and university organizations to support the project.
10	Allocate funds appropriately	Determine level of budget detail needed; Include budget and narrative; Make sure to budget only allowable items.
11	Sustain the project after the grant period	Describe the sustainability of the project after the funding ends.
12	Disseminate the EBP project	Describe the plan for disseminating outcomes

evidence in combination with other evidence may indicate enough potential to fund the proposed EBP project (see Chapter 1, Figure 1-2).

To obtain funding, the team will need to describe the conceptual framework or theories supporting the practice change. A theoretical framework helps to illustrate the mechanisms and the concepts upon which the practice change is based. The reviewers of the funding proposal use this conceptual understanding to anticipate the variables of the EBP project, how the practice change is designed, and to assess the adequacy of the measurement and data analysis plans. When the literature support is weak for the practice change, the conceptual framework becomes more important for making the case for funding due to the sound theoretical explanation and clear scientific principles.

Now the interprofessional team is ready to highlight the purposes or aims of the interprofessional EBP project, particularly relating these goals to answering the PICO question and any sub-questions. Because of the conceptual framework, the interprofessional team is able to logically define and operationalize the variables of the project. Participant recruitment processes are delineated, particularly highlighting fairness and ensuring that the recruitment process does not violate the privacy of potential participants. The participants selected for the EBP project are described in terms of inclusion and exclusion criteria and as having to complete IRB-approved consent processes when applicable. Determination of sample size is statistically supported in terms of a power analysis in the case of research designs and is appropriate for balancing the depth and breadth of the data in qualitative designs. Assignment of participants to groups is described as convenience or randomization in the case of quantitative research designs. Procedures for implementing the practice change within a specific context are listed, including the needed expertise and training to carry out the procedures.

Both fidelity and outcome measurement tools are described in terms of their standardization, validity, reliability, scoring, and interpretation of the scores. It may be best to list the measurement tools and their characteristics in a table that also includes the frequency of measurement, such as pre-, post-, and follow-up testing. When using published or proprietary outcome measures in the evaluation plan, the team gives credit to researchers and includes permission from the publisher to use an instrument or to adapt a measure for the interprofessional EBP project. Finally, in this section of the proposal, the team discusses the data analysis plans involving the appropriate statistics or strategies guiding the inductive coding processes to explicate themes.

The proposal must also provide the timeline for completion, making conservative estimates regarding the timeline for each action step while also completing the project within the grant period. A management plan for the interprofessional EBP project addresses the roles and responsibilities of team members in conducting the project and the manner that the qualifications of each team member are sufficient for completing their assigned responsibilities according to the protocol. In addition, the interprofessional team highlights for the reviewers the capacity and resources of the organization in terms of in-kind contributions and the infrastructure needed for a project of the size and scope the team is proposing in the funding application. This infrastructure might include technical support from the IT department and other personnel the health care organization or university pays to work on the project. It is important to demonstrate the sustainability of the project change once the grant is completed.

The budget for the project itemizes all of the costs of the project, without going over the total funds available per award from the funding source. Typical costs included are personnel wages and benefits, equipment and supply costs, printing/copying and mailing expenses as needed, travel funds and other dissemination costs as warranted, and monies to hire outside consultants and statisticians. The interprofessional team reviews the budget guidelines about the types of expenses the funders will pay and the aspects of the budget they will not fund. For instance, some grants pay salaries but do not pay benefit costs of project personnel. Once the team has completed the detailed budget, the team should also include a brief budget justification narrative that explains the specific expenses within the budget. The last step in creating the funding proposal is to include a set of letters of support from key personnel within the organization as well as from outside organizations. The team includes the resume or curriculum vitae of each person working on the project.

MENTOR CHALLENGES

The mentor challenge occurring when navigating micro and macro contexts (discussed in Chapter 3) relates to the ethical decision making when designing the EBP project, applying to the IRB, and submitting grant proposals. The interprofessional team is juggling both externally and internally driven requirements for the ethical design of EBP projects and is often navigating two different IRBs as well. The mentor must learn these project approval and funding processes and may need help from experts to ensure the design of the project adequately protects human subjects. Grant and IRB submission deadlines require the mentor to work with the team to create efficient and effective work processes. This is particularly important for team members so that they will be able to complete any required education or training (e.g., CITI training prior to submitting the IRB application as well as prior to the grant applications). Both of these application processes necessitate teamwork to provide complete proposals in the preferred format and on the strict schedule of the IRB or of the funding agency. Some teams may struggle to identify sources of funding compatible with the project's intent, leading the mentor and program coordinator to facilitate critical team discussions about budgetary constraints and funding opportunities.

Another challenge may occur when the interprofessional team selects the PI for the project. The interprofessional team has to balance the requirements the IRB and the funder might have for the PI, particularly in terms of making sure the PI possesses verifiable research experience or a record of accomplishment for completing EBP projects. The clinical scholar and other members may not have this experience, which often causes the faculty member to assume the PI role. It could be that the health care organization requires the PIs of all studies to be employees. In this case, the EBP program coordinator for the health care institution might have to be the PI.

Mentor Techniques and Mentor Supports

Essential mentor techniques, previously discussed in Chapter 3 include anticipating what might happen, teaching, providing resources, and providing structure. All of these mentor techniques apply given most team members have little experience with IRB and grant writing processes. During this phase of project design, grant funding, and IRB submission for approval, the mentor focuses these techniques on critical team issues related to time management and proactive communication. Team members may struggle with the ethical issues related to their designs, which requires effective problem solving with mentors, program coordinators, and outside experts, such as representatives from the IRB and methodologists. Program coordinators support mentors through inquiry about IRB processes and due dates early in the planning phase of the project in order to advise the team about the project timeline. Mentors should facilitate a team brainstorming session about potential funding sources as soon as the EBP project topic has been determined. Identifying funding sources early brings attention to the due dates for funding applications. The project timeline should incorporate the need for extra time to deal with inevitable delays from the IRB and the grant processes. Often submitting to the IRB and grant funders requires the team to take on extra work and to meet more often within a short period. The mentor will have to ensure that members are completing work on time, are asking for help when struggling, and are communicating carefully about their design questions and concerns. Program coordinators offer timely supports to the mentor and interprofessional teams, particularly when ethical decision making related to project design requires informed problem solving beyond the expertise of the mentors.

Summary

The design phase is not complete until the team secures IRB approval when indicated. EBP projects are more successful if the team identifies funding sources for the interprofessional EBP project and determines whether the project should be implemented as an evaluation of a pilot practice change using pragmatic designs, such as a quality improvement approach, or using an explanatory research design. Regardless of the design, the interprofessional team considers the potential ethical issues related to protection

of human subjects in order to include strategies to maintain confidentiality, minimize risk, and create transparency for the participants' decision making about giving consent. The involvement of IRBs in providing review of the EBP project is clear when the team chooses a research design but is often unclear when choosing non-research designs. Strategies to make this decision about IRB involvement and level of review were provided. However, consultation with the chair of the IRB is often the best way for the team to make decisions about an IRB application for a non-research EBP project. Writing grant proposals for funding often incorporates some of the information prepared for the IRB, such as informed consent and descriptions of protecting confidentiality of the data. A discussion of content to include in a grant highlighted the slight difference in explanation needed when asking for external funding for an EBP project compared to submitting funding requests for research projects. As the team completes the design phase of the work, the team begins to look forward to the actual implementation of the EBP pilot of a practice change or a research study.

Reflection Questions

1. What might be the ethical issues inherent in the EBP practice project and how will the team modify the design to address these concerns?

2. Describe at least three potential sources of outside funding for an EBP project and develop a preliminary plan to explore the requirements of these sources.

References

Arnstein, P., Broglio, K., Wubrman, E., & Kean, M. B. (2011). Use of placebos in pain management. *Pain Management Nursing, 12*(4), 225-229. doi:10.1016/j.pmn.2010.10.033

Benz, J., & Sendelbach, S. (2014). *Evidence-Based Fellowship Program: A collaboration between Abbott Northwestern Hospital and St. Catherine's University.* Paper presented at the IPE Summit at St. Catherine University, St. Paul, MN.

Blanco, M. A., & Lee, M. Y. (2012). Twelve tips for writing educational research grant proposals. *Medical Teacher, 34,* 450-453.

Bruce, S., & Paxton, R. (2002). Ethical principles for evaluating mental health services: A critical examination. *Journal of Mental Health, 11*(3), 267-279. doi:10.1080/09638230020023651.

Cacchione, P. Z. (2011). When is institutional review board approval necessary for quality improvement projects? *Clinical Nursing Research, 20*(1), 3-6. doi:10.1177/1054773810395692

Carter, S. M., Rychetnik, L., Beverly, L., Kerridge, I. H, Baur, L., Bauman, A., ... Zask, A. (2011). Evidence, ethics, and values: A framework for health promotion. *American Journal of Public Health, 101,* 465-472. doi:10.2105/AJPH.2010.195545.

Cerfolio, R. J., Bass, C., & Katholi, C. R. (2001). Prospective randomized trial compares suction versus water seal for air leaks. *Annals of Thoracic Surgery 71*, 1613-1617. doi:PII S0003-4975(01)02474-2

Coughlin, S. M., Emmerton-Coughlin, H. M., & Malthaner, R. (2012). Management of chest tubes after pulmonary resection: a systematic review and meta-analysis. *Canadian Journal of Surgery, 55*(4), 264-270. doi:10.1503/cjs.001411

Emanuel, E. J., Wendler, D., & Grady, C. (2000). What makes clinical research ethical? *Journal of the American Medical Association, 283*(20), 2701-2711.doi:10.1001/jama.283.20.2701

Ernst, E. (2000). The role of complementary and alternative medicine. *British Medical Journal, 321*(4), 1133-1135. doi:10.1136/bmj.321.7269.1133

Gondolf, E. W. (2000). Human subject issues in batterer program evaluation. *Journal of Aggression, Maltreatment & Trauma, 4*(1), 273-297. doi:10.1300/j146v04n01_12

Han, S., Hur, M., Buckle, J., Choi, J., & Lee, M. (2006). Effect of aromatherapy on symptoms of dysmenorrhea in college students: A randomized placebo-controlled clinical trial. *The Journal of Alternative and Complementary Medicine, 12*(6), 535-541. doi:10.1089/acm.2006.12.535

Hardicre, J. (2014). An overview of research ethics and learning from the past. *British Journal of Nursing, 23*(9), 483-486. doi:10.12968/bjon.2014.23.9.483

Inouye, S. K., & Fiellin, D. A. (2005). An evidence-based guide to writing grant proposals for clinical research. *Annals of Internal Medicine, 142*, 274-282. doi:10.7326/0003-4819-142-4-200502150-00009

Institute of Medicine. (2001). *Crossing the quality chasm: A new health system for the 21st century*. Washington, DC: The National Academy Press. www.nap.edu/catalog/10027.htm.

Kumar, S., Grimmer-Somers, K., & Huges, B. (2010). The ethics of evidence implementation in health care. *Physiotherapy Research International, 15*, 96-102. doi:10.1002/pri.479

Lindenauer, P. K., Benjamin, E. M., Naglieri-Prescod, D., Fitzgerald, J., & Pekow, P. (2002). The role of institutional review board in quality improvement: A survey of quality officers, institutional review board chairs and journal editors. *American Journal of Medicine, 113*(7), 575-579. doi:10.1016/S0002-9343(02)01250-0.

Loi, C. X., & McDermott, R. J. (2010). Conducting program evaluation with Hispanics in rural settings: Ethical issues and evaluation challenges. *American Journal of Health Education, 41*(4), 252-256. doi:10.1080/19325037.2010.1059 9151

Lynn, J., Baily, M. A., Bottrell, M., Jennings, B., Levine, R. J., Davidoff, F.,... James, B. (2007). Ethics of using quality improvement methods in health care. *Annals of Internal Medicine, 146*, 666-673. doi:10.7326/0003-4819-146-9-200705010-00155

Millum, J., & Grady, C. (2013). The ethics of placebo-controlled trials: Methodological justifications. *Contemporary Clinical Trials, 36*(2), 510-514. doi:10.1016/j.cct.2013.09.003

Moyers, P. A., Finch Guthrie, P. L., Swan, A. S., & Anderson Sathe, L. (2014). *Interprofessional evidence-based clinical scholar program: Learning to work together. American Journal of Occupational Therapy, 68*, S23-S31. doi:10.5014/ajot.2014.012609

Neff, M. (2008). Institutional review board consideration of chart reviews, case reports, and observational studies. *Respiratory Care, 53*(10), 1350-1353.

Newhouse, R. P., Petit, J. C., Poe, S., & Rocco, L. (2006). The slippery slope: differentiating between quality improvement and research. *The Journal of Nursing Administration, 36*(4): 211-219). doi:10.1097/00005110-200604000-00011

Ni, C., Hou, W., Kao, C., Chang, M., Yu, L., Wu, C., & Chen, C. (2013). The anxiolytic effect of aromatherapy of patients awaiting ambulatory surgery: A randomized controlled trial. *Evidence-based Complementary and Alternative Medicine,* Article ID 927419, 5 pages, doi:10.1155/2013/927419

Ogrinc, G., Nelson, W. A., Adams, S. M. & O'Hara, A. E. (2013). An instrument to differentiate between clinical research and quality improvement. *IRB: Ethics and Human Research, 35*(5):1-7.

Petersen, L. A., Simpson, K., SoRelle, R., Urech, T., & Chitwood, S. S. (2012). How variability in the institutional review board review process affects minimal-risk multisite health services research. *Annals of Internal Medicine, 156,*(10), 728-735. doi:10.7326/0003-4819-156-10-201205150-00011

Platteborze, L. S., Young-McCaughan, S., King-Letzkus, I., McClinton, A., Halliday, A., & Jefferson, T. C., (2010). Performance improvement/research advisory panel: A model for determining whether a project is a performance or quality improvement activity or research. *Military Medicine, 175*(4), 289- 291. doi:10.7205/milmed-d-09-00087

Proctor, E. K., Powell, B. J., Baumann, A. A., Hamilton, A. M., & Santens, R. L. (2012). Writing implementation research grant proposals: Ten key ingredients. *Implementation Science, 7*, 1-13. doi:10.1186/1748-5908-7-96

Seale, J. K., & Barnard, S. (1999). Ethical consideration in therapy research. *British Journal of Occupational Therapy, 62*(8), 371-375. doi:10.1177/030802269906200808

Titler, M. G., Kleiber, C. Steelman, V. J., Rakel, B. A., Budreau, G., Everett, L. Q. , & Goode, C. J. (2001). The Iowa model of evidence-based practice to promote quality care. *Critical Care Nursing Clinics of North America, 13*(4), 497-509.

U.S. Department of Health and Human Services. (2009). Human subjects research (45 CFR 46). Retrieved from http://www.hhs.gov/ohrp/humansubjects/guidance.

United States Food and Drug Administration. (2014). Applications for FDA approval to market a new drug. Code for Federal Regulations, 21(5), 314.126, Adequate and well controlled studies. http://www.accessdata.fda.gov/scripts/cdrh/cfdocs/cfcfr/CFRSearch.cfm?fr=314.126

Supplemental materials for this chapter are available online.
Please refer to the sticker in the front of the book and enter the access code provided.

Planning and Implementing the Interprofessional Evidence-Based Practice Project

Patricia L. Finch-Guthrie, PhD, RN

CHAPTER TOPICS

- Implementation science
- Theoretical framework guiding implementation
- Pre-planning phase and the diagnostic analysis
- Implementation planning phase
- Sustainability planning phase
- Mentor challenges
- Mentor techniques and mentor supports

PERFORMANCE OBJECTIVES

After reading this chapter, the interprofessional evidence-based practice team will be able to do the following:

1. Define implementation and differentiate the concept from other similar evidence-based concepts, such as translation, diffusion, and dissemination.

2. Conduct a diagnostic analysis that includes a stakeholder analysis, factors that affect the uptake of change, staff attitudes and readiness, and the implementation climate of the organization.

3. Design an implementation plan involving the phases of pre-implementation, implementation, and sustainability to address the common barriers to change.

4. Create a positive, problem-solving approach for implementing a practice change.

Designing an interprofessional evidence-based practice (EBP) project not only involves delineating the project evaluation plan, obtaining institutional review board approval, and applying for grant support (Chapters 10 and 11), but also includes planning the actual implementation of the intervention, program, or strategy for a specific setting. Research informs health care professionals about new, more effective interventions, treatments, and care processes;

Moyers, P. A., & Finch-Guthrie, P. L.
*Interprofessional Evidence-Based Practice:
A Workbook for Health Professionals* (pp 183-195).
© 2016 Taylor and Francis Group.

however, clinicians are often unable to implement these better practices. Inappropriate care continues to occur in many health care systems because of the gap between research and practice and the difficulty clinicians have in using evidence-based interventions (McGlynn et al., 2003). Glasgow et al. (2012) found that only modest gains occur for patient outcomes because most efficacious treatments are not widely implemented, even within a single health care organization. Solomon (2010) asserted that advancing a science for implementation is an urgent, ethical issue because of the dismal uptake of evidence-based interventions. Furthermore, Solomon postulated that effective implementation strategies for integrating well-tested interventions in practice would substantially improve the health of millions of people.

Implementation is an essential EBP phase, and without understanding the nature of implementation, an interprofessional EBP team risks having an unsuccessful project. Ideally, an interprofessional team should use strategies for implementation based on well-tested implementation theories known to assist with changing practice. However, the science of implementation is relatively new, and it is often unclear why a change works well in one institution and does not work in another setting. In addition, some researchers have developed implementation science more fully within their respective disciplines compared to others (Clark, Park, & Burke, 2013). Thus, variation in understanding this phase of EBP may exist among the members of the interprofessional team. The purpose of this chapter is to help the interprofessional EBP team anticipate the most common issues for implementing an EBP project and to equip the team with implementation science principles for addressing challenges.

IMPLEMENTATION SCIENCE

To appreciate the complexity of the implementation phase of EBP, the interprofessional team needs to understand the concepts of implementation and implementation science. According to Fixsen, Naoom, Blasé, Friedman, and Wallace (2005) in an extensive systematic review on implementation, researchers use the term *implementation* inconsistently. In some studies, *implementation* means initiating the intervention or putting it into effect, and in other studies, *implementation* refers to specific methods designed to expand the use of an intervention so that it has a far-reaching effect on society (p. 4). Often, authors use the terms *implementation, translation, diffusion,* and *dissemination* interchangeably. While these terms are interrelated, they describe different aspects of the process for changing practice.

Translation science is a broader concept that incorporates diffusion, implementation, and dissemination as strategies for translating knowledge from empirical evidence

into practice (Nieva et al., 2005). The Canadian Institutes of Health Research (CIHR) defines knowledge translation as a "dynamic and iterative process that includes the synthesis, dissemination, exchange, and ethically sound application of knowledge to improve health, provide more effective health services and products, and strengthen the health care system" (CIHR, n.d., para. 1). Knowledge translation decreases the research–practice gap as a result of actively engaging those who created the new practice with those who will use the new intervention (Zidarov, Thomas, & Poissant, 2013).

Rabin and Brownson (2012) defined diffusion as the "passive, untargeted, unplanned, and uncontrolled spread of new interventions" (p. 25). Diffusion is the least intense form of knowledge transfer and tends to be more gradual. According to Rogers (2010), diffusion refers to the adoption and spread of an innovation across time and individuals within a specific social system. Each individual engages in his or her own innovation decision that includes five processes. The knowledge phase occurs when the person becomes aware of an innovation. The persuasion phase involves an individual developing a favorable or unfavorable attitude toward an innovation. The decision phase includes activities that culminate in a choice to adopt or reject an innovation. The last two phases include implementation, where the individual actually puts the innovation into use, and confirmation, which occurs when the person evaluates the results of adopting the new practice. Understanding the diffusion process is important for planning implementation strategies that will positively affect each phase of an individual's adoption of a new practice. Roger's diffusion model stresses the importance of knowledge translation occurring at the individual level within a social system or group. However, the model does not directly address knowledge transfer at the organizational level, which is a significant aspect of knowledge translation (Zidarov et al., 2013).

Implementing a new practice within an organization that the interprofessional team deems appropriate after appraising and synthesizing the literature is also part of translation science. Effective implementation requires using well-tested strategies known to facilitate change. Eccles and Mittman (2006) defined *implementation science* as the "scientific study of methods to promote the integration of research findings and evidence-based interventions into healthcare policy and practice, hence to improve the quality and effectiveness of health services and care" (Implementation Science section, para. 2). Schillinger (2010) described implementation in a similar manner and wrote, "implementation is the use of strategies to adopt and integrate evidence-based health interventions and change practice patterns within specific settings" (p. 1).

In the Iowa model (Titler & Everett, 2001), the implementation process, although not explicitly identified, most likely occurs within three action steps in the model (see Chapter 1, Figure 1-2). Specifically, the implementation process is required when developing a pilot of a practice change that was supported with sufficient evidence, when planning a research study testing an intervention that did not have sufficient evidence to pilot a change, and when permanently adopting an effective piloted practice change or tested intervention. In each instance of the Iowa model (Titler & Everett), planning occurs to ensure the intervention is in use prior to testing or evaluating effectiveness (see Chapter 13) and making decisions about next steps (see Chapter 14).

Dissemination, the last interprofessional EBP phase, which is also part of translation science, is the targeted distribution of information and results from conducting an EBP study or project (see Chapter 15). Dissemination is slightly different from the implementation phase of EBP in that it is concerned with implementing EBP interventions on a broader scale. Dissemination includes strategies that facilitate other departments within an organization, other institutions and settings, and the larger health care community to adopt the new practice.

THEORETICAL FRAMEWORK GUIDING IMPLEMENTATION

The implementation of an intervention requires a coordinated team effort for proactively addressing potential barriers and identifying facilitators that ensure adoption of the new practice. A high rate of adoption is necessary before measuring and analyzing outcomes; otherwise, it is impossible to determine the effectiveness of the intervention. Variable adoption of a new practice is more likely to produce negative outcomes. Practice integration requires planning throughout the implementation process that proactively prevents problems. However, unanticipated problems still occur, making a problem-solving perspective critical that consists of a rapid cycle process of ongoing planning, doing, and checking. Effective interprofessional teams should expect to encounter implementation problems, but should have the view that these issues stimulate creative thinking and ultimately contribute to the effectiveness of an innovation.

Using an implementation model that clearly identifies the actual steps for implementation and translating knowledge into practice is important to ensure a successful practice change (Zidarov et al., 2013). Implementation is a complex process, and models help to facilitate a shared understanding among team members regarding the multiple factors and processes involved, assist with predicting change-related outcomes, and reinforce the need for a multicomponent strategy to ensure success. Plastow's (2006) EBP model for change developed for allied health professionals describes an eight-step implementation process, which guides the discussion in the rest of this chapter.

The first two steps in the model are initiating and identifying the change, which involve creating awareness of a problem, identifying practice variation or a new technique or practice, and clearly describing the intended change. These two steps are really part of the interprofessional EBP phases covered extensively in Chapters 7 through 9 of this book. This chapter focuses on the next steps for implementation, which include conducting a diagnostic analysis, planning the implementation, designing the implementation strategy, and initiating the implementation cycle. Chapters 13 through 15 more extensively address the last two steps in the implementation model involving evaluation and determining future action.

All of the interprofessional team members assist with creating the implementation plan and with developing strategies to monitor and evaluate the implementation. The general planning phases of implementation include pre-planning that occurs prior to implementing the project, implementation planning that occurs during the implementation of the project, and planning for sustaining the change that occurs before ending the project. Table 12-1 lists and defines each phase of the implementation process and describes essential activities.

PRE-PLANNING PHASE AND THE DIAGNOSTIC ANALYSIS

The goal of the pre-planning phase is for the interprofessional EBP team to develop a realistic view about implementation in which the major activity is conducting a diagnostic analysis and gaining support for implementation. The pre-planning phase relies heavily on team members from the partnering health care institution to translate institutional policies or processes as they relate to the project and to identify internal stakeholders who have significant influence on the success of the EBP project.

Stakeholder Analysis

Stakeholders are best described as anyone whom a change in practice will directly or indirectly affect and are individuals or groups who may facilitate or block the actual implementation of the EBP project (Everett & Titler, 2006). Effectively involving stakeholders requires a systematic approach or stakeholder analysis. Interprofessional team members from the health care organization are essential for identifying internal stakeholders to determine the level of influence and support for the EBP project. However, all team members assist in identifying external stakeholders, such as patient or professional organizations/societies that may provide financial or other types of resources (e.g., materials, equipment, and education modules). The interprofessional team conducts an analysis of the stakeholders for the following important reasons:

TABLE 12-1

IMPLEMENTATION PLANNING PHASES

IMPLEMENTATION PHASE	DEFINITION	ESSENTIAL ACTIVITIES
Pre-planning phase	Planning that occurs prior to initiation of a project, focused on activities for preparing for full implementation. This planning phase is about developing a realistic view about implementation.	1. Stakeholder analysis 2. Engage stakeholders in the planning process 3. Factor analysis affecting the uptake of change 4. Identify potential barriers for implementation (see Table 11-1) 5. Identify strategies to address the barriers (see Table 11-1) 6. Readiness and Attitudes Assessment of staff's readiness to change 7. Implementation climate of the organization 8. Literature review for implementation studies regarding the intervention conducted in other organizations 9. Establish an overall project timeline 10. Obtain leadership support 11. Develop a communication plan 12. Identify educational needs 13. Determine the resources needed for implementation 14. Identify fidelity measures using both formative and summative evaluation processes
Implementation phase	Ongoing planning that starts with initial staff education and ends with full implementation. This planning phase is about responding to feedback, evaluation, concerns, and issues. The team is planning, doing, checking, and acting.	1. Develop and implement staff initial education, address concerns and issues identified during staff education 2. Communicate clear expectations about the change, the date when it will launch 3. Deploy resources 4. Implementation cycle: Rapid cycle of change, make corrections, and re-evaluate 5. Provide coaching and at the elbow support 6. Provide opportunities for ongoing feedback, addressing needs and concerns 7. Initiate fidelity measures and respond to adherence and competency rates
Sustainability phase	Planning that focuses on continuing the intervention for the long term. This planning phase is about making the change permanent.	1. Adherence often diminishes overtime, requires periodic monitoring of adherence 2. Ensure change is hardwired into workflow 3. Provide ongoing education as indicated, focusing on new staff 4. Continue to refine the intervention 5. Ensure long-term leadership and support

TABLE 12-2

STAKEHOLDER ANALYSIS

NAME/ROLE	IMPORTANCE/INFLUENCE	IMPACT	PERCEIVED ATTITUDES AND RISK	SUPPORT NEEDED/EXPECTATIONS	SUPPORT ABLE TO PROVIDE	RESPONSIBLE TEAM MEMBER
John Master Unit Manager	High importance High Influence	Minimal impact on role, high impact on unit practice, will change assessments currently being done	Has given support for the project and sees the value. Believes will need significant planning.	Expects to be involved in planning, needs the team to plan staff education, wants to craft communication to staff.	Knows staff on the health care organization unit, understands who the informal leaders are, will assist with getting them involved	Sally Jensen Clinical Scholar

- Involving stakeholders early in the implementation process is essential for developing their sense of ownership of the practice change.

- Practitioners are more likely to adopt a new practice when they assist with determining the use and implementation of a new practice.

- Sustainability of a practice change is highly dependent on stakeholders.

- Including stakeholders in the decision making for implementation enhances learning about the practice change for both the interprofessional EBP team and the stakeholders.

- Working with stakeholders builds organizational capacity for change.

A stakeholder analysis determines the stakeholders' level of interest, potential role in the implementation of the project, and level of influence with other stakeholders. Table 12-2 is an example of a stakeholder analysis tool developed from a review of the literature (Jepsen & Eskerod, 2009; Olander & Landin, 2005; Registered Nurses' Association of Ontario, 2010; Varvasovsky & Brugha, 2000). The analysis categories in the tool include the name and role of the stakeholder in the organization, the importance and degree of influence the stakeholder has regarding the practice change, the impact of the change on the role and attitudes of the stakeholder, and the risk the stakeholder perceives in implementing the practice change. The tool also includes the stakeholder's expectations about the support the project requires and the support the stakeholder is willing to provide.

The interprofessional team works closely with those stakeholders who not only are supportive of the change, but who have high importance and influence for implementing the project. These individuals are potential opinion leaders who may strongly influence adoption. In addition, the interprofessional EBP team targets those stakeholders whom they identify as having high importance and influence but who indicate they are not supportive or have reservations about the project. The interprofessional EBP team needs to address the concerns of those individuals to ensure successful implementation. Securing stakeholder input includes asking and then *listening* to each stakeholder's opinion and perception of the recommended practice change. Several key questions to ask stakeholders include the following:

- How will you decide whether the EBP practice change is successful and produces the desired results?

- What service delivery or process concerns do you have regarding implementation of the practice change that will affect complete adoption?

- Who do you think needs to champion the implementation of the EBP practice project?

- Who in the organization will influence the implementation of the proposed EBP project?

- What type and level of cooperation do you feel the team needs from selected stakeholders? Does the team need the full support from some stakeholders or does the team simply need to know that staff will support the EBP practice project?

- What do you think are the essential steps for implementing this EBP project successfully?

- What can you do to facilitate this change in practice?

Factors Affecting the Uptake of Change

Many believe problems associated with implementing EBP interventions largely result from contextual factors (macro- and micro-contexts) or the interaction of those factors, such as leadership, health care culture, and equipment and technology (Titler, 2010). Thus, a major goal of implementation is achieving full adoption through strategies that address contextual factors and their interactions. Titler and Everett (2001) developed the translation research model, which maintains that, in order to improve the rate and extent of adoption, those implementing an intervention need to focus on the characteristics of the intervention, the communication processes that assist with implementation, and also the social systems and the needs of the user.

The Ottawa model of research use identifies that adoption of an intervention is dependent on the attributes of the intervention, characteristics of potential adopters, and the factors of the practice environment (Graham, Logan, Tetroe, Robinson, & Harrison, 2008). Table 12-3 outlines known factors or barriers of implementation and matches them with potential strategies from the implementation science literature. For instance, a major facilitator or barrier to change implementation is the nature of the intervention itself. According to Rogers' (2010) diffusion of innovation theory, adoption occurs more readily when clinicians and practitioners perceive the new approach as compatible with not only their values, but also current systems. In addition, adoption is enhanced when the clinician or practitioner discovers the relative advantage of the new approach compared to current practice. An interprofessional team facilitates adoption when simplifying the intervention, creating ways that practitioners and clinicians can easily try the new method, and ensuring clinicians will observe others using the intervention successfully (Rogers, 2010). When practitioners within an organization observe their colleagues struggling with a new intervention, this visual will quickly curtail their planned adoption.

Due to lack of understanding of the intervention's core components, the team may find that results similar to the outcomes of the pilot change project are not achievable when widely adopting the intervention (Fixsen et al., 2005). For example, the team may have identified an intervention as patient teaching for the practice change project. During the pilot, a small group of experts conducted the patient teaching; however, with wide adoption in the health care organization, perhaps all of the staff conduct patient teaching after a short in-service. More than likely there will be differences in outcomes because part of the intervention in this example is actually the expertise of those performing the teaching.

Attitudes and Readiness for Change

Organizational change also depends on changing the behaviors of individuals (Damschroder et al., 2009). The characteristics of individuals affecting change include knowledge and beliefs about the change; self-efficacy regarding abilities to use the new intervention; the individual's stage of change; and identification with the department, unit, and organization. One well-known theory addressing individual change is Prochaska's and Velicer's (1997) trans-theoretical model in which individuals go through different stages: pre-contemplation (no awareness of the need to change), contemplation (awareness of the need to change), preparation (planning for change), action (implementing the change), and maintenance (sustaining the change). The objective for the interprofessional EBP team is to understand the stage of readiness for change of individuals who will be adopting the intervention, and to target strategies designed to move the individual from one stage to the next.

Rogers' (2010) diffusion theory classifies members of a social system regarding their degree of innovativeness (i.e., innovators, early adopters, early majority, late majority, and laggards). Innovators are those individuals who take risks and like to explore new ways of doing things. Innovators are important members to have on an interprofessional EBP team because of their excitement about innovations that may improve care. Early adopters serve as informal opinion leaders in the change process and are typically not in a formal leadership position (Grimshaw, Eccles, Lavis, Hill, & Squire, 2012; Prior, Guerin, & Grimmer-Somers, 2008; Zidarov et al., 2013). Medves et al. (2010), in a systematic review regarding dissemination and implementation of practice guidelines, identified input from local opinion leaders as a factor in guideline use. Thus, it is important for the interprofessional EBP team to identify early adopters who can assist with implementation and who will lead the majority of the staff (i.e., early and late majority) in making the change.

The early majority, while not necessarily leading the change, chooses to make the change through a deliberate process and have important networks helpful in facilitating change. The late majority makes the change primarily because of peer pressure or out of necessity (e.g., older equipment is discontinued). The laggards are the most skeptical and generally wait to change until the intervention is successful. Laggards may not adopt the new practice, which may dramatically affect patient outcomes. Individuals who are extremely skeptical significantly delay implementation because of focusing on what could go wrong with the new intervention. Communication, relationship building and collaboration, engagement, and staff education are common strategies for creating change in individuals (Damschroder et al., 2009; Meyers et al., 2012).

TABLE 12-3

IMPLEMENTATION BARRIERS AND STRATEGIES

BARRIER	SOURCE	STRATEGY	SOURCE
Culture	Brennan, Bosch, Buchan, & Green, 2012; Shojania & Grimshaw, 2005; Zidarov et al., 2013	Identify fit with culture and social norms; align project goals and objectives with mission, vision, strategic plan, and organizational resources; and assess organizational readiness.	Damschroder et al., 2009; Plastow, 2006; RNAO, 2012; Rogers, 2010; Titler & Everett, 2001
Leadership	Francke, Smit, de Veer, & Mistiaen, 2008; Moulding, Silagy, & Weller, 1999	Identify leaders for support, involve them in the process, ask them to assist with issues, identify opinion leaders (early adopters) and change agents, and develop a local team to lead the change	Fixsen et al., 2005; Gifford, Davies, Edwards, & Graham; 2006; Grol & Grimshaw, 2003; McCormack et al., 2013; Menon, Korner-Bitensky, Kastner, McKibbon, & Straus, 2009; RNAO, 2012; Rogers, 2010; Zidarov et al., 2013
Education	Haines, Kuruvilla, & Borchert, 2004; Koh, Manias, Hutchinson, Donath, & Johnston, 2008; Shojania & Grimshaw, 2005; Zidarov et al., 2013	Brief unit huddles, seminars, in-services, at the elbow education, ongoing consultation and coaching, question and answer sessions, rounds, simulations, return demonstrations, interactive education, super-users/local experts	Achterberg, Schoonhoven, & Grol, 2008; Davis et al., 1999; Fixsen et al., 2005; Forsetlund et al., 2012; Myers et al., 2012; Menon et al., 2009; Moulding et al., 1999; Plastow, 2006
Intervention	Glasgow, 2003; Grol & Grimshaw, 2003; Francke et al., 2008	Clarification of core intervention components, simplify steps, address useability and trialability, manualized, adequately packaged	Damschroder et al., 2009; Glasgow & Emmons, 2007; Fixsen et al., 2005; Plastow, 2006; Rogers, 2010; Titler & Everett, 2001
Communication	Morrison & Milliken, 2000; Moulding et al., 1999	Determine target audience, use normal site communication processes: key meetings, e-mails, posters, newsletters, blogs, reminders, ongoing communication. Prevent information overload	Damschroder et al., 2009; Grol & Grimshaw, 2003; Haines et al., 2004; Menon et al., 2009; Moulding et al., 1999; RNAO, 2012; Rogers, 2010; Titler & Everett, 2001
Equipment and space	Hutchinson & Johnston, 2006; Koh et al., 2008; Shojania & Grimshaw, 2005; Zidarov et al., 2013	Identification of materials and equipment, deploy equipment, ensure routine access, create decision support, and assess and address space needs	Achterberg et al., 2008; Fixsen et al., 2005; Moulding et al., 1999; RNAO, 2012
Policies	Grol & Grimshaw, 2003; Haines et al., 2004; Hutchinson & Johnston, 2006; Shojania & Grimshaw, 2005	Developing/revising policies and guidelines, matching the guideline to the problem, and making the changes accessible. Identify external policy or regulation support or issues	Achterberg et al., 2008; Menon et al., 2009; Plastow, 2006; RNAO, 2012; Zidarov et al., 2013

(continued)

TABLE 12-3 (CONTINUED)

IMPLEMENTATION BARRIERS AND STRATEGIES

BARRIER	SOURCE	STRATEGY	SOURCE
Stakeholders/ users	Brennan et al., 2012; Cabana et al., 1999; Grol & Grimshaw, 2003	Identifying key stakeholders; understanding needs, values, beliefs, attitudes, and concerns; assess readiness/motivation, garner strong support, assess user qualifications, understand the social systems	Achterberg et al., 2008; Fixsen et al., 2005; Plastow, 2006; RNAO, 2012; Rogers, 2010; Titler & Everett, 2001; Zidarov et al., 2013
Patients/clients	Francke et al., 2008; Grol & Grimshaw, 2003; Haines et al., 2004; Koh et al., 2008	Obtain input from patients/clients and families, and identify patients/clients appropriate for the intervention	Achterberg et al., 2008; Damschroder et al., 2009; Haines et al., 2004; Plastow, 2006; RNAO, 2012
Systems/work flow/workload or time	Francke et al., 2008; Grol & Grimshaw, 2003; Zidarov et al., 2013	Develop systems to support the new practice: computer supports and alerts, reminders, documentation systems, embed in workflow, decrease time involved, and substitute tasks	Fixsen et al., 2005; Grol & Grimshaw, 2003; RNAO, 2012; Zidarov et al., 2013
Cost/financial disincentives/ resources	Grol & Grimshaw, 2003; Haines et al., 2004; Koh et al., 2008; Shojania & Grimshaw, 2005	Determine start-up and ongoing costs, budget planning, human resource needs, in-kind support; identify cost savings; and address reimbursement and liability issues	Achterberg et al., 2008; Damschroder et al., 2009; Haines et al., 2004; RNAO, 2012
Evaluation	Haines et al., 2004	Evaluating patient clinical outcomes and experience, staff adherence/experience, performance feedback, formative and summative evaluation planning, audit	Achterberg et al., 2008; Damschroder et al., 2009; Fixsen et al., 2005; Grol & Grimshaw, 2003; Haines et al., 2004; Meyers et al., 2012; Plastow, 2006; RNAO, 2012; Zidarov et al., 2013

Implementation Climate

Implementation climate is a critical aspect of organizational readiness that includes the tension for change and whether the organization perceives the change as necessary or as a priority. The presence of a learning environment, routine use of rewards and incentives, and a high level of commitment to change are important elements for a positive implementation climate (Damschroder et al., 2009). Meyers, Durlak, and Wandersman (2012) recommend conducting an intervention fit assessment in which a determination occurs regarding the degree to which the intervention meets the organizational needs, mission, vision, values, priorities, and strategic plan.

Leadership engagement is critical in ensuring organizational readiness (Moser, Deluca, Bond, & Rollins, 2004). In contrast, leaders who are resistant to an EBP change have a negative effect on implementation (Parahoo & McCaughan, 2001). The interprofessional EBP team needs to engage the most appropriate leaders for the project early in the implementation process. An analysis of internal organizational strengths, weaknesses, opportunities, and external threats (SWOT) is a common method for examining the change factors of an organization, department, or unit (McCluskey & Cusick, 2002). The analysis helps the team focus on organizational strengths for facilitating change, while at the same time addressing weaknesses and eliminating threats that will negatively affect outcomes. Another method is for the team to analyze driving and restraining forces for the proposed change with the goal of eliminating or mitigating the restraining forces while enhancing driving forces (Heward, Hutchins, & Keleher, 2007; Lewin, 1951). When examining institutional climate and readiness, the interprofessional team uses systems thinking to understand how each aspect of a change may potentially influence and interact with processes across multiple levels of an organization (Holmes, Finegood, Riley, & Best, 2012).

IMPLEMENTATION PLANNING PHASE

The focus for the implementation planning phase is to ensure fidelity of the intervention and respond to feedback, concerns, and issues. This phase of the process involves the major strategy of rapid cycle change, which includes planning, doing, checking, and acting (Kendrick, Klossner, & Haubrick, 2010; Kilo, 1998). When using rapid cycle change, team members make immediate small corrections, implementing changes, and re-evaluating results.

Fidelity Outcomes

When an interprofessional team is conducting an EBP project, the team needs to consider two different types of outcomes. The first outcome is whether the new intervention is effective and has improved patient care (Chapter 10), and the second outcome focuses on whether the caregiver is using the new intervention as intended. The team cannot determine the first outcome if they do not know whether clinicians or practitioners adopted the intervention as designed. The team should not expect positive outcomes without full implementation (Bernfeld, 2001; Fixsen et al., 2005; Institute of Medicine, 2001). According to Schillnger (2010), fidelity is defined as "the adherence of actual treatment delivery to the protocol originally developed or the degree program developers implement programs as intended" (p. 2). Lower levels of fidelity may account for the difference in research results compared to practice outcomes for the same intervention.

Breitenstein et al. (2010) described fidelity as having two elements: adherence and competence. Adherence is useful for determining the rate and degree of adoption for the new practice. To understand the elements of adherence, the interprofessional team could view the intervention as having a dose, like a medication, in which the team clearly identifies what constitutes a dose, the frequency for delivering the dose, and the duration of and type of contact needed with each patient. Based on the administration requirements for the full intervention, the team develops a treatment protocol or guideline. A lack of an equivalent treatment dose across conditions and populations occurs (Bellg et al., 2004) due to the following:

- A large number of patients and families who still receive treatment and services based on the old approach or protocol
- A significant number of patients and families who receive an incomplete dose (partial intervention) of the treatment

Measures of adherence quantify the occurrence of the required intervention and process components. Examples of adherence measures include the percent of appropriate patients receiving the new intervention, the timing of administration, the actual dose (i.e., full or partial), and identification of the most commonly missed intervention components. A variety of data collection methods for fidelity exists, such as audits of patient records, observations, and user and patient feedback.

While adherence addresses the adoption of the intervention, competence focuses on the quality of applying the intervention (Breitenstein et al., 2010). Competence includes not only technical competence, but also clinical judgement regarding when and how to use the intervention given individual patient circumstances. Measures of competence include pre- and post-tests for knowledge acquisition and application, as well as successful completion of simulated experiences and direct practice observations. Implementation fidelity measures involving adherence and competency provide a feedback loop so that the interprofessional team is able to clarify and improve the intervention, provide ongoing staff education, and streamline processes for intervention delivery.

Designing the Implementation Strategies

The interprofessional team needs to use multifaceted implementation strategies to ensure full adoption of an intervention (Grimshaw et al., 2001; Medves et al., 2010; Prior et al., 2008). Traditionally, didactic education is often the only strategy organizations use for changing practice. Unfortunately, staff education, while necessary, is not sufficient on its own to change practice (Allery, Owen, & Robling, 1997; Davis et al., 1999; Forsetlund et al., 2012; Zidarov et al., 2013). While practice guidelines have the potential to improve outcomes, their actual use is variable. However, guidelines are successful when coupled with multifaceted implementation strategies (Grol, 2001; Medves et al., 2010; Prior et al., 2008).

Fixsen et al. (2005) identified through an extensive review of the literature the core implementation strategies or drivers that create *high-fidelity practitioner behavior,* which occurs when using the new intervention consistently (p. 28). These core implementation components include careful staff selection based on the needed qualifications for using the intervention, pre-service training, consultation and coaching at the point of care, staff and program evaluation, facilitative administrative support, and system interventions (Anderson, Finch Guthrie, Kraft, Reicks, & Skay, 2015; Kelleher, Moorer, & Makie, 2012; Lopez et al., 2002; McCleary, Ellis, & Rowley, 2004). It is critical that the interprofessional EBP team develop an overall work plan that addresses each phase of implementation, with clearly assigned responsibilities, project timelines, and time for reviewing and modifying the plan at every team meeting. Discussing progress on the implementation plan for which every team member has a role is part of the team briefing process that occurs during regular meetings.

SUSTAINABILITY PLANNING PHASE

Sustainability is the degree an intervention continues to produce benefits over time after concentrated support is withdrawn (Rabin & Brownson, 2012). With the sustainability phase, the focus is on maintaining and institutionalizing change, making it part of the natural workflow (Shediac-Rizkallah & Bone, 1998). Sustainability is dependent on codifying the new practice in policies and on thoroughly training staff. Including education into staff orientation and competency evaluations assists with maintaining the change. Implementation adherence often dissipates over time. Thus, the interprofessional team should continue to monitor adherence measures that correlate with the intervention outcome. For example, if using an assessment tool correlates with a patient outcome, then monitoring the completion rate is an appropriate adherence measure. Innovation champions and leaders leave an organization; thus, ensuring continued leadership support is important. The interprofessional EBP team may need to transition work to influential organizational committees that integrate the innovation into work plans. Chapter 14 discusses in more depth the sustainability planning that occurs as the interprofessional team ends the EBP project.

MENTOR CHALLENGES

In general, implementation may not necessarily proceed smoothly, at least initially, but with a continuous project improvement approach, the issues become less frequent. The interprofessional EBP program coordinators and the mentors should set a matter-of-fact tone that implementation problems are common and solvable. The goal is for the interprofessional team members to avoid perceptions that implementation occurs effortlessly and that, when problems occur, there is a crisis. The mentor focuses the team on monitoring data and measuring fidelity to assist with identifying root causes for implementation problems. With this focus, the team targets solutions to address the most salient implementation issues. During implementation, knowing each team member's strengths (e.g., project management, quality improvement, information technology, or staff education) is an important strategy for assigning implementation roles that fit with the level of expertise of each team member.

A common and often the most difficult mentor and interprofessional team challenge is staff resistance to the change process. Resistance that is unanticipated and poorly managed can derail even the best interprofessional EBP project. Resistance often indicates a lack of understanding, knowledge, skills, or resources to carry out a project. It is not uncommon for those developing a practice change to underestimate the learning in which they have engaged compared to learning of those who have not had direct involvement. Thus, the team may misjudge the communication and training that others need. Ongoing staff communication and education lessens resistance for changing practice.

Resistance is more likely with those individuals who represent the late majority or laggards as described in Rogers' (2010) diffusion theory. Engaging opinion leaders and coaches to work with staff is an effective approach. Listening to staff and ensuring they have a voice in the change is essential to ensure that both patient and staff benefit from changing practice. Often, staff concerns relate to their apprehension about an increased workload, which makes it critical to design an intervention that is easy to perform.

Another common challenge for an interprofessional team is running out of time or funding prior to project completion. Poorly defined projects are susceptible to scope creep, which is an inadvertent increase in the project activities without planning for increases in time and budget. The mentor and the program coordinator's expertise with interprofessional EBP is important for assisting teams in narrowing the project to a well-defined practice change and in clearly identifying resource needs for keeping to the time line.

MENTOR TECHNIQUES AND MENTOR SUPPORTS

Unexpected problems or issues are common, but well-known strategies are available for the project coordinators and mentors to ensure team success. The main success principles are as follows:

- Staying positive, adopting a problem-solving approach
- Educating the interprofessional EBP team regarding implementation
- Keeping the interprofessional team members engaged throughout implementation, assigning responsibility for each action on the implementation work plan
- Planning that addresses known barriers and facilitators of implementation
- Conducting a stakeholder analysis to garner support and ensure involvement in the implementation process, and to identify early adopters as opinion leaders
- Analyzing the factors affecting the uptake of change and matching these factors with appropriate change strategies
- Analyzing the implementation climate of the organization, involving leaders in the readiness assessment, and using systems-level thinking

- Planning that addresses ongoing feedback about the implementation process to ensure high fidelity of the intervention

- Planning for project sustainability

- Reframing setbacks and problems as learning experiences and opportunities

SUMMARY

Implementation is a crucial part of the interprofessional EBP process that requires a proactive approach for addressing known barriers to change. An interprofessional EBP team is successful with implementing a practice change when the entire team engages in pre-implementation, implementation, and sustainability planning phases. Mentors and program coordinators who engage in reflective and deliberative mentoring are effective in encouraging EBP teams to assume a problem-solving posture throughout the project. Part of the pre-planning phase includes conducting a diagnostic analysis that assists the team in garnering support needed to put the new intervention into practice. During pre-implementation, the team develops a plan that addresses known barriers to change. The interprofessional team focuses on achieving fidelity of the intervention during the implementation phase. Adherence to the intervention and staff competency is necessary to achieve an improvement in patient outcomes. In sustainability planning, the interprofessional EBP team works to embed the practice change fully into the workflow and routine practices of clinicians and practitioners.

REFLECTION QUESTIONS

1. What barriers to change are the most difficult to address and prevent? Discuss your reasoning.

2. If you were to engage in implementation in your practice area, what implementation strategies would be the most effective in your setting? Discuss your reasoning.

REFERENCES

Achterberg, T. V., Schoonhoven, L., & Grol, R. (2008). Nursing implementation science: How evidence-based nursing requires evidence-based implementation. *Journal of Nursing Scholarship*, 40(4), 302-310. doi:10.1111/j.1547-5069.2008.00243.

Allery, L. A., Owen, P. A., & Robling, M. R. (1997). General practice. *British Medical Journal*, 314(22), 870-874.

Anderson, M., Finch Guthrie, P., Kraft, W., Reicks, P., & Skay, C. (2015). Universal pressure ulcer prevention bundle with WOC nurse support. *Journal of Wound Ostomy Continence Nurse*, 42(3), 217-225. doi:10.1097/won.0000000000000109

Bellg, A. J., Borrelli, B., Resnick, B., Hecht, J., Minicucci, D. S., Ory, M., ... Czajkowski, S. (2004). Enhancing treatment fidelity in health behavior change studies: Best practices and recommendations from the NIH behavior change consortium. *Health Psychology*, 23(5), 443-451. doi:10.1037/0278-6133.23.5.443

Bernfeld, G. A. (2001). The struggle for treatment integrity in a "dis-integrated" service delivery system. In G.A. Bernfeld, D.P. Farrington, & A.W. Leschied (Eds.), *Offender Rehabilitation in practice: Implementing and evaluating effective programs* (pp. 167-1888). London, UK: Wiley.

Breitenstein, S. M., Gross, D., Garvey, C. A., Hill, C., Fogg, L., & Resnick, B. (2010). Implementation fidelity in community-based interventions. *Research in Nursing & Health*, 33, 164-173. doi: 10.1002/nur.20373

Brennan, S. E., Bosch, M., Buchan, H., & Green, S. E. (2012). Measuring organization and individual factors thought to influence the success of quality improvement in primary care: A systematic review. *Implementation Science*, 7(121), 1-19. doi:10.1186/1748-5908-7-121

Cabana, M. D., Rand, C. S., Powe, N. R., Wu, A. W., Wilson, M. H., Abboud, P. C., & Rubin, H. R. (1999). Why don't physicians follow clinical practice guidelines? *Journal of American Medical Association*, 282(15), 1458-1465. doi:10.1001/jama.282.15.1458

Canadian Institutes of Health Research. (n.d.). Knowledge translation. Ottawa, Canada: CIHR. Retrieved at www.cihr-irsc.gc.ca/e/39033.html#Knowledge-Action.

Clark, F., Park, D. J., & Burke, J. P. (2013). Dissemination: Bringing translational research to completion. *American Journal of Occupational Therapy*, 67, 185-193. doi:10.5014/ajot.2013.006148

Damschroder, L. J., Aron, D. C., Keith, R., Kirsh, S. R., Alexander, J. A., & Lowery, J.C. (2009). Fostering implementation of health services research findings into practice: A consolidated framework for advancing implementation science. *Implementation Science*, 4, 50. doi:10.1186/1748-5908-4-50.

Davis, D., Thomson O'Brien, M. A., Freemantle, N., Wolf, F. M., Mazmanian, P., & Taylor-Vaisey, A. (1999). Impact of formal continuing medical education: Do conferences, workshops, rounds, and traditional continuing education activities change physician behavior of health care outcomes? *Journal of American Medical Association*, 282(9), 867-874. doi:10.1001/jama.282.9.867

Eccles, M. P., & Mittman, B. S. (2006). Welcome to implementation science. *Implementation Science*, 1, 1.

Everett, L. Q., & Titler, M. G. (2006). Making EBP part of clinical practice: The Iowa model. In R.F. Levin & H. R. Feldman (Eds.), *Teaching evidence-based practice in nursing* (pp. 295-324). New York, NY: Springer Publishing Company.

Fixsen, D. L., Naoom, S. F., Blasé, K. A., Friedman, R. M. & Wallace, F. (2005). *Implementation research: A synthesis of the literature.* Tampa, FL, University of South Florida, Louis de la Parte Florida Mental Health Institution, The National Implementation Research Network (FMHI Publication #231).

Forsetlund, L., Bjorndal, A., Rashidian, A., Jamtvedt, G., O'Brien, M. A., Wolf, F. M.,...Oxman, A.D. (2012). Continuing education meetings and workshops: Effects on professional practice and health care outcomes. *The Cochrane Library* (11). Retrieved at www.thecochranelibrary.com.

Francke, A. L., Smit, M., de Veer, A. J., & Mistiaen, P. (2008). Factors influencing the implementation of clinical guidelines for health care professionals: A systematic meta-review. *BC Medical Informatics and Decision Making, 8*(38). doi:10.1186/1472-6947-8-38.

Gifford, A. W., Davies, B., Edwards, N., & Graham, D. I. (2006). Leadership strategies to influence the use of clinical practice guidelines. *Nursing Leadership, 19*(4), 72-88. doi:10.12927/cjnl.2006.18603

Glasgow, R. E. (2003). Translating research to practice: Lessons learned, areas for improvement, and future directions. *Diabetes Care, 26,* 2451-2456. doi:10.2337/diacare.26.8.2451

Glasgow, R. E., & Emmons, K. M. (2007). How can we increase translation of research into practice? Types of evidence needed. *Annual Review of Public Health, 28,* 413-433. doi:10.1146/annurev.publhealth.28.021406.144145

Glasgow, R. E., Vinson, C., Chambers, D., Khoury, M. J., Kaplan, R. M., & Hunter, C. (2012). National Institutes of Health approaches to dissemination and implementation science: Current and future directions. *American Journal of Public Health, 102*(7), 1274-1281. doi:10.2105/ajph.2012.300755

Graham, I. D., Logan, J., Tetroe, J., Robinson, N., & Harrison, M. B. (2008). Models of implementation in nursing (pp. 231-243). In N. Cullum, D. Ciliska, R.B. Haynes, S. Marks (Eds.), *Evidence-based nursing.* Oxford, UK: Blackwell Publishing Ltd.

Grimshaw, J. M., Eccles, M. P., Lavis, J. N., Hill, S. J., & Squires, J. E. (2012). Knowledge translation of research findings. *Implementation Science, 750.* http://www.implementation-science.com/content/7/1/5

Grimshaw, E. M., Shirran, L., Thomas, R., Mowatt, G., Fraser, C., Bero, L.,...O'Brien, M.A. (2001). Changing provider behavior: An overview of systematic reviews of interventions. *Medical Care, 39*(8), II2-II45. doi:10.1097/00005650-200108002-00002

Grol, R. (2001). Success and failures in the implementation of evidence-based guidelines for clinical practice. *Medical Care, 39*(8 supplement 2), 1146-1154. doi:10.1097/00005650-200108002-00003

Grol, R., & Grimshaw, J. (2003). From best evidence to best practice: Effective implementation of change in patients' care. *Lancet, 362,* 1225-1230. doi:10.1016/s0140-6736(03)14546-1

Haines, A., Kuruvilla, S., & Borchert, M. (2004). Bridging the implementation gap between knowledge and action for health. *Bulletin of the World Health Organization, 82*(10), 724-732.

Heward, S., Hutchins, C., & Keleher, H. (2007). Organizational change—key to capacity building and effective health promotion. *Health Promotion International, 22*(2), 170-178. doi:10.1093/heapro/dam011

Holmes, B. J., Finegood, D. T., Riley, B. L., & Best, A. (2012). Systems thinking in dissemination and implementation research. In R. C. Brownson, G. A. Colditz, and E. K. Proctor (Eds.), *Dissemination and Implementation Research in Health.* New York, NY: Oxford University Press.

Hutchinson, A. M., & Johnston, L. (2006). Beyond the barriers scale: Commonly reported barriers to research use. *Journal of Nursing Administration, 36*(4), 189-199. doi:10.1097/00005110-200604000-00008

Institute of Medicine Committee on Quality of Health Care in America. (2001). *Crossing the quality of chasm: A new health system for the 21st century.* Washington, DC: National Academy Press.

Jepsen, A. L., & Eskerod, P. (2009). Stakeholder analysis in projects: Challenges in using current guidelines in the real world. *International Journal of Project Management, 27,* 335-343. doi:10.1016/j.ijproman.2008.04.002

Kelleher A. D., Moorer A., & Makic, M. F. (2012). Peer-to-peer nursing rounds and hospital-acquired pressure ulcer prevalence in a surgical intensive care unit: a quality improvement project. *Journal of Wound Ostomy Continence Nursing, 39*(2), 90-94. doi:10.1097/won.0b013e3182435409

Kendrick, K., Klossner, J., & Haubrick, K. (2010). Implementing projects using the rapid-cycle approach. *Journal of Nursing Administration, 40*(3), 135-139.doi:10.1097/nna.0b013e3181d042d6

Kilo, C. M. (1998). A framework for collaborative improvement: Lessons from the Institute for Healthcare Improvement's Breakthrough Series. *Quality Management in Health Care, 6*(4), 1-14. doi:10.1097/00019514-199806040-00001

Koh, S. S., Manias, E., Hutchinson, A. M., Donath, S., & Johnston, L. (2008). Nurses' perceived barriers to the implementation of a fall prevention clinical practice guideline in Singapore hospitals. *BMC Health Services Research, 8*(105). doi:10.1186/1472-6963-8-105

Lewin, K. (1951). *Field theory in social science.* New York, NY: Harper Row.

Lopez, M., Delmore, B., Ake, J. M., Kim, Y. R., Golden, P., Bier, J., & Fulmer, T. (2002). Implementing a geriatric resource nurse model. *Journal of Nursing Administration, 32*(11), 577-585. doi:10.1097/00005110-200211000-00005

McCleary L., Ellis, J., & Rowley, B. (2004). Evaluation of the pain resource nurse role: a resource for improving pediatric pain management. *Pain Management Nursing, 5*(1), 29-36. doi: org/10.1016/j.pmn.2003.08.001

McCluskey, A., & Cusick, A. (2002). Strategies for introducing evidence-based practice and changing clinician behavior: A manager's toolbox. *Australian Occupational Therapy Journal, 49,* 63-70. doi:10.1046/j.1440-1630.2002.00272.x

McCormack, B., Rycroft-Malone, J., DeCorby, K., Hutchinson, A. M., Bucknall, T., Kent, B., ... Wilson, V. (2013). A realist review of interventions and strategies to promote evidence-informed healthcare: A focus on change agency. *Implementation Science, 8*(107), 1-12.

McGlynn, E. A., Asch, S. M., Adams, J., Keesey, J., Hicks, J., DeCristofaro, A., & Kerr, E. A. (2003). The quality of health care delivered to adults in the United States. *New England Journal of Medicine, 348,* 2635-2645. doi:10.1056/nejm200311063491916

Medves, J., Godfrey, C., Turner, C., Paterson, M., Harrison, M., MacKenzie, L., & Durando, P. (2010). Systematic review of practice guideline dissemination and implementation strategies for healthcare teams and team-based practice. *International Journal of Evidence-Based Healthcare, 8,* 79-89. doi:10.1111/j.1744-1609.2010.00166.x

Menon, A., Korner-Bitensky, N., Kastner, M., McKibbon, K. A., & Straus, S. (2009). Strategies for rehabilitation professionals to move evidence-based knowledge into practice: A systematic review. *Journal of Rehabilitation Medicine, 41,* 1024-1032.doi:10.2340/16501977-0451

Meyers, D. C., Durlak, J. A., & Wandersman, A. (2012). The quality implementation framework: A synthesis of critical steps in the implementation process. *American Journal of Community Psychology, 50,* 462-480. doi:10.1007/s10464-012-9522-x

Meyers, D. C., Katz, J., Chien, V., Wandersman, A., Scaccia, J. P., & Wright, A. (2012). Practical implementation science: Developing and piloting the quality improvement tool. *American Journal of Community Psychology, 50,* 481-496. doi:10.1007/s10464-012-9521-y

Morrison, E. W., & Milliken, F. J. (2000). Organizational silence: A barrier to change and development in a pluralistic world. *The Academy of Management Review, 25*(4), 706-725. doi:10.5465/amr.2000.3707697

Moser, L., DeLuca, N., Bond, G., & Rollins, A. (2004). Implementing evidence-based psychosocial practices: Lessons learned from statewide implementation of two practices. *The International Journal of Neuropsychiatric Medicine, 9*(12), 926-936.

Moulding, N. T., Silagy, C. A., & Weller, D. P. (1999). A framework for effective management of change in clinical practice: Dissemination and implementation of clinical practice guidelines. *Quality in Health Care, 8,* 177-183. doi:10.1136/qshc.8.3.177

Nieva, V. F., Murphy, R., Ridley, M., Donaldson, N., Combes, J., Mitchell, P.,...Carpenter, D. (2005). From science to service: A framework for the transfer of patient safety research into practice. In K. Henriksen, J. B. Battles, E. S. Marks (Eds.), *Advances in Patient Safety: From Research to Implementation,* (Volume 2: Concepts and Methodology). Rockville, MD: Agency for Healthcare Research and Quality (US); 2005 Feb. Retrieved at http://www.ncbi.nlm.nih.gov/books/NBK20521/.

Olander, S., & Landin, A. (2005). Evaluation of stakeholder influence in the implementation of construction projects. *International Journal of Project Management, 23,* 321-328. doi:10.1016/j.ijproman.2005.02.002

Parahoo, K., & McCaughan, E. M. (2001). Research utilization among medical and surgical nurses: A comparison of their self-reports and perception of barriers and facilitators. *Journal of Nursing Management, 9,* 21-30.

Plastow, N. A. (2006). Implementing evidence-based practice: A model for change. *International Journal of Therapy and Rehabilitation, 13*(10), 464-469.

Prior, M., Guerin, M., & Grimmer-Somers, K. (2008). The effectiveness of clinical guideline implementation strategies—a synthesis of systematic review findings. *Journal of Evaluation in Clinical Practice, 14,* 888-897.

Prochaska, J. O., & Velicer, W. F. (1997). The transtheroretical model of health behavior change. *American Journal of Health Promotion, 12,* 38-48. doi:10.4278/0890-1171-12.1.38

Rabin, B. A., & Brownson, R. C. (2012). Developing the terminology for dissemination and implementation research. In R. C. Brownson, G. A. Colditz, and E. K. Proctor (Eds.), *Dissemination and implementation research in health.* New York, NY: Oxford University Press. doi:10.1093/acprof:oso/9780199751877.003.0002

Registered Nurses' Association of Ontario. (2012). *Toolkit: Implementation of best practice guidelines* (2nd ed.). Toronto, Canada: Registered Nurses' Association of Ontario.

Rogers, E. M. (2010). *Diffusion of Innovations* (4th ed.). New York, NY: The Free Press.

Schillinger, D. (2010). An introduction to effectiveness, dissemination and implementation research. In P. Fleischer & E. Goldstein (Eds.), *UCSF Clinical and Translational Science Institute (CTSI) Resource Manuals and Guides to Community-Engaged Research.* San Francisco, CA: Clinical Translational Science Institute Community Engagement Program, University of California San Francisco. Retrieved at http://ctsi.ucsf.edu/files/CE/edi_introguide.pdf.

Shediac-Rizkallah, M. C., & Bone, L. R. (1998). Planning for the sustainability of community-based health programs: Conceptual frameworks and future directions for research, practice and policy. *Health Education Research, 13*(1), 87-108. doi:10.1093/her/13.1.87

Shojania, K. G., & Grimshaw, J. M. (2005). Evidence-based quality improvement: The state of the science. *Health Affairs, 24*(1), 138-150. doi:10.1377/hlthaff.24.1.138

Solomon, M. Z. (2010). The ethical urgency of advancing implementation science. *The American Journal of Bioethics, 10*(8), 31-44. doi:10.1080/15265161.2010.494230

Titler, M. G., & Everett, L. Q. (2001). Translating research into practice: Considerations for critical care investigators. *Critical Care Nursing Clinics of North America, 13*(4), 587-604.

Titler, M. G. (2010). Translation science and context. *Research and Theory for Nursing Practice, 24*(1), 35-55.

Varvasovszky, Z., & Brugha, R. (2000). A stakeholder analysis. *Health Policy and Planning, 15*(3), 338-345. doi:10.1093/heapol/15.3.338

Zidarov, D., Thomas, A., & Poissant, L. (2013). Knowledge translation in physical therapy: From theory to practice. *Disability and Rehabilitation, 35*(18), 1571-1577. doi:10.3109/09638288.2012.748841

Supplemental materials for this chapter are available online.
Please refer to the sticker in the front of the book and enter the access code provided.

Evaluating and Analyzing the Interprofessional Evidence-Based Practice Project

Mark Blegen, PhD, FACSM and Penelope A. Moyers, EdD, OT/L, FAOTA

CHAPTER TOPICS

- Level of evidence and the project results
- From PICO question to project question
- Data collection, preparation, and cleaning
- Common statistical terminology
- Summarizing the data
- Analyzing the data
- Mentor challenges
- Mentor techniques and supports

PERFORMANCE OBJECTIVES

By the end of this chapter, the mentors and interprofessional team members will be able to do the following::

1. Develop a data management plan that ensures confidentiality and reduces error arising from missing data and from data entry.

2. Perform simple descriptive analysis of the data using measures of central tendency, variability, population parameters, and graphs and charts.

3. Select the appropriate statistical analysis with support of a statistician.

4. Interpret statistical results and determine clinical significance.

Think about how far the team has come with the interprofessional evidence-based practice (EBP) project. Teams and partnerships have been developed, roles have been clarified; in turn, everyone has been a leader, a learner, a mentor, a data collector, a motivator, and a coach. Much time and energy have gone into the interprofessional EBP

Moyers, P. A., & Finch-Guthrie, P. L.
Interprofessional Evidence-Based Practice:
A Workbook for Health Professionals (pp 197-213).
© 2016 Taylor and Francis Group.

project, and now it is time to analyze the data and evaluate the results of the project in order to produce a recommendation about a potential practice change to the health care organization. In reviewing the Iowa model (Titler et al., 2001) presented in Chapter 1, the team is now evaluating the process and outcomes of the EBP change pilot in order to answer the question, "Is this change appropriate for adoption in practice?"

Being confident in the practice recommendation arises from knowing the project was well-designed and was implemented with fidelity. The project also produced error-free data through careful data collection and management strategies. Finally, through appropriate data analysis and interpretation within the confines of the project's limitations, the team can be sure that the recommendations arising from the EBP project are both valid and accurate.

The goal of this chapter is not to present an in-depth discussion of data analysis and statistical reasoning because other texts are more appropriate for that kind of learning. Instead, the goal is to familiarize the interprofessional team members who are not comfortable with research methodologies, and statistical analysis and reasoning to have at least a common language in communicating with their statistician and with other team members who are taking the lead on this aspect of the interprofessional EBP project task. Understanding what the data indicate about the practice change is powerful, and all clinicians and practitioners should gain basic knowledge of statistical reasoning in order to engage in EBP appraisal and in analysis and evaluation of the interprofessional EBP project.

LEVEL OF EVIDENCE AND THE PROJECT RESULTS

The team gathered evidence through the data collected from the interprofessional EBP project. The team wants to arrive at the appropriate conclusions based on the data; therefore, it is important to understand the hierarchy of evidence so that appropriate consideration is given to the type of evidence the EBP project produced (Chapter 9). Recall that the study design determines the strength of the evidence. Consequently, if the interprofessional team in their project randomized study participants to a control group and an intervention group, level I type of evidence is produced where cause and effect questions are addressed (Dearholt & Dang, 2012). The results from the interprofessional EBP project answer the question of whether the intervention led to the change in the outcome. If it was not possible to randomize or there was no control group, then the level of evidence the project produced was at level II. The interprofessional EBP project may have involved a nonexperimental design, or level III evidence, such as an observational study, or the project may have incorporated a

quality improvement study, or level V evidence. Recall that it is not enough to focus on the level of evidence produced; the interprofessional team is also expected to report the quality of their evidence from the project. For example, the quality of the interprofessional EBP project with a randomized control design depends on internal validity such that there is reduction in potential bias and measurement error so there is generalizability of the results from the study sample to the population.

Other chapters of this book focused on the literature search that linked to the development of the PICO (i.e., population/problem, intervention, comparison, and outcome) question (Chapter 7), and then sought, appraised, and synthesized evidence in the literature to answer the PICO question once developed (Chapters 8 and 9). If the evidence was not found to answer the PICO question, or the evidence found was not strong enough to lead to an unequivocal recommendation to adopt an intervention, the interprofessional team might have chosen to conduct some type of effectiveness research study or implement a quality improvement project (Chapter 10). With stronger evidence, the interprofessional team would have decided to conduct a pilot implementation project before deciding to adopt the practice change throughout the organization or to targeted areas of the organization (Chapter 12).

This chapter advances the understanding of the key concepts related to data analysis, interpretation, and project evaluation upon completion of the implementation phase of the interprofessional EBP project. Statistics involve the methods of "collecting, summarizing, presenting, analyzing, and drawing conclusions" from a set of data (Petrie, 2006, p. 1125). These topics can be overwhelming and confusing to many novice evidence-based practitioners and clinicians; however, this chapter brings a level of clarification and understanding that leads the interprofessional EBP project to success. Although this chapter appears near the end of the text, be assured that data analysis and project evaluation have their roots in the very beginnings of the interprofessional EBP project. Understanding study design, methodology, and statistics lays the foundation for a successful interprofessional EBP project.

FROM PICO QUESTION TO PROJECT QUESTION

As part of the interprofessional EBP process, a PICO question was developed. This question translated a practice problem into an answerable question (Petrie, 2006) as illustrated in Table 13-1. Perhaps the evidence from the literature only weakly answered the PICO question, leading the interprofessional team to develop an effectiveness research study examining a walking program and its effect on fear of falling. The first term to understand in interpreting the

TABLE 13-1

PICO QUESTION TO EVIDENCE-BASED PRACTICE PROJECT QUESTION

PICO QUESTION	COMPONENTS OF THE PICO	RESULTS OF APPRAISAL AND SYNTHESIS *(Dearholt & Dang, 2012)*	EBP PROJECT QUESTION	EBP PROJECT VARIABLES
For community dwelling and sedentary older adults, what is the effect of walking on the fear of falling compared to elders who engage in minimal physical activity?	P: Community dwelling sedentary older adults I: Walking C: Minimal physical activity O: Fear of falling	Two level II studies weakly supported walking programs for community dwelling older adults in reducing fear of falling. One of those level II studies at quality medium supported daily walking for 30 minutes while the other level II study at quality low involved walking three times per week for 45 minutes. Both studies had small effect sizes.	Will a daily walking program of 30 minutes in community dwelling and sedentary older adults decrease the fear of falling compared to older adults who engage in minimal physical activity?	Independent variable: daily 30-minute walking program versus no walking program for sedentary adults who engage in minimal physical activity Dependent variable: fear of falling

interprofessional EBP project is the concept of a variable, which is a measurable characteristic that varies within a population or a sample. In this example project, there is an independent variable, or the variable the team manipulates. In other words, there are two categorical levels of the independent variable, meaning one group of sedentary, community-dwelling adults participated in the walking program and the other group did not and continued to engage in a sedentary lifestyle as had been their habit. The participants in the EBP study were placed randomly or by convenience into these two categories. The dependent variable is the outcome that was measured. Fear of falling is the outcome of interest in this particular interprofessional EBP project and was measured with some instrument possessing the characteristics of being reliable (i.e., consistently measures fear of falling in the same way), valid (i.e., actually measures fear of falling), and sensitive to change (i.e., picks up relatively small degrees of change in the levels of fear).

The way in which variables in the interprofessional EBP project are studied is related to the type of design. For example, the interprofessional team may simply want to describe the frequency or percentage of older adults in their 70s and 80s who have a decreased fear of falling after walking 30 minutes daily for 1 month. A correlational study would determine the relationship between two variables (e.g., as walking speed increases, fear of falling decreases), while a predictive study would determine how some variables together or singularly predict the outcome of another variable (e.g., age of the community-dwelling older adult and time in the week spent walking for 1 month predict fear of falling).

DATA COLLECTION, PREPARATION, AND CLEANING

Answering the EBP project question depends on an appropriate design to accomplish the goals of the EBP interprofessional project and implementation of the project according to plan. Before analysis of the collected data and evaluation of the project can proceed, however, the interprofessional team must first have confidence in the quality of the data. The integrity of the data management process throughout the study is critical in terms of protecting the confidentiality of the participants (see Chapter 11), as well as to prevent misplaced, lost, missing, erroneous, or corrupted data. Data entry, data management, and data cleaning present wonderful opportunities for engaged and interested students who desire to learn more about the research process to play an invaluable role in the success of the interprofessional EBP project.

Data Management

Both during the data collection and analysis phases of the interprofessional EBP project, data confidentiality and security are of critical importance. Data protection and confidentiality were discussed in Chapter 11 as they are closely tied to the protection of human subjects and research ethics. A central tenant of ethical research is that collected data is either anonymous or confidential. Confidentiality is achieved when the interprofessional team removes the participant's name and replaces the participant identifier with a number known only to the fewest members

TABLE 13-2		
DATA SECURITY QUESTIONS		
CATEGORY	**DOES EVERYONE ON THE INTERPROFESSIONAL TEAM, ESPECIALLY THE PRIMARY INVESTIGATOR, UNDERSTAND THE FOLLOWING:**	√
General	Role and responsibility for data security?	
	Policies of the health care organization and university on data security for research even if the data are de-identified or anonymous?	
	Policies of the IRB for research data security even if the data are de-identified or anonymous?	
	The data management processes for the study, including data security?	
	What to do if a security breach occurs?	
	Informed consent requires that human research subjects must understand where data are going and authorize the arrangements.	
	The requirement of the team to sign data confidentiality agreements with the health care organization?	
Data Storage	Where to find all the data for the study? (includes paper, electronic, and mobile devices [including external hard drives, flash drives and smart devices])	
	Who is managing the data infrastructure for the study?	
	Who has access to the data for the study?	
	How is the data for the study secured?	
	The policies for storing social security numbers?	
	The policies for encryption and whether data can be stored only on health care organization computers or mobile devices, or may be housed on the university encrypted data servers and mobile devices if there is a data sharing collaborative agreement that leads to appropriate security?	
	The policies for using software, such as cloud services, survey tools, social media, and mobile apps to collect, store, and access data?	
	The policies for protecting video and audio data security?	

of the team as possible, such as a research assistant and the primary investigator (PI) on the grant. The codes matching participant identifiers are maintained separately from the data and are ultimately destroyed once the research is completed. The study design should minimize the use of identifying patient information through de-identification whenever possible, particularly in terms of Social Security numbers.

The data management plan, similar to what Duke University has outlined for their institutional review board (IRB) in terms of data security (http://docr.som.duke.edu/sites/docr.som.duke.edu/files/documents/rdsp_submission_instructions.pdf), should address these key questions (Table 13-2). Collected data must be secure, protected, and confidential at all times. This security is best accomplished in consultation with the IRB that typically has data management policies, and in consultation with the information technology team of the university or health care organization in obtaining advice about the physical security of the data, especially protected health information. There are standard procedures to reduce the possibility of the project having a security breach of the data (i.e., storing confidential data on the health care organization owned network servers that are encrypted and backed up regularly; or restricted/confidential information stored on *approved* mobile computing devices that are encrypted).

Data Entry

Either the interprofessional team members enter data into statistical programs, or if the team does not have access to this resource, team members should enter data into a spreadsheet to give to the statistician. The standard entry for data is that each variable is entered into a column, and each row represents the data from a particular participant or case, also sometimes called a *record* (Portney & Watkins, 2009). The code number of the participant should be the first column when the data are not anonymous, or the

TABLE 13-3

SAMPLE COLLECTED DATA

SUBJECT NUMBER	GENDER	EXERCISE	HEART RATE	SYSTOLIC BLOOD PRESSURE	DIASTOLIC BLOOD PRESSURE
001	F	Y	62	24	74
002	F	Y	14	110	88
003	F	N	71	114	80
004	—	N	68	126	220

TABLE 13-4

CLEANED SAMPLE DATA

SUBJECT NUMBER	GENDER	EXERCISE	HEART RATE	SYSTOLIC BLOOD PRESSURE	DIASTOLIC BLOOD PRESSURE
001	F	Y	62	124	74
002	F	Y	74	110	88
003	F	N	71	114	80
004	F	N	68	126	78

record number when the data are anonymous. Creating this code/record number column will ensure the PI and the research assistant are able to track down missing data, or replace incorrect data with the correct data. The first row of the spreadsheet usually lists the name of the variables in each column. The data for each research participant is entered beginning in the second row. Each research participant's information on each variable is subsequently entered into the correct row under the corresponding column. The point of intersection of the row and column is referred to as a *field* (Portney & Watkins). A participant's case has several fields of data depending on the number of variables.

Statistical software often includes a second view of the data that becomes the codebook. The codebook, or another spreadsheet, includes the full name of the variable, (e.g., gender), the label of the value, (e.g., male or female), and the value (e.g., male = 0, female = 1). The codebook helps the interprofessional team interpret correctly the data that is entered into the spreadsheet.

Data Cleaning

Another aspect of data management is the cleaning of collected data. *Cleaning* refers to the process of correcting or removing any inaccurate information in the data set. The interprofessional team should clean the data as it is collected rather than waiting until the end of the study. When the interprofessional team pays careful attention to the data

and creates strategies to ensure their integrity, the team avoids several potential hazards in the interprofessional EBP project. For example, consider an interprofessional EBP project that is investigating the influence of exercise on resting heart rate and blood pressure (Table 13-3). A quick review of the data set demonstrates potential issues. A systolic blood pressure of 24 mm Hg is reported for subject 001, while a resting heart rate of 14 is recorded for subject 002. There are obvious inaccuracies throughout the data set that need to be either corrected or removed. However, what is not known is why the data are in error. Is it because of poor instrumentation (i.e., the sphygmomanometer was not working appropriately) or human error (i.e., the reported systolic blood pressure of subject 001 was actually 124, not 24)?

In addition, the gender variable for subject 004 is missing. In terms of missing information, this could occur because the team member could not obtain the information, information was not entered, the team members forgot to collect the data, or the participant would not or did not provide the information. Missing data should be obtained when possible to avoid problems of analysis and interpretation. When the data are lost to the study, the data should not be recorded as a zero. Some statistical programs will show a period as a missing variable. Thus, the cleaned data set now appears in Table 13-4. By carefully cleaning the data as it is collected, both instrumentation issues and human errors are alleviated. Finally, cleaning the data

TABLE 13-5	
DATA CLEANING STRATEGIES	
Create table stating expected values	For all dependent variables, create a quick reference guide to the acceptable range (see Table 13-6)
Review data as they are collected	As data are collected, refer to the quick reference guide and establish whether the data point is acceptable.
Use two team members to enter data	Working together, enter collected data into database (i.e., one team member can read the data and another can enter it).
Record which team member collected data	Initial the collected data so that if questions exist, errors can be quickly traced.
Use simple statistical techniques to find errors in data	Determine possible ranges for all variables (e.g., there are only 7 days in 1 week).

TABLE 13-6		
QUICK REFERENCE GUIDE OF RANGES FOR VARIABLES		
VARIABLE NAME	**VARIABLE TYPE**	**VALID VALUES**
Gender	Character	M or F
Exercise	Character	Y or N
Resting heart rate (bpm)	Numeric	40 to 200
Resting systolic blood pressure (mm Hg)	Numeric	80 to 200
Resting diastolic blood pressure (mm Hg)	Numeric	60 to 120

throughout the project removes the tedious task of cleaning huge amounts of data upon conclusion of the project. See Table 13-5 for data cleaning strategies and Table 13-6 for a sample quick reference guide to define the possible range of scores for each variable, which will aid the research assistants in cleaning the data. Once the data have been collected, prepared, and cleaned, statistical analysis begins.

COMMON STATISTICAL TERMINOLOGY

A basic understanding of common statistical terms enables the interprofessional team members to engage in dialogue with the statistician to fully understand the analysis of the interprofessional EBP project data. Without this shared mental model, team members will also be unsure of how to interpret the data analysis in order to make a recommendation to the health care organization about the practice change.

A sample is defined as a random subset of the population, with the population being an entire entity (Portney & Watkins, 2009, p. 143). For example, all of the nurses in a given health care organization represent a population,

while a sample would be a randomly selected smaller number of nurses from that group. When conducting a research study, samples are used to represent the population.

Numerical variables are those that have specific values associated with them (e.g., cholesterol), while categorical variables are those that place individuals into distinct categories (i.e., nurses, physicians, and exercise physiologists). Within these numerical groups of variable types is even more specificity as to the nature of the data (see Table 13-7 for a discussion of nominal, ordinal, and interval/ratio data). Understanding the type of data gathered for each variable forms the basis of determining the appropriate statistical analysis.

SUMMARIZING THE DATA

Summarizing the data is a key step in data analysis with the goal being to reduce all of the collected individual data so that it can be readily understood. This summary is often presented visually in the form of graphs and figures. Another summary method is using descriptive statistics.

TABLE 13-7

VARIABLE TYPE

VARIABLE TYPE	DEFINITION	EXAMPLE
Nominal	Data that can only be in one category	Colors
Ordinal	Data that can be placed in a natural order (i.e., 1 to 10); however, the distinction between values is not always the same	Ranking of hospitals (i.e., #1, #2, #3, etc.)
Interval or discrete	Data that are in order and where difference between values is equivalent	Temperature
Ratio or continuous	Data that are in order and have a meaningful zero	Number of falls per 1000 patient days

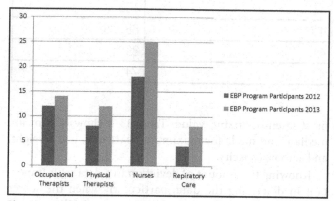

Figure 13-1. Participants in EBP program.

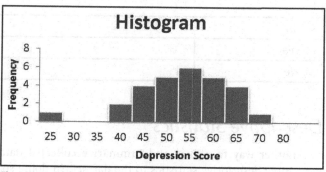

Figure 13-2. Histogram of scores on depression scale.

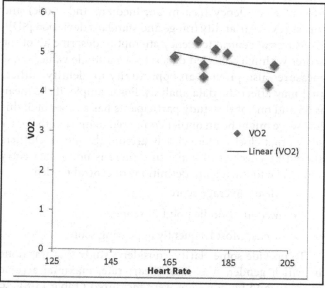

Figure 13-3. Scatterplot showing relationship between two variables.

Visual Representation

A quick and easy way to summarize reduced data is to generate a frequency distribution or "the frequency of occurrence of each observation or group of observations" (Petrie, 2006, p. 1125). See Figure 13-1 for a bar chart representing the frequency in each categorical variable. A pie chart is another way to visually present frequency data. A histogram in Figure 13-2 shows the frequency of each score on the Y-axis and the measured variable—in this case a depression score—on the X-axis. The histogram shows the shape of the data. In Figure 13-2, the data are symmetrical and is a bell-shaped curve or a normal distribution. In other words, most of the scores fall in the middle of the scale, while fewer scores are on either end of the curve. A curve can be asymmetrical, where a positive skew (i.e., skewed to right) shows the data falling mostly on the left with fewer scores on the right. A negative skew (i.e., skewed to left) would show most of the data on the right with fewer scores on the left. Whether the distribution of a variable is normal is important in determining the type of statistic to use to complete the data analysis.

Scatterplots provide an excellent way to display the relationship between numerical variables (Green & Salkind, 2008). By simply plotting two variables against one another, relationships can be quickly identified when the data points approximate a diagonal line, such as in Figure 13-3. In this example, the relationship between heart rate and maximum rate of oxygen consumption (VO_2) during incremental exercise shows an inverse relationship, as one variable goes up (heart rate), the other variable, VO_2, goes down. A positive relationship shows that both variables increase together. A negative relationship between two numbers is one in which a decrease in the value of one number results in a decrease in the value of the other number.

TABLE 13-8

CALCULATING MEAN, MEDIAN, AND MODE

GENDER (M OR F)	MAXIMUM HEART RATE (BPM)	AEROBIC CAPACITY (L/MIN)	BODY WEIGHT (KG)
M	180	5.1	101
M	200	4.7	98
F	198	4.2	74
F	176	4.4	62
M	184	5.0	110
M	174	5.3	74
F	166	4.9	80
M	176	4.7	106
Mean	181.75	4.78	88.125
Median	178	4.8	89
Mode	176	4.7	74

Descriptive Statistics

Another way to reduce and summarize collected data is to apply descriptive statistics to the dataset. In doing so, important characteristics of the data can be quantified. The descriptive statistics used most often include measures of central tendency (i.e., mean, median, and mode) and measures of variability (range and standard deviation [SD]). Measures of central tendency attempt to describe all of the scores within a collected data set with a single value. These measures also provide an opportunity to identify outliers that may affect the data analysis. For example, if the mean is 55 and one of the study participants has a score of 5, this low score might be an outlier compared to most of the other scores that cluster more closely around the mean. Outliers should be checked to make sure there is not a data entry error. The following are definitions of central tendency:

- *Mean*: Average score
- *Median*: Middle point of scores
- *Mode*: Most frequently appearing score

To provide some clarity, consider a study that was done in which gender, maximum heart rate, maximal aerobic capacity, and body weight were measured (Table 13-8). To describe the data, measures of central tendency summarize each set of scores with one value. To calculate the mean, the scores within a data set are summed (i.e., maximum heart rate) and divided by the number of scores in the set. To find the median, arrange a given set of scores (i.e., aerobic capacity) in value order and identify the middle value. When the data set contains an even number of values, identify the middle two values, and the median is the value between them. In order to determine the mode, simply identify the most often-occurring value. Table 13-8 shows the mean, median, and mode for maximum heart rate, body weight, and aerobic capacity.

Knowing the amount of deviation in a data set is important in describing the data, particularly when the scores spread widely from the mean. When this variability occurs, the mean may not be a good representation of the data. The mean is affected from extreme scores where the median is not affected. The range and SD are the most common measures of variation and are defined as follows:

- *Range*: Difference between the smallest and largest values
- *SD*: Amount of variability in the values relative to the mean

By calculating the range, a reference point is gained for interpreting the data. Although not terribly useful, if the calculated range for a data set is greater than an expected range of values, this could indicate an error in the data. Calculating the SD helps determine the spread of scores away from the mean score. If the SD = 2 and the mean is 10, then a score that is one SD above the mean would be 12, and the score that is one SD below the mean would be 8. The majority of the scores in a normal distribution would fall within two SDs from the mean in either direction, or in the example would be between the scores of 6 and 14. In addition, if the SD were larger than the mean, this would indicate that the data are spread out and the mean may not be the best measure of central tendency. The mean is more precise when the scores are close to the mean within two SDs on either side of the mean. For instance, if the mean score of 10 had an SD of 1, this would be more precise when compared to an SD of 2.

TABLE 13-9

APPROPRIATE STATISTICAL ANALYSES FOR FINDING DIFFERENCES AMONG GROUPS

NOMINAL DATA (COUNTING/ FREQUENCIES)	ORDINAL DATA (LIKERT SCALES OR RANKED DATA)	INTERVAL/RATIO DATA (ADDED & SUBTRACTED)
[2 groups]	*[2 groups]*	*[2 groups]*
{> 2 groups}	*{> 2 groups}*	*{> 2 groups}*
Independent Groups where no group member is in more than one group		
[Chi-square or Fisher's Exact Test]	[Mann-Whitney U test]	[Student t or Independent t-test]
{Chi-square}	{Kruskal-Wallis}	{Analysis of variance (ANOVA)}
Dependent Groups where a group member is in more than one group (pre-test/post-test)		
[McNemar test]	[Wilcoxon signed rank test]	[Dependent or Paired-t test]
{Cochran Q}	{Friedman}	{Repeated Measures ANOVA}
Choose the column that represents the type of data collected, and then simply choose the statistic that represents the number and type of groups to identify the appropriate statistical analysis. (For example, our sample project collected interval/ratio data and had two groups where there were different participants in each group. Therefore, the analysis would use an independent t-test.)		

Parameter estimation of the population values based on the sample characteristics can also help give insight into the collected data. Estimating parameters include calculations of standard error of the mean (SEM) and confidence intervals (CIs). When a random sample has been used in a study, it is hoped that the sample mean equals the population mean. Because there is error in sampling, there is a difference between the sample and population means. A lower SEM indicates a smaller difference between the sample and population means, thus identifying the preciseness of the sample data. In addition to the SEM, the CI can be used to determine a range of values that contains the true population mean with 95% certainty. In other words, the population's mean would fall within two SDs of the sample mean in either direction. The larger the range in the CI, the less precise the sample mean is in estimating the population mean.

ANALYZING THE DATA

Calculating central tendency, variability, and parameter estimates provides keen insight into understanding the collected data. These are simple ways to get to know the data, which also lead to more in-depth statistical analysis. The goal of the interprofessional EBP project is to answer the PICO question and to make a practice recommendation, either involving a new course of action or providing confirmation that the existing practice should continue. In order to make this recommendation, statistical analyses must be completed on the collected data. By conducting the

appropriate analysis and evaluating the results properly, the team is assured of making the correct recommendation.

The key step in analyzing the collected data is to choose the appropriate statistical analysis linked to the PICO question and the project question being asked. In a PICO question, typically there is a group receiving the intervention and a group receiving usual and customary interventions. This means the statistical analysis focuses on the differences in scores among the groups. To select the correct analysis method (Table 13-9), the statistician will need to know how many comparison groups exist, such as two or three or more. Refer back to the data presented in Table 13-8. Maximum heart rate, aerobic capacity, and body weight values are shown for a group of men and women. Not only is the number of groups important in selecting the analysis, but also the type of groups involved. In Table 13-8, there are two independent groups represented (men and women). *Independent groups* refer to the fact that participants can only be in one group, whereas in dependent groups, the same people are in the groups (e.g., pre-test, post-test, and 6-month follow-up).

Another factor in selecting the statistic for analysis is the type of data (nominal, ordinal, or interval/ratio) collected for each variable. In Table 13-8, maximum heart rate is interval/ratio data. Consequently, if the interprofessional team wanted to discern the difference in heart rate between men and women engaged in an intensive activity, one would select the independent *t* test. However, the statistics in the right-hand column of Table 13-9 for interval/ratio data are referred to as *parametric*, which means certain assumptions have to be met in order to use them. Primarily, the data have to be normally distributed or shaped like a bell-shaped curve. The EBP team members should analyze the distribution of the data through histograms for each of the variables with interval/ratio data. If the data are skewed, then the more appropriate statistics are those used for ordinal data.

Working with a statistician helps the interprofessional EBP team further clarify statistical tools needed for the analysis; however, building on an understanding of variable types, choosing the appropriate statistical analysis need not be overwhelming. The EBP practice team should use the following checklist to ensure appropriate statistical analyses for finding differences are chosen:

- Does the analysis require understanding differences among groups?
- What is the data type for each variable?
- How many groups are there?
- What kinds of groups were involved: independent or dependent?
- Are the assumptions of the statistical test met?

Other analysis methods are chosen if the interprofessional EBP team is interested in the relationship between variables. In this case, correlational statistics are chosen depending on the type of data collected for each variable. Likewise, if interested in prediction, the interprofessional team may want to know if a variable or several variables predict the outcome measure. Again, depending on the data type for each variable will determine the type of regression statistic the statistician recommends to the group.

Interpreting Data

Upon the conclusion of the statistical analysis, proper interpretation must take place in terms of understanding the meaning of the results. The alpha level the interprofessional team selected prior to the start of data collection provides a comparison for determining statistical significance. The alpha level is the probability that the difference found between groups occurred because of chance. Typically, the alpha level is set at either .05 (i.e., five times out of 100 a difference is due to chance), or at .01 (i.e., one time out of 100 a difference is due to chance). The team compares the probability of their results occurring due to chance with the alpha level, and if their finding is equal to or smaller than the alpha level, a significant difference is found. Finding a statistical difference informs the interprofessional team members that they can reject the null hypothesis that there is no difference between groups. When the null hypothesis is rejected, then the alternative hypothesis can be accepted that there is a difference between groups.

Setting the alpha level involves a trade-off in terms of what kind of interpretation error might be made. Type I errors occur when you incorrectly reject a true null hypothesis, often as a result of an alpha level being too large; whereas, a type II error occurs when incorrectly accepting the null hypothesis, often as a result of an alpha level being too small. Type II errors are prevented with a large sample size where the statistical test has enough power to find a difference if there is one. In fact, statisticians conduct a power analysis for the interprofessional EBP project to help the interprofessional team determine the sample size needed. It is inappropriate and unethical to run an effectiveness research study or an EBP change project evaluation when the sample size is such that there will not be an opportunity to find a difference if one exists.

Statistical Significance

Typically, the statistician provides the interprofessional team the printouts of the statistical analysis and helps the team interpret the results when needed. Consider a study comparing the systolic blood pressure between women who choose to participate in yoga and those who do not. The statistician conducted a t test to find the difference in systolic blood pressure between the two groups. Recall that the t test finds differences between two groups where the data type for the variable of interest is interval/ratio and the groups are independent. See Table 13-10A for an example table the statistician might provide. The table indicates that the mean systolic blood pressure of women in yoga (group one) was lower than the mean heart rate of women who did not attend yoga (group two). However, the mean for the women not in yoga was more precise than the mean for systolic blood pressure for women in yoga as indicated by the SD for each group or the variability statistic. When examining each group's SEM, the sample mean for women not in yoga had a mean that was a better parameter for the population mean compared to the women in yoga.

The question though is what does this mean in terms of whether the two sets of data really have differences in variability around their means. The Levene's test for equality of variances is examining the hypothesis that there is no difference in variability between the two sets of data. In other words, do the two groups have scores that vary in the same way around the mean? The result of the Levene's test is F = 1.250 (Table 13-10B). To interpret this result, the probability of the result that there is no difference in variability between the two groups is provided as the significance (Sig), or $p = .278$. The p value is compared to the alpha level in terms of whether it is larger than the alpha level or smaller than the alpha level. In this case, the p value is much larger than the .05 alpha level, so the null hypothesis is accepted. In other words, any difference in variability between the two groups occurred due to error almost 30 times out of a 100.

Examining variability between the two data sets was important as there are two t test results that can be used—one for when the variability of the data is the same in the two groups, and the other when the two groups have different variability. The two-tailed t test is read from the variability assumed row of Table 13-10B. A two-tailed test

TABLE 13-10A				
SAMPLE GROUP STATISTICS FOR SYSTOLIC BLOOD PRESSURE				
GROUP	N	MEAN	STANDARD DEVIATION	STANDARD ERROR MEAN
1.00	10	117.0000	8.75595	2.76887
2.00	10	131.0000	6.12826	1.93793

TABLE 13-10B									
DIFFERENCE IN SYSTOLIC BLOOD PRESSURE FOR WOMEN IN YOGA (GROUP 1) AND THOSE NOT IN YOGA (GROUP 2)									
	LEVENE'S TEST FOR EQUALITY OF VARIANCES	T-TEST FOR EQUALITY OF MEANS							
								95% CONFIDENCE INTERVAL OF THE DIFFERENCE	
	F	Sig	t	df	Sig (2-tailed)	Mean Diff.	Std Error Difference	Lower	Upper
BP equal variances assumed	1.250	.278	-4.14	18	.001	-14.00	3.379	-21.1	-6.89
BP equal variances not assumed			-4.14	16.11	.001	-14.00	3.379	-21.6	-6.83

means there is not a directional hypothesis where you are asking whether one group's mean is higher or lower than the other group's mean. Instead, the two-tailed test just determines whether there is a difference between the two groups. The result is that $t = -4.14$, indicating the mean systolic blood pressure of the women who were not in yoga (a larger number) is subtracted from the blood pressure of women who attended yoga (a smaller number). The p value is .001, meaning that the difference in systolic blood pressure between the two groups occurred due to chance only one time out of 1,000. Consequently, the women attending yoga had a significantly different systolic blood pressure than did the women who did not attend yoga. The null hypothesis is rejected.

The mean difference in systolic blood pressure is –14.00 with a 95% CI of ± 7.1 (lower bound is –21.1 and the upper bound is –6.90) where the real mean difference for the population is somewhere in this range. Notice that a mean difference of 0 is not in this CI. For instance, if the CI for the mean difference was ± 18, the lower bound for the difference would be –32 with an upper bound of 4. A

mean difference of 0 would be in that interval indicating the two groups did not differ in systolic blood pressure because there was a possibility that the mean difference in the population could be no difference. Table 13-11 has statistical notation examples of several statistics. To interpret, go back to Table 13-9 to decide the type of data and the number and type of groups for which the test statistic would be used, then interpret the results using a .05 and then a .01 alpha level. Which test found differences between and among groups? Did the alpha level make a difference in the interpretation?

In the preceding example, two independent groups (women participating in yoga and women who did not participate in yoga) were compared using an independent t test when examining differences in blood pressure. Often in clinical research, there are more than two groups being compared, and thus a different statistic must be used. In the case of more than two groups, an analysis of variance (ANOVA) is the statistic of choice given one has interval/ratio data, independent groups, and symmetrical data. For example, a physical therapist wants to determine whether

TABLE 13-11

STATISTICAL INTERPRETATION

STATISTIC	STATISTICAL NOTATION	SIGNIFICANCE	ALPHA = .05 REJECT NULL? YES OR NO	ALPHA = .01 REJECT NULL? YES OR NO
Chi square	$X^2 = 3.84$	$p = .05$	Yes	No
	$X^2 = 6.635$	$p = .01$	Yes	Yes
Independent t test	$t = 2.228$	$p = .05$	Yes	No
	$t = 3.169$	$p = .01$	Yes	Yes
ANOVA	$F = 3.35$	$p = .05$	Yes	No
	$F = 5.49$	$p = .01$	Yes	Yes

TABLE 13-12A

TEST FOR ANALYSIS OF VARIANCE

NPRS; ANOVA	SUM OF SQUARES	DF	MEAN SQUARE	F	SIG.
Between groups	62.550	3	20.850	36.261	.001
Within groups	9.200	16	.575		
Total	71.750	19			

TABLE 13-12B

HOMOGENEITY OF VARIANCE

LEVENE STATISTIC	DF1	DF2	SIG.	F
	3	16	.509	.805

there are differences in pain based on a chosen treatment plan using the numeric pain rating scale (NPRS). The three treatment plans were stretching, manual therapy, and cold therapy. In addition, a control group received no treatment; thus, the number of groups in the physical therapist's research project was four. In order to test for statistical difference, an ANOVA is appropriate.

Upon completion of data collection for the physical therapist's project on pain, the data were analyzed. Similar to the study on women and yoga, the statistician in the pain study gathered descriptive statistics and conducted a test for homogeneity of variance, or put simply, to determine whether each group's data look similar. The statistician wants to ensure that there are no differences in variability among the groups. To check homogeneity of variance, the statistician once again used the Levene's test and determined that the group data does not significantly vary from one group to the next (Table 13-12A). Table 13-12B shows this in that the Levene statistic is 0.805 and the significance value is 0.509. With a level of significance greater than 0.05, the groups do not statistically differ in variability. The ANOVA was then completed, and a significant difference was identified between treatment groups. This difference between groups can be identified by the significance value of .001 in Table 13-12A.

However, when dealing with more than two groups, other statistical tests are needed to determine which groups were significantly different from all or one of the other groups. In other words, was there a difference between the manual therapy and the control, the stretching and the cold therapy, or perhaps the manual therapy and cold therapy? An additional statistical test that is completed in order to make this determination is called a *post hoc analysis*, which are *t* tests corrected for error when multiple *t* tests are used.

TABLE 13-13

TUKEY POST HOC

(I)GROUP	(J) GROUP	MEAN DIFFERENCE (I-J)	STD. ERROR	SIG.	95% CONFIDENCE INTERVAL	
					Lower Bound	Upper Bound
Stretching	Manual therapy	4.00000	.47958	.838	-.9721	1.7721
	Cold therapy	-3.00000*	.47958	.001	-4.3271	-1.6279
	Control	-3.60000*	.47958	.001	-4.9721	-2.2279
Manual therapy	Stretching	-.40000	.47958	.838	-1.7721	.9721
	Cold therapy	-3.40000*	.47958	.001	-4.7721	-2.0279
	Control	-4.0000*	.47958	.001	-5.3721	-2.6279
Cold therapy	Stretching	3.00000*	.47958	.001	1.6279	4.3721
	Manual therapy	3.40000*	.47958	.001	2.0279	4.7721
	Control	-.60000	.47958	.605	-1.9721	.7721
Control	Stretching	3.60000*	.47958	.001	2.2279	4.9721
	Manual therapy	4.00000*	.47958	.001	2.6279	5.3721
	Cold therapy	.60000	.47958	.605	-.7721	1.9721

For this example, a common post hoc test, Tukey, was chosen. The statistician gives advice regarding the best post hoc test to use as some of these tests control the error rate more stringently than do others, thereby making it harder to find a difference. Table 13-13 displays the treatments in the far left column, with each treatment plan being compared to others. In the first box, stretching is compared to the other three groups (manual therapy, cold therapy, and control). Looking across the table to the significance column (Sig.), the following values appear: .838 (comparing stretching to manual therapy), .001 (comparing stretching to cold therapy), and .001 (comparing stretching to control). Based on this post hoc analysis, stretching decreased pain when compared to both cold therapy and the control condition. This process can be repeated to determine differences in each of the treatment plans.

Clinical Significance

The interprofessional EBP team cannot determine whether the intervention should be fully implemented in the health care organization until the difference between the group receiving the intervention from the group receiving the usual and customary care is also analyzed in terms of clinical significance. Clinical significance has to do with a meaningful difference where the participants notice the effect of the intervention in the outcome of interest. The minimal clinically important difference (MCID) is "the smallest difference in score in the domain of interest which patients perceive as beneficial and which would mandate, in the absence of troublesome side effects and excessive cost, a change in the patient's management" (Wright, Johnson, & Cook, 2014, p. 186).

If the sample size in the effectiveness research study is large enough, small differences among groups are statistically significant. A statistically significant result may not mean the patient really feels or is aware of the change in a way that makes a difference to him or her (i.e., there is no clinical significance because the MCID score is low). For instance, what if there is a significant difference on a measure of pain between two treatment groups? This difference might not be clinically meaningful if both groups scored in the "normal" range on the measure or the intervention produced a small benefit with large side effects.

In addition, clinical difference depends on the size of the measurement scale. With a large range of score possibilities, such as 100 points, would a significant difference of 2 points really be clinically significant (Baicus & Caraiola, 2008)? Abbott and Schmitt (2014) in physical therapy used the 15-point global rating of change (GROC) as the recommended reference standard (Terwee et al., 2010) for determining minimally clinically important differences in other outcome measures. These outcome measures were compared across three levels of change of the GROC (i.e., somewhat better, moderately better, and quite a bit better) for a population of patients with musculoskeletal disorders. These kinds of studies provide those who use the studied outcome measures a reference point for determining the MCID for a similar population.

Figure 13-4. Effect size calculation and interpretation.

The effect size is expressed as a d-index when the outcome measured is continuous level data and is calculated with the following formula:

$$d\text{-index} = \frac{\text{Mean of intervention group} - \text{Mean of control or comparison group}}{\text{Standard deviation}}$$

*There are different formulas for calculation of effect size based on measurement properties of the outcome measured; interpretation, however, is the same for the d-index.

The criteria are as follows (Cohen, 1988):

- Small effect = 0.20
- Medium effect = 0.50
- Large effect = 0.80

The interprofessional team should consider using the 95% CI to determine the quality of evidence that their intervention study produced. According to Atkinson and Nevill (2001), an intervention is deemed clinically significant as long as the following two conditions are satisfied: (a) the CI excludes zero, as described previously; and b) the lower limit of the CI must be equal to or greater than the smallest MCID or beneficial effect. Portney and Watkins (2009) indicated that this smallest worthwhile effect signifies an important rather than a trivial difference (p. 871).

The interprofessional team should be cautioned to avoid strictly interpreting the CI as just described (Wilkinson, 2014, p. 493). For instance, according to the example Wilkinson described, what if the intervention had a CI in which the smallest beneficial improvement (lower number in the range) was –3 degrees for ankle flexion? The conclusion would have to be the intervention might be of little use given such a small change, especially since there was a reduction in range. However, the team should examine the entire CI interval, in which the mean difference of the population in ankle flexion ranged from –3 to 10 degrees. In this CI range, as indicated previously, there is possibility of a negative result where the ankle range of motion worsens. In addition, there is a possibility of no difference in the intervention group. More importantly, however, most of the mean difference in the population lies above the smallest beneficial improvement rather than below it.

Would this intervention then warrant further study? With strict interpretation of the CI, the interprofessional team might not recommend further study given that no statistical differences were found between the groups and that there was a chance for a small worthwhile effect, including a worsening of the outcome. The possibility of the intervention having potential for further study in this case should be examined carefully before rejecting a potentially effective intervention outright. There is still a possible change of 10 degrees in ankle flexion that could be important, especially if verified with further study the conditions under which this stronger outcome occurs.

Another way to interpret the CI is to determine whether the effectiveness or the evaluation study produced a mean difference with a narrow CI, which is stronger evidence compared to a study with a wider CI. A wide CI indicates the sample's mean difference between groups is less precise in estimating the population mean difference (McNeely & Warren, 2006).

Another strategy to understand the clinical significance is to determine the magnitude of the difference between the group outcomes. The theme of clinical significance so far is that knowledge of whether results are statistically significant is not sufficient to inform decisions about an intervention for a health care organization. Just because the mean difference was greater in the group that received the intervention does not indicate that every participant who received the intervention had a better outcome than did every person in the control or comparison group. If this were the case, the interprofessional team would not hesitate but to recommend the intervention. Inevitably, there is overlap in outcomes between those who received the intervention and those who did not. Examining effect size is useful in determining whether the intervention produced a strong enough difference in the outcome when compared to the other groups (Portney & Watkins, 2009). Figure 13-4 provides information about how to calculate and interpret the effect size for continuous data (Green & Salkind, 2008). The formula tells the interprofessional team that the larger the mean difference between groups and the smaller the variability in outcomes among subjects, the larger the effect size.

MENTOR CHALLENGES

The key to mentoring as it relates to the EBP project is the mentor encouraging the members to stay connected as a team throughout the data analysis and project evaluation process. The mentor encourages all team members to take responsibility for ensuring that the data is accurate and complete as well as for the reasonableness of the data interpretation and the soundness of the recommendations given to the health care organization. The team that does not work together creates a situation in which few individuals, often

TABLE 13-14

MENTORING CHALLENGES AND TECHNIQUES

MENTORING CHALLENGES	MENTOR TECHNIQUES
Data collection	Appropriately train each member of team in methodology for data collection.
Data management	Clean data as you go. Secure data in password protected computer, behind firewalls, locked cabinet.
Not wanting to take time to clean data	Train each member in data collection to ensure accuracy, completeness, and consistency. Clean data as you go; do not wait until the end of data collection.
Passing data cleaning onto others	Share the responsibility and engage the entire team in reviewing the data entry. Own the project knowing each team member wants the project to be carefully done given the patient centeredness.
Not understanding data	Ask the statistician to work with the team to ensure learning and understanding. Choose a statistician or other knowledgeable team members and experts who can translate the information into common language.
Disappointment in results	No significant difference? Understand that clinical significance is more important and learn how to use CIs to determine potential of the intervention for further study. Determining whether the intervention is not useful is important as long as there were no fatal flaws in the study design, issues of fidelity in implementing the intervention, and sampling (randomization and an appropriate sample size). Unexpected results? Take time to figure out why they might make sense and what you might do differently in the future.

the clinical scholar and the mentor, become overwhelmed with the responsibility the team inappropriately placed upon them. A situation such as this could lead to serious problems with the data, such as improper entry, coding errors, and incorrect analyses. Working as a team prevents these issues and ensures that the data are trustworthy.

Not many on the team are statistical experts, thus the team needs to share knowledge and resources with each other. Faculty may be able to provide this leadership in working with the statistician. However, the entire team needs to consult with the statistician in that every member has valuable insight about the design of the interprofessional EBP project. Team members have knowledge of the methods for collecting and managing the data. More than likely, the team has completed some analysis leading them to better understand what the statistician is saying. Typically, the team has explored the shape of the data on each variable and has determined central tendency, variability, and estimates of the population parameters. Mentors and faculty should ensure that the team members understand the information the statistician is sharing and the decisions the team needs to make about data analysis and interpretation. When examining the data analysis involving tables, figures, charts, and statistical notations and their values, team members who are not as confident might become easily intimidated. The mentor needs to

lower the anxiety team members may feel through ensuring that the team has experts to clarify the statistics in a language everyone can understand.

MENTOR TECHNIQUES AND SUPPORTS

Table 13-14 describes some of the common mentoring challenges and possible mentor techniques to address these mentor challenges. For instance, often, the interprofessional EBP team is disappointed if the results are not statistically significant and could believe all their work was wasted. In this instance, the mentor technique is for the mentor to work with the team to examine the fidelity of the intervention throughout the project pilot, as well as determine the threats to internal validity that might have occurred. Perhaps some of the participants in the control group inadvertently received the intervention. If the interprofessional team determines the threats to internal validity were reasonable given the typical lack of control over variables in a real-world situation, the team may examine the CIs to determine whether the majority of the results indicated there was improvement even though the mean difference could have been zero.

TABLE 13-15

STRATEGIES FOR SUCCESS

MENTORING SUPPORTS	MENTOR TECHNIQUES
Provide learning resources so every team member learns about the nuances of their data collection strategies.	Set up appropriate data collection methods that allow for seamless transition to data analysis. Train every team member to accurately and appropriately collect data.
Work with the mentor to set up a spreadsheet or database prior to data collection.	Show team members how to enter data carefully into a spreadsheet. Have team members engage in meticulous cleaning of the data.
Provide references to statisticians and help the mentor determine the cost of the consultation and ways to manage the cost.	Ensure that any potential costs of hiring a statistician (if not a member of the team or in some way affiliated with the project) are included in any budgets and/or grants.
Instill an approach of constant problem solving with the mentor.	Constantly employ a problem-solving attitude as a role model to the team.
Provide the mentor and team with education about types of data and relationship to the analysis.	Determine the level of measurement as a team for the outcome variable. Find outcome instruments with scores and supports for interpreting results in terms of clinical significance.
Show the mentor and team members how to interpret descriptive statistics.	Interpret descriptive statistics as a team and develop visual displays of the data.
Teach the team how to select the appropriate statistics, but provide the team with verification of statistical reasoning with a statistician, particularly if complicated statistics are required.	Work with the team and the statistician to select the analysis methods and to ensure the team members understand the rationale.
Ensure that everyone understands statistical results.	Encourage the team to ask questions about the statistical results. Check their understanding and provide information in understandable language.
Provide the mentor and team with ways to determine clinical significance as a basis for the practice recommendation to the health care organization.	Work with the team to analyze CIs and effect sizes. Ensure that there are experts on the team who understand and can explain the minimum clinical worthwhile effect of the outcome measure.

The mentor needs support from the program coordinators to work with the team during this difficult time of data analysis and interpretation and in determining the final recommendations of the interprofessional EBP project. Program coordinators may provide the mentor and the team access to a statistician who can confirm the analysis or provide alternative suggestions while simultaneously avoiding the tendency to run too many statistical tests in order to fish for a significant result. Any suggestion from the statistician has to be appropriate given the data. Table 13-15 outlines the mentor challenges and the corresponding supports the program coordinators should provide.

SUMMARY

This chapter covered the topics of data management and security, promoting careful collection and storage of data to ensure confidentiality. Possible mistakes in data collection and entry into spreadsheets and databases were described. Team members are cautioned to prevent missing values through careful collection of the data. Team members were encouraged to "clean" the data as they are collected and entered. Providing research assistants with a data guide is helpful in determining whether the data values are consistent with the ranges expected for the outcome measure. Looking for extreme outliers in the data is another way to decide whether to go back and check a data value for accuracy. The process for setting up the data spreadsheet along with ways for the team to work together to avoid data entry errors were discussed.

Basic data analysis methods were outlined, particularly focusing on visual displays of data and on descriptive statistics and population parameters. Team members are instructed in how to get to know their data. Statistical terminology was reviewed as a precursor for understanding how statistics are chosen for the data analysis. Statistical significance in comparison to pre-set alpha levels helps the team to make the decision whether to accept or reject a null hypothesis. Clinical significance was identified as the important component of determining the ultimate recommendation to the health care organization about the potential intervention. Chapter 14 describes how the team should wrap up the project and make recommendations to the health care organization. Chapter 15 discusses the ways to disseminate the recommendations based on the project analysis.

REFLECTION QUESTIONS

1. What is your plan to advance your knowledge of research design and analysis?
2. How will you maximize your learning about data management through this interprofessional EBP project?

REFERENCES

Abbott, J. H., & Schmitt, J. (2014). Minimum important differences for the patient specific functional scale, 4 region-specific outcome measure, and the Numeric Pain Rating Scale. *Journal of Orthopaedic and Sports Physical Therapy, 44,* 560-564. doi:10.2519/jospt.2014.5248

Atkinson G., & Nevill, A. M., (2001). Selected issues in the design and analysis of sport performance research. *Journal of Sports Science, 19*(10), 811-27. doi:10.1080/026404101317015447

Baicus, C., & Caraiola, S. (2008). Effect measure for qualitative endpoints: Statistical versus clinical significance, or "how large the scale is?" *European Journal of Internal Medicine, 20,* e124-e125. doi:10.1016/j.ejim.2008.10.002

Dearholt, S. L., & Dang, D. (2012). *Johns Hopkins nursing evidence-based practice: Model and guidelines* (2nd ed.). Indianapolis, IN: Sigma Theta Tau International.

Green, S. B., & Salkind, N. J. (2008). *Using SPSS for Windows and Macintosh. Analyzing and understanding data* (5th ed.). Upper Saddle River, NJ: Pearson Prentice Hall.

McNeely, M. L., & Warren, S. (2006). Value of confidence intervals in determining clinical significance. *Physiotherapy Canada, 58,* 205-211. doi:10.3138/ptc.58.3.205

Petrie, A. (2006). Statistics of orthopaedic papers. *Journal of Bone and Joint Surgery, 88 b,* 1121-1136. doi:10.1302/0301-620x.88b9.17896

Portney, L. G., & Watkins, M. P. (2009). *Foundations of clinical research: Applications to practice* (3rd ed.). Upper Saddle River, NJ: Prentice Hall Health.

Terwee, C. B., Roorda, L. D., Dekker J., Bierma-Zeinstra, S. M., Peat G., Jordan, K. P.,... de Vet, H. C. (2010). Mind the MIC: large variation among populations and methods. *Journal of Clinical Epidemiology, 63,* 524-534. http://dx.doi.org/10.1016/j.jclinepi.2009.08.010

Titler, M. G., Kleiber, C. Steelman, V. J., Rakel, B. A., Budreau, G., Everett, L. Q., & Goode, C. J. (2001). The Iowa model of evidence-based practice to promote quality care. *Critical Care Nursing Clinics of North America, 13*(4), 497-509.

Wilkinson, M. (2014). Clinical and practical importance vs statistical significance: Limitations of conventional statistical inference. *International Journal of Therapy and Rehabilitation, 21*(10),488-494. doi:10.12968/ijtr.2014.21.10.488

Wright, A., Johnson, J., & Cook, C. (2014). Do the reported estimates of minimal clinically important difference scores amongst hip-related patient-reported outcome measures support their use? *Physical Therapy Reviews, 19*(3), 186-195. doi:10.1179/1743288x14y.0000000134

Wrapping Up the Interprofessional Evidence-Based Practice Project

Penelope A. Moyers, EdD, OT/L, FAOTA

CHAPTER TOPICS

- Benefits of a wrap-up process
- Identifying final tasks and assigning responsibility
- Implementing and monitoring final task completion
- Reconciling budgets
- Ensuring sustainability of the practice change
- Final evaluation
- Final reports
- Celebration
- Mentor challenges
- Mentor techniques and supports

PERFORMANCE OBJECTIVES

At the conclusion of the chapter, the program coordinators, mentors, and team members will be able to do the following:

1. Develop and implement a wrap-up plan for the evidence-based practice project or for the interprofessional evidence-based practice program.

2. Write an evidence-based practice project or interprofessional evidence-based practice program report.

3. Implement appropriate processes to enhance sustainability of the practice change and sustainability of the interprofessional evidence-based practice program.

4. Plan and conduct a celebration for project and program conclusion.

Moyers, P. A., & Finch-Guthrie, P. L.
*Interprofessional Evidence-Based Practice:
A Workbook for Health Professionals* (pp 215-228).
© 2016 Taylor and Francis Group.

Now that the evidence-based practice (EBP) project has been implemented and evaluated as described in Chapters 11 through 13, it is necessary for the team members, mentors, and the program coordinators to perform a final inventory of their projects, or in case of the program coordinators, the program tasks. The purpose of the inventory is to ensure that the interprofessional team identifies all the details that remain outstanding in order to design a corresponding plan to complete project tasks and activities of the interprofessional EBP program (Snyder, 2011). Without engaging in this critical close-out or wrap-up process, teams run the risk of disbanding prior to full project completion, often leaving the mentors and program coordinators in the thankless position of figuring out how to address the remaining tasks, including those tasks necessary for sustaining the practice change and for sustaining the interprofessional EBP program. When improper wrap-up happens, it is often very difficult to motivate team members who believe they are finished to expend the extra effort to complete the remaining tasks, particularly when most of the team members are no longer available. The better alternative is to include a wrap-up process as a part of the interprofessional EBP phases where everyone on the team is clear about how the project needs to be properly finished. This wrap-up plan should determine the supports needed to sustain the practice change in the health care organization.

Team members may become impatient with these details as the project draws to a close, being anxious to move on. Consequently, the mentors and program coordinators will need to take extra care in keeping all involved and accountable for completion of the final activities of the project and of the interprofessional EBP program, which includes devising and implementing supports for practice change sustainability within the health care organization. It is also important that team members take the time to celebrate their success and receive recognition for their work. Properly saying goodbye to all who have given so much to the work is important in order to avoid leaving people with a lack of fulfillment and feelings of dissatisfaction that may negatively influence future involvement with interprofessional EBP.

BENEFITS OF A WRAP-UP PROCESS

To convince the team and to help the mentors and program coordinators manage wrap-up, consider the following benefits (Richman, 2006) to a carefully planned ending process:

- Allows team members, mentors, and program coordinators to reflect on and communicate about team performance
- Ensures all final reports (e.g., institutional review board [IRB] and grants) for the projects and the program are completed and disseminated to the appropriate stakeholders or program sponsors
- Facilitates financial reporting of grant budgets and return of unspent funds if indicated
- Enhances sustainability of the practice change through provision of needed organizational supports and leadership involvement
- Ensures stakeholder satisfaction with project and program results
- Provides time to gather data about the project and program processes in order to determine future interprofessional EBP program improvements that enhance program sustainability
- Identifies team and mentor learning outcomes

Typically, requirements of projects and the program are considered met when the goals and objectives are either met or surpassed. These critical success factors are reflected in the implementation and evaluation plans of the project and of the program. In addition, the team charter also outlined team expectations. It is important for mentors and program coordinators to help teams differentiate between successfully completing the project versus achieving positive results of the project. Projects are successful even when projects end with results that show the practice change did not improve patient outcomes as hypothesized, particularly when the team can indicate that interventions were implemented with fidelity. Often, projects produce results that were unintended but highly important to discover. For instance, perhaps the project goal was to implement an aromatherapy protocol to reduce pain for persons with traumatic injuries. Maybe the results were not definitive due to difficulty obtaining enough patients who consented to participate within the time frame available. Perhaps the team learns that the older patient population tended to refuse aromatherapy due to distrust of complementary medicine interventions compared to the study consent rate of younger patients. The team may thus recommend that a subsequent practice change study or quality improvement effort focus on a population of younger age due to data trends indicating greater potential participation of this group.

Sometimes, the most influential results are the products that are generated from the project work, such as measurement processes and tools, changes in electronic health record documentation fields or processes, protocol development, and training programs and manuals. Perhaps the team discovers potential for future success as indicated in the aromatherapy example, leading the organization to continue the work through other mechanisms over a longer time period. Wrap-up should involve, when appropriate, the transition of the team's work to a work group or standing committee of the health care organization in order to enhance sustainability of the work and of any important practice change.

There are instances when projects are closed without reaching goals due to uncontrollable external pressures from the organizational sponsors or context (e.g., employee labor disputes, organizational budget shortfalls, organizational reorganizations, etc.). In these cases, the program coordinators and mentors must work closely with the teams to salvage certain parts of the project. Often the scope of the original project can be narrowed to still allow achievement of important results. Any project scope change, however, requires the team to consult with stakeholders. Requests made to the IRB to modify the project protocol must also occur. Failure to follow through on projects after participants have given consent is potentially a serious ethical dilemma. Care must be exercised when stopping a study prematurely in order to follow processes required by the IRB to properly notify participants. Grant agencies have to be contacted immediately, not only when return of unused funds is expected, but also in some cases if the full amount must be returned.

The project wrap-up and program completion process is a cycle that includes the following: identifying final tasks, assigning team member responsibility for task completion, implementing the wrap-up plan, reconciling project and program budgets, putting in place the sustainability supports from the implementation plan for the practice change and for continuation of the interprofessional EBP program, and monitoring the wrap-up cycle (Figure 14-1). The wrap-up process is circular until the project/program is completed and team members and program coordinators write final reports. The concept of wrap-up can be distilled down to the following main points:

- Wrap-up takes time and must be included as a part of the work plan.

- All projects end, but the most satisfying ending is one that is planned.

- Wrap-up of projects and programs follows a series of predetermined steps that include fostering sustainability of a practice change and of the interprofessional EBP program.

- Wrap-up always includes study of lessons learned so that future interprofessional EBP programs and projects will benefit.

- Celebration is an important aspect of wrap-up and should not be skipped or minimized.

IDENTIFYING FINAL TASKS AND ASSIGNING RESPONSIBILITY

Teams need to meet to discuss and inventory the status of their project relative to the implementation and evaluation/analysis plans. In order to make adjustments to deadlines and the timeline, inventorying remaining tasks

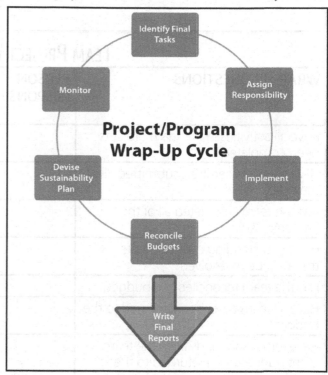

Figure 14-1. Wrap-up cycle.

should occur in a timely manner and is most useful when it is incorporated as a regular project or program check-up (Baker & Baker, 2000). One of the last checkups should occur no later than 1 month from the project or program completion deadline with a final checkup 1 week before conclusion. Program coordinators similarly need to check with each other to determine the outstanding activities of the program that remain. Tables 14-1 and 14-2 provide teams, mentors, and program coordinators with a checklist to help determine the unfinished steps of the projects and the program, respectively. Note that one or more team members are assigned responsibility to ensure task completion, and a program coordinator is assigned responsibility to assure program completion.

IMPLEMENTING AND MONITORING FINAL TASK COMPLETION

Note that in Tables 14-1 and 14-2, there are columns in which to add additional resources. Considering needed resources is an important determination for proper wrap-up given that the team is facing a hard stop to the project. Consequently, the team may need additional resources to speed up the completion process or may need additional resources if the team plans to keep working beyond the program end date. Program coordinators need to work with the mentors and the team members to assist in obtaining needed resources when possible or to devise a different

TABLE 14-1				
TEAM PROJECT WRAP-UP TASKS				
WRAP-UP QUESTIONS	**PERSON RESPONSIBLE**	**ADDITIONAL RESOURCES NEEDED**	**DATE TO BE COMPLETED**	**ACTUAL DATE COMPLETED**
Have all activities in the team projects been completed?				
Have all team members submitted all of their assigned work?				
Has the team completed all of the deliverables?				
Has all outstanding commitments for the team been resolved?				
Has the team reconciled the budget?				
Have all team costs been charged to the budget?				
Have remaining funds from the team grant budget been returned to the granting agency?				
Have final team project reports been prepared and distributed?				
Has the "client" (e.g., hospital unit or clinic managers) of the team project accepted the final results/product?				
Has the team made arrangements with the project stakeholders to transition the project for full implementation?				
If applicable, has a final report to the IRB and/or grant funders been submitted for the team?				
Has the team recognized and celebrated the work of the project?				

strategy to finish the work if resources cannot be obtained. If the team plans to work past the program end date, the sponsors of the program and other stakeholders will need to be involved in the decision, particularly if health care staff are paid for their work on the project, and given that faculty and students may have competing work preventing them from continuing on the team.

Mentors and team members need to guard against the tendency to rush to completion, thereby failing to solve problems thoroughly or carefully. Monitoring of the final wrap-up plan requires daily supervision from mentors and program coordinators and from other team member leaders and those team members assigned key wrap-up tasks. There may be a need to schedule additional ad hoc team meetings to solve problems and communicate about progress made on the wrap-up plan. Teams that are comfortable with communication technologies will find it easier to schedule these ad hoc meetings.

RECONCILING BUDGETS

How the team project was funded will determine who has the lead responsibility for reconciling the project budget. Some projects are funded through one or both sponsoring organizations and may be assigned to an existing department budget or a new organizational budget account. In these instances, the program coordinators may be the budget managers when funding occurs as a single budget inclusive of all the project expenses of all the teams and

TABLE 14-2				
PROGRAM TASK WRAP-UP				
PROGRAM WRAP-UP QUESTIONS	**PERSON RESPONSIBLE**	**ADDITIONAL RESOURCES NEEDED**	**DATE TO BE COMPLETED**	**ACTUAL DATE COMPLETED**
Have all activities in the program been completed?				
Have mentors completed all of their assigned work?				
Have all outstanding commitments for the program been resolved?				
Have all of the deliverables of the program been completed?				
Have all of the data from the program outcome measures been gathered and analyzed?				
Have the grant/organizational budgets of the program been reconciled?				
Have all costs been charged to the program budget?				
Have remaining funds from the program grant budget been returned to the granting agency?				
Have program coordinators and mentors documented lessons learned?				
Has a final program project report been prepared and distributed?				
If applicable, has a final report for the evaluation of the program been submitted to the IRB and/or to grant funders?				
Has the program sponsors accepted the results/recommendations of the program evaluation?				
Has the program recognized and celebrated the efforts of all team members, mentors, and staff?				
Have both partner organizations met their agreements in the Memorandum of Understanding?				

of the entire program. In this situation, a team member or the mentor should assume the project budget liaison role to work with the program coordinators on managing the specific expenses of the project.

In terms of grant-funded projects, the principal investigator (PI) identified in the grant is responsible for submitting final financial reports, as well as for turning in final expense requests to meet the terms of the award. Typically, the PI has to work with the appropriate organizational office charged to manage grant awards, such as an office of sponsored research. These sponsored program offices have budget reconciliation procedures the PI must follow, including submission of a checklist similar to the one in Table 14-3.

TABLE 14-3

GRANT BUDGET RECONCILIATION CHECKLIST

BUDGET RECONCILIATION CHECKLIST	DATE COMPLETED	NOTES
Meet with Office of Sponsored Programs for final budget meeting 1 to 3 months prior to project completion.		
Contact grant funder to receive approval for any budget line item adjustments.		
Plan final allowable purchases prior to grant ending date, unless permission received from funder to extend the grant time line.		
Submit request to funder if project meets requirements for cost extensions (additional money over a given time period).		
Submit all final receipts for payment and determine that wages are being paid appropriately.		
Set final date for budget close out and last date for expenditures and adjustments.		
Check with sponsored program office for achievement of zero balance or make arrangements with funder to return remaining balance.		
Work with Human Resources to ensure payment of personnel ends with budget close-out.		
Work with appropriate offices to close-out copying or document services codes, organizational credit cards, etc.		

ENSURING SUSTAINABILITY OF THE PRACTICE CHANGE

According to the Iowa model (see Chapter 1, Figure 1-2) (Titler et al., 2001), the team along with the appropriate stakeholders have arrived at a critical decision point when an EBP change pilot is completed. After a practice change pilot, the team members and relevant stakeholders answer the following questions in order to make the appropriate decision (Dearholt & Dang, 2012):

- Do the team members recommend implementing the pilot interventions or products into practice as a permanent change for the site of the pilot within the health care organization (*maintaining the change*)?
- Do the team members recommend extending the pilot interventions or products beyond the original site to the rest of the health care organization (*extending the change*)? And if so, when (*timing of the change*)?

- Do the team members recommend ending the pilot project because of insignificant statistical and clinical findings, as well as recommend ways to ensure that quality of care is continually monitored and new knowledge is examined as it becomes available (*stopping the change*)?
- Do the team members recommend redesign of the change pilot for retesting on the same or another unit of the health care organization (*redesigning the change*)?

Team members should discuss with stakeholders the process and criteria they will use to make decisions regarding next steps after EBP practice change pilot completion (Stetler, 2001). Decision-making criteria may include the statistical and clinical significance (effect size and confidence intervals) of the findings, the degree that project goals were met, staff and patient feedback, cost of the intervention or change, patient satisfaction and outcomes, and acceptability and usability of the intervention (Owen, Glanz, Sallis, & Kelder, 2006).

If the team and its stakeholders decide the practice change should be fully implemented, whether system-wide or within a particular unit of the organization, the team members will need to work with the health care organization to begin the process within a proposed time period of assuring the practice change is implemented and is sustainable. As you learned in Chapter 12, sustainability of the intervention is part of the implementation plan. When wrapping up the project, the interprofessional team revisits the sustainability plan originally developed throughout implementation of the intervention, ensures that identified actions were implemented, and identifies if more is needed and further planning is required. To foster the sustainability phase of implementation, the team and the health care organizational stakeholders consider strategies to address the common factors contributing to poor sustainability of a practice change (Doyle et al., 2013; Doyle & Bennett, 2014; Gitlin, 2013; South, 2004; Virani, Lemieux-Charles, Davis, & Berta, 2009). The following lists those factors addressed in the implementation plan that if not also revisited in the wrap-up plan may degrade a practice change over time:

- Adequate time and the most appropriate methods for teaching the practice change to all staff involved

- Identification of facilitators for and removal of barriers to implementing the practice change

- Supportive work flow processes that promote habitual use in practice

- Available supplies and equipment

- Leadership support given through supervision and recognition

Another way to think about the sustainability phase of a practice change is to determine strategies to embed the new practice within the institutional memory of the organization (Virani et al., 2009). The team should consider where the information about the practice change is stored and who will need to access this stored information. Policies and procedures may need writing along with training manuals and self-paced training programs to be housed within the health care organization's learning platform (Melnyk, 2012). Physician order sets may need revision to ensure the practice change becomes routine. Documentation fields in the electronic health record also provide cues to implement the new practice. Practice huddles with practice change champions or dialogues with peers (Maas et al., 2015) prompt discussions about the practice change and promote problem solving for smoother implementation. Leaders will need to consider adding the practice change as an expectation for employee evaluation and performance review. Consideration of recognition for early practice change adopters should occur. Refresher and booster training sessions may be needed periodically to prevent staff from reverting back to previous practices. Providing staff, including physicians, with information about patient outcome improvements is a highly effective reminder about why the change is important to patients, to the practices of physicians and other providers, and to the health care organization.

The interprofessional EBP team will not have time and may not have the authority to ensure that all these factors are addressed with the sustainability phase of their recommended practice change implementation plan, particularly if the change is targeted as a system-wide change because of the successful pilot. However, the interprofessional team likely developed many sustainability strategies as a part of implementation of the practice change during the pilot (see Chapter 12). It is important for the team to work with key practice and leadership groups, such as clinical practice committees, quality improvement committees, the medical department, educators, and other relevant departmental leaders, such as pharmacy, the emergency department, laboratory and imaging, informatics and information technology, admissions, rehabilitation, respiratory therapy, homecare, and purchasing. The goal is to ensure these committee members receive all the training materials, proposed policies and procedures, and information about needed equipment and supplies and their cost. In some health care organizations, there may be a specific organizational structure to manage system-wide practice changes, such as a project management office or a quality improvement office (Stevens et al., 2015). In this situation where the responsibility for leading the practice change is clear, the sustainability phase of the implementation plan may be somewhat easier to manage given the infrastructure and experience of such an office within an organization.

Chapter 15 discusses internal dissemination of the practice change results as an important process to promote the sustainability phase of the implementation plan. Because the interprofessional EBP team developed detailed plans to implement the practice change within a single unit, clinic, or department, these implementation plans are a valuable resource to practice and leadership committee members. Because of the pilot, the interprofessional EBP team will be able to report other needed strategies that would improve translation into practice. Perhaps they learned that rounding regularly with staff members who are implementing the practice change would be helpful for a prescribed period of time. Health care organizational staff on the interprofessional EBP team should consider volunteering to serve as practice change champions, offering to provide ongoing training and coaching as the system adopts, implements, and sustains the change.

FINAL EVALUATION

The final evaluation for the program includes determination of lessons learned in order to improve future interprofessional EBP programs and the team project experience. There is a need to determine the effect of the program on advancing the interprofessional competencies and on stimulating positive beliefs of team members and mentors related to teams and to interprofessional EBP. Each team and its mentor will want to schedule time for a lessons learned session. Program coordinators will want to set aside time for post-testing with the survey tools, such as those originally described in Chapter 1.

Lessons Learned

Mentors should lead a discussion session near the end of the project with their team members about the lessons learned as a part of carrying out the project from start to finish (Thurston & King, 2004). The program coordinators need to lead a similar discussion with the mentors, and the program coordinators should also engage in a separate discussion among themselves. Lessons-learned dialogues should start with team members, then mentors, and should end with program coordinators. This discussion sequence helps compile the lessons learned in a more thorough way with one discussion session building upon another. A lessons-learned session could be done with all the program's teams simultaneously in such a way that dialogue from one team triggers identification of lessons learned of another team. It is important for the mentors and the program coordinators to note the differences in lessons learned that also occur among the teams. Each team functioned differently, and consequently the lessons learned should reflect these unique team experiences as well. Here are some examples of team, mentor, and program coordinator questions to stimulate these lessons learned discussions.

Team Discussion

- What did we learn about the interprofessional EBP question formation, literature search, and appraisal and synthesis processes that if we had it to do over again, we would change what we did?
- What did we learn about the interprofessional EBP project design, implementation, and evaluation processes that if we had it to do over again, we would change what we did?
- What tools and resources would have made our interprofessional EBP project easier to design, implement, and complete?
- What preparation for interprofessional EBP and implementation science tasks would have enabled team members to perform more effectively and efficiently?
- Were there preventable surprises for which we were unprepared as team members that mentors and program coordinators should address?
- What valuable lessons did we learn that would help the health care organization sustain the practice change?

- What did we learn about interprofessional EBP and what do teams need to know more about regarding highly effective teams?
- What did we learn about the cultures of the two organizations that hindered and facilitated the work of the team?

Mentor Discussion

- How might I have been better prepared for interprofessional EBP in order to mentor my team?
- What would have helped me improve my mentor techniques in order to assist my team in problem solving?
- What mentor supports from the program coordinators would have increased my effectiveness and efficiency as a mentor?
- What tools and resources should have been available to me in order to mentor my team through the interprofessional EBP and implementation science processes?
- Were there preventable surprises for which I was unprepared as a mentor that program coordinators should address?
- What did I need to help the organization create ways to widely implement and sustain the practice change?
- What did I learn about interprofessional EBP and what do mentors need to know more about regarding highly effective teams?
- What did I learn about the cultures of the two organizations that hindered and facilitated the mentoring of the team?

Program Coordinator Discussion

- How might I have been better prepared for interprofessional EBP and implementation science in order to mentor the mentors and team members?
- How might I have improved my use of mentor supports with the mentors and team members?
- What tools and resources should have been available to me from the program sponsors to run the program more efficiently and effectively?
- How would changing the design of the program better support the mentors and the teams?
- Were there preventable surprises for which I was unprepared as a program coordinator that program sponsors should address?
- Were there preventable surprises the program sponsors experienced that program coordinators should address?

- What did we need from the program sponsors to assist in widespread practice change adoption and sustainability?

- What did we learn about interprofessional EBP and what do program coordinators need to know more about regarding highly effective teams?

- What did we learn about the cultures of the two organizations that hindered and facilitated the mentor supports of the team?

Results from the lessons learned discussions should be shared with the program sponsors and should be incorporated into the program design adjustments prior to offering the program to another cohort of health care organizational staff and university faculty and students (Moyers, Finch Guthrie, Swan, & Sathe, 2014). For instance, Moyers et al. learned that the educational sessions needed to be carefully timed with the work progression of the teams, educational sessions needed to include additional information on project management for implementation and on dissemination, selection of students should be partially based upon having at least 1 year of availability to the program and upon ability to use the interprofessional EBP project work as assignments within their coursework, and 6-month interprofessional EBP projects were not effective in terms of impacting the health care organization's ability to implement the recommendation. Typical program design changes include the following:

- Adding, deleting, and modifying interprofessional EBP education sessions

- Modifying the timing of program activities to better accommodate learning

- Shortening or lengthening the program

- Establishing methods for focusing projects earlier and faster

- Adding, deleting, and modifying the use of communication technologies

- Changing the program evaluation plan

- Increasing or decreasing the program budget

- Changing team member recruitment strategies

- Communicating more clearly the team member expectations prior to participation

- Adding, deleting, or modifying mentor training processes

- Developing additional team interprofessional EBP and implementation science tools

- Preparing strategies to better assist the teams and mentors address the issues of practice change sustainability

Program Outcomes

Program coordinators should have selected measurement tools prior to the conclusion of the program to enable pre- and post-testing of specific learning outcomes (see Chapter 1). Table 14-4 provides a method for comparing results. The measures listed in the table were used in the program evaluation of an interprofessional EBP program involving North Memorial Medical Center in Robbinsdale, Minnesota, and St. Catherine University, St. Paul, Minnesota (Moyers et al., 2014). Moyers et al. found that there were significant positive changes in the terminology subscale of the Evidence-Based Practice Profile (McEvoy, Williams, & Olds, 2010), but no change in the Evidence-Based Practice Belief Scale (Melnyk, Fineout-Overholt, & Mays, 2008) as the interprofessional EBP program participants seemed to have entered the program with strong beliefs. There were also significant positive changes on the Attitudes Toward Interprofessional Teamwork and Education Scale (Curran, Sharpe, & Forristall, 2007). In addition to these quantitative approaches, the program coordinators may want to use qualitative methods to analyze data from the program coordinator and mentor field notes to explicate key program themes.

Some programs include in their budgets money for an outside program evaluator. The program evaluator may conduct team member individual and group interviews, along with interviews of mentors, program coordinators, and sponsors. Regardless of the program evaluation plan, the need will be to ensure full participation of everyone from the interprofessional EBP program in the evaluation processes. Participation in the interprofessional EBP program evaluation is often complicated when team members end their involvement early. Program coordinators will want to ensure the team members who leave early have an opportunity to give program feedback for the portion of the program in which they participated.

Interprofessional Evidence-Based Practice Program Sustainability

The program coordinators should always be considering issues of sustainability of the interprofessional EBP program in terms of the viewpoints of both sponsoring organizations. Programs are more likely to continue when taking the following actions:

- Addressing attrition of key team members during program implementation, such as obtaining a new mentor when the previous mentor leaves the program prematurely

- Adding and training new program coordinators as the program expands or prior to expected transitions

TABLE 14-4

PROGRAM OUTCOME MEASUREMENT

INSTRUMENT	REFERENCE	PRE-PROGRAM RESULTS	POST-PROGRAM RESULTS	INTERPRE-TATION
Terminology subscale from the *Evidence-Based Practice Profile*	McEvoy et al., 2010			
The Evidence-Based Practice Belief Scale	Melnyk et al., 2008			
The Attitudes Toward Interprofessional Teamwork and Education Scale, faculty and student versions. Two subscales: Attitudes Toward Interprofessional Health Care Teams and The Attitudes Toward Interprofessional Education	Curran et al., 2007; Curran, Sharpe, Forristall, & Flynn, 2008			
Frequencies of grants obtained, papers submitted for publication, number of papers published, numbers of juried presentations, and number of products developed.	Moyers et al., 2014	Not applicable		
Course Evaluations of Educational Sessions	Typically developed within the program	Not applicable		
Attendance of Participants		Not applicable		
Field Notes	See Chapter 3 for form	Not applicable		
Team Member Interviews		Not applicable		

- Building a cadre of clinical scholars or EBP fellows and encouraging them to volunteer in future programs as mentors (Melnyk, Fineout-Overholt, Giggleman, & Cruz, 2010)

- Keeping previous interprofessional EBP team members updated about new project opportunities and program roles, such as asking previous team members to share their experience as a part of new team member recruitment

- Consistently collecting interprofessional EBP program outcomes to demonstrate the effect and benefits of the program, particularly tracking grants obtained and their amounts, numbers of publications and presentations, types of practice change products developed, and impact of the practice change on patient outcomes and satisfaction scores (Moyers et al., 2014)

- Conducting long-term follow-up with students and staff to determine how the program has influenced

their engagement in EBP and implementation science, as well as to determine the effect on seeking higher graduate degrees

- Informing new organizational leaders on both sides of the partnership about the program and its outcomes

- Developing more permanent systems and infrastructure for the program on both sides of the partnerships, such as improved access to EBP resources, including databases

- Embedding the program EBP tasks as coursework for students within relevant university courses and graduate student projects, and developing an associated honors program for undergraduate health profession students recognizing their participation in the interprofessional EBP program (Zeegers & Barron, 2009)

- Identifying resource needs prior to each interprofessional EBP program launch to determine how available funding supports program design and

TABLE 14-5	
FINAL PROJECT/PROGRAM REPORT	
PROJECT REPORT	**PROGRAM REPORT**
An overview of the project	An overview of the program
A summary of results as compared to the project goals and objectives, and study questions or hypotheses	A summary of accomplishments as compared to the program goals and objectives
Final financial accounting with a narrative discussing any budget variances	Summary of program evaluation results and interpretation
Recommendations for project implementation throughout health care organization if applicable	Final financial accounting with a narrative discussing any budget variances
Issues of the project that require further work or resolution	Issues of the program that require further work or resolution
Recommendations for practice change sustainability	Recommendations for program revisions
Special acknowledgement of team members	Special acknowledgement of team members and mentors

planned program outcomes, thereby ensuring the expectations of program sponsors are realistic given the proposed budget

- Regularly reviewing the partnership contract to identify changes in roles and responsibilities and any other issues the organizations wish to address, such as pending organizational changes that if not discussed might impact the program

FINAL REPORTS

Final reports of the project typically include those disseminated to the stakeholders, IRB, and grant funders. The program coordinators are responsible for creating reports for the program sponsors about the success of the program. Report forms are typically available from the IRB to which the project was submitted. Grant funders may also provide a final report form. If forms are not provided, Table 14-5 provides a sample of what should be included in either the project or the program final report.

CELEBRATION

Celebration of project success at the team level and at the program level should occur regularly as small wins happen and prior to program conclusion when project teams have met or surpassed their goals and objectives (Brown et al., 2010). Mentors should encourage teams to design their own final celebrations that are consistent with the team's culture and style of being together. Some teams will want to go to a restaurant, go to a team member's home for dinner, order

food for their final meeting, or award themselves with a special trip or team visit to a sporting event, movie, or theater. Mentors need to watch out for teams that do not want to celebrate, claiming they are too busy to take time for these fun activities. Celebrations are crucial for full closure and for promoting a sense of accomplishment. Consequently, mentors may have to enable a team celebration. Some teams may not have had a satisfactory experience and will not want to celebrate given their lack of success or dissatisfaction with each other. The mentor in this case should work with the program coordinator to engage the team in some type of reflection that at least highlights the small successes that were overlooked because of their negative viewpoints. In cases in which teams choose not to celebrate, the program recognition process becomes more important.

The interprofessional EBP program should include an ending event or ceremony for officially closing the program for the cohort. The organizational sponsors should be invited to the celebration where mentors and team members are recognized and are given a chance to speak about their experiences. Most team members also want to thank the sponsors for the opportunity they were given to participate. Special food, awards, and professional continuing education certificates can be provided at the event. Many organizations will want to designate each team member as an organizational interprofessional EBP fellow, scholar, or graduate so that the team member can include this designation on his or her curriculum vitae or resume. Mentors should also receive designation as an interprofessional EBP mentor or as an advanced interprofessional EBP fellow or scholar. Some program coordinators will create an event where the work of the teams is on display as posters or as a component in a special local conference for the communities of both organizations.

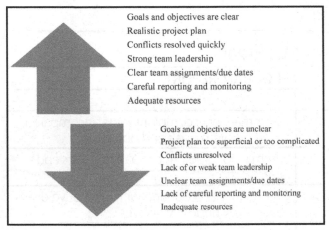

Goals and objectives are clear
Realistic project plan
Conflicts resolved quickly
Strong team leadership
Clear team assignments/due dates
Careful reporting and monitoring
Adequate resources

Goals and objectives are unclear
Project plan too superficial or too complicated
Conflicts unresolved
Lack of or weak team leadership
Unclear team assignments/due dates
Lack of careful reporting and monitoring
Inadequate resources

Figure 14-2. Project success factors.

MENTOR CHALLENGES

Mentors have to be aware of the characteristics of successful projects. Understanding these characteristics will help mentors increase the likelihood that the team meets or surpasses the goals and objectives of the interprofessional EBP project (Figure 14-2). The mentor's role along with support from the program coordinators is to prevent projects from missing deadlines, going over budget, using too many resources of the partnering organizations, or leaving the participants in the interprofessional EBP program and the project stakeholders unhappy with the experience and the outcomes of the projects. Projects with these types of outcomes usually signal poor project management. The goal is to complete the interprofessional EBP project on time and on budget as well as to meet the quality standards of the team, project stakeholders, and program sponsors (Crawford & Cabanis-Brewin, 2006).

MENTOR TECHNIQUES AND SUPPORTS

The main strategies for the team and mentors to use for successful project completion involves setting project goals, planning carefully to determine completion dates and to assign responsibility, and holding each other accountable for assigned work completed according to criteria and deadline. When projects are not carefully monitored to adjust budget and deadlines, the likelihood of having a successful outcome is diminished. The mentor must work with team members to keep them focused on tasks and to problem solve when deadlines are not met. Mentors should consult with program coordinators regarding needs for mentor supports often during this phase of the interprofessional EBP project. Teams approaching a hard and fast deadline often experience unexpected disruptions, which

lead to high anxiety about being able to finish. Project coordinators should have designated resources in reserve (e.g., avenues to obtain volunteers to help finish data collection or entering data into spread sheets), when possible, to address these last-minute problems.

Mentors may need to discern how faculty on the teams plan to help students finish their aspects of the project and to make sure the student meets the criteria for the respective health professions program from which the student might be receiving credit. Students should be expected to share the results of their work with the team and with the clinical scholar, such as when the student creates a separate poster for presentation to a class. Clinical scholars feel accountable for the results of their project idea and want to make sure students are representing the work to other students accurately and in a professional way. Faculty need to ensure the student work is truly representative of the students' contribution to the interprofessional EBP project.

Program coordinators should work with mentors to determine the best way to assess the team during wrap-up. How the mentors and their teams decide to use team performance assessments during the wrap-up phase depends on the team and communication assessment purposes (see Chapters 4 and 5). Routine assessment of team performance throughout the project is preferable; however, if the team has not engaged in assessment of its performance and the contribution of team members, wrap-up should introduce only certain types of team and communication assessments. In those situations where there has not been steady use of team assessments, team performance assessment during wrap-up should be focused on whether the interprofessional EBP project met the learning goals of the team and each team member, as well as on the positive performance of each team member.

It is difficult for team members to give and receive negative feedback from their team members during wrap-up when there has not been a history for the team to conduct team assessments. Wrap-up is a time when there are no longer ways to foster significant improvement in each member's contribution to the interprofessional EBP project, and more likely the team risks hard feelings as the team members finish the interprofessional EBP program if feedback is too focused on problem behaviors. If the team has been using these team assessments all along, the team members are familiar with the team and communication assessments and are used to receiving and responding to feedback about performance. As a result, team performance has the potential of getting even better during the wrap-up phase. The team assessments during wrap-up can build on previous team performance improvements and can focus on the task demands of wrap-up and the micro- and macro-contexts that support team performance during wrap-up. Positive project completion is more likely to occur as the function of the team's steady improvement throughout the experience as well as during wrap-up.

SUMMARY

In this chapter, the wrap-up process was delineated along with tools to ensure thorough completion of the projects and of the interprofessional EBP program. Wrap-up involves predetermined steps and is incorporated as a formal process of any project and of any interprofessional EBP program. The objective is to ensure that project and program reports are completed and that project stakeholders and funders as well as program sponsors are satisfied with the work. Excellent documentation of the project and of the program will ensure that the projects can transition to full implementation in the health care organization when indicated, or will enable the program to be properly revised and funded before additional cohorts experience the next offering of the program. Compilation of lessons learned guides the improvement of the interprofessional EBP processes and tools for future interprofessional EBP programs.

REFLECTION QUESTIONS

1. Think about how you will address the wrap-up issues of the EBP project and outline a plan.

2. Reflect about your level of participation in the interprofessional EBP project program and determine how you might improve your role as a team member, EBP scholar, or mentor during the wrap-up phase of the project.

REFERENCES

Baker, S., & Baker, K. (2000). *The complete idiot's guide to project management* (2nd ed.). Indianapolis, IN: Alpha Books.

Brown, J. B., Lewis, L., Ellis, K., Beckhoff, C., Stewart, M., Freeman, T., & Kasperski, M. J. (2010). Sustaining primary health care teams: What is needed? *Journal of Interprofessional Care, 24,* 463-465. doi:10.3109/13561820903417608

Crawford, J. K., & Cabanis-Brewin, J. (2006). *Optimizing human capital with a strategic project office.* Boca Raton, FL: Auerbach Publication.

Curran, V. R., Sharpe, D., & Forristall, J. (2007). Attitudes of health science faculty towards interprofessional teamwork and education. *Medical Education, 41,* 892-896. http://dx.doi.org/10.1111/j.1365-2923.2007.02823.x.

Curran, V. R., Sharpe, D., Forristall, J., & Flynn, K. (2008). Attitudes of health science students toward interprofessional teamwork and education. *Learning in Health and Social Care, 7,* 146-156. http://dx.doi.org/10.1111/j 1473-6861.2008.00184.x

Dearholt, S. L., & Dang, D. (2012*). Johns Hopkins nursing evidence-based practice: Model and guidelines* (2nd ed.)., Indianapolis, ID: Sigma Theta Tau International Honor Society of Nursing.

Doyle, C., Howe, C., Woodcock, T., Myron, R., Phekoo, K., McNicholas, C., ... Bell, D. (2013). Making change last: applying the NHS institute for innovation and improvement sustainability model to healthcare improvement. *Implementation Science, 8,* 1-10. doi:10.1186/1748-5908-8-127

Doyle, S. D., & Bennett, S. (2014). Feasibility and effect of a professional education workshop for occupational therapists' management of upper-limb poststroke sensory impairment. *American Journal of Occupational Therapy, 68,* e74-e83. http://dx.doi.org/10.5014/ajot.2014.009019

Gitlin, L. N. (2013). Introducing a new intervention: An overview of research phases and common challenges. *American Journal of Occupational Therapy, 67,* 177-184. http://dx.doi.org/10.5014/ajot.2013.006742

Maas, M. J. M., van der Wees, P. J., Braum, C., Koetsenruitjer, J., Heerkens, Y. F., van der Vleuten, C. P. M., & Nijhuis-van der Sanden. (2015). An innovative peer assessment approach to enhance guideline adherence in physical therapy: Single-masked, cluster-randomized controlled trial. *Physical Therapy, 95,* 600-612. doi:10.2522/ptj.20130469

McEvoy, M. P., Williams, M. T., & Olds, T. S. (2010). Development and psychometric testing of a trans-professional evidence-based practice profile questionnaire. *Medical Teacher, 32,* e373-e380. http://dx.doi.org/10.3109/0142159X.2010.494741.

Melnyk, B. M. (2012). Achieving a high-reliability organization through implementation of the ARCC model for systemwide sustainability of evidence-based practice. *Nursing Administration Quarterly, 36,* 127-135. doi:10.1097/NAQ.0b013e318249fb6a

Melnyk, B. M., Fineout-Overholt, E., Giggleman, M., & Cruz, R. (2010). Correlates among cognitive beliefs, EBP implementation, organizational culture, cohesion, and job satisfaction in evidence-based mentors from a community hospital system. *Nursing Outlook, 58,* 301-308. http://dx.doi.org/10.1016/j.outlook.2010.06.002.

Melnyk, B. M., Fineout-Overholt, E., & Mays, M. Z. (2008). The Evidence-Based Practice Beliefs and Implementation Scales: Psychometric properties of two new instruments. *Worldviews on Evidence-Based Nursing, 5,* 208-216.

Moyers, P. A., Finch Guthrie, P. L, Swan, A. R., & Sathe, L. A. (2014). Interprofessional evidence-based clinical scholar program: Learning to work together. *American Journal of Occupational Therapy, 68,* S23-S31. doi:10.5014/ajot.2014.012609

Owen, N., Glanz, K., Sallis, J.F., & Kelder, S.H. (2006). Evidence-based approaches to dissemination and diffusion of physical activity interventions. *American Journal of Preventative Medicine, 31*(4S), S35-S44.

Richman, L. (2006). *Improving your project management skills.* New York, NY: American Management Association.

Snyder, B. (2011). *Everything's a project. 70 lessons from successful project-driven organizations.* Centennial, CO: Rock Creek Publishing.

South, S. (2004). The 360° nature of change implementation and the essential three Ds for successful and sustainable change. *Clinical Leadership and Management Review, 18,* 107-111.

Stetler, C. B. (2001). Updating the Stetler model of research utilization to facilitate evidence-based practice. *Nursing Outlook, 49,* 272-279. doi:10.1067/mno.2001.120517

Stevens, J. M., Bise, C. G., McGee, J. C., Miller, D. L., Rockar Jr., P., & De litto, A. (2015). Evidence-based practice implementation: Case report of the evolution of a quality improvement program in a multi-center physical therapy organization. *Physical Therapy, 95,* 588-599. doi:10.2522/ptj.20130541

Thurston, N. E., & King, K. M. (2004). Implementing evidence-based practice: Walking the talk. *Applied Nursing Research, 17,* 239-247. doi:10.1016/j.apnr.2004.09.003

Titler, M.G. C., Steelman, V.J., Rakel, B. A., Budreau, G., Everett, L.Q., Buckwalter, K.C.,...Goode, C. (2001). The Iowa Model of evidence-based practice to promote quality care. *Critical Care Nursing Clinics of North America, 13*(4), 497-509.

Virani, T., Lemieux-Charles, L., Davis, D. A., & Berta, W. (2009). Sustaining change: Once evidence-based practices are transferred, what then? *Healthcare Quarterly, 12,* 89-96.

Zeegers, M., & Barron, D. (2009). Honours: A taken-for-granted pathway to research? *Higher Education, 57,* 567-575.

Disseminating the Interprofessional Evidence-Based Practice Project

Susan M. Hageness, DNP, RN, AHN-BC, CNE and Patricia L. Finch-Guthrie, PhD, RN

CHAPTER TOPICS

- Dissemination models and theories
- Developing a dissemination plan
- Identifying the dissemination audience and end users
- Selecting the right communication venue
- Mentor challenges
- Mentor techniques and mentor supports

PERFORMANCE OBJECTIVES

At the conclusion of this chapter, interprofessional team members will be able to do the following:

1. Create an effective dissemination plan for the evidence-based practice project.

2. Use strategies to identify and engage potential audiences and end users in learning about the evidence-based practice project findings and products.

3. Identify professional venues and apply effective strategies to disseminate successfully the evidence-based practice project findings and products.

Dissemination, which is part of the broader concept of translation science as outlined in Chapter 12, is the process of spreading information in a targeted manner about an effective intervention, program, or strategy with the purpose of increasing use to achieve a greater impact (Schillinger, 2010). Dissemination is different from the implementation phase of evidence-based practice (EBP) because the focus is on communication and dispersion of a practice change to the larger health care community. Like implementation, there is a growing science around dissemination. Dearing and Kee (2012) define dissemination science as "the study of how EBPs, programs, and policies can best be communicated to an inter-organizational societal sector of potential adopters and implementers to produce

Moyers, P. A., & Finch-Guthrie, P. L.
Interprofessional Evidence-Based Practice:
A Workbook for Health Professionals (pp 229-242).
© 2016 Taylor and Francis Group.

uptake and effective use" (p. 55). The goal of dissemination is to replicate positive outcomes in both similar and dissimilar settings, as well as to increase the potential impact of the change, or what may be referred to as *scaling up*. Milat, King, Bauman, and Redman (2012) identified that transferring an intervention outside of the original implementation site and conditions involves a change in scale in which suitability for dissemination is related to the intervention's potential effectiveness, efficiency, and cost savings. Overall, the goal is to benefit substantially more people than would occur without the dissemination process.

At one time, the narrow view of dissemination included primarily publishing research findings where the expectation was for practicing clinicians to automatically seek out this research and to initiate the recommendations. In addition, many researchers and clinicians have not viewed dissemination as their responsibility outside of possibly publishing their results (Kreuter, Casey, & Bernhardt, 2012). Unfortunately, publishing as the only method of dissemination does not lead to widespread use of innovations because of being a gradual and passive process for improving the quality of health care. Failure to spread innovations has had negative consequences. Studies indicate due to the lack of translating new findings into practice that a significant number of patients do not receive the recommended care, that care quality varies substantially, and that patients frequently receive unneeded care or care that increases the risk for harm (Grimshaw, Eccles, Lavis, Hill, & Squires, 2012; Grol, 2001; McGlynn et al., 2003).

Dissemination requires advanced planning that is action-oriented, especially since it takes approximately 17 years for 14% of original research to reach patient care (Balas & Boren, 2000; Green, Ottoson, Garcia, & Hiatt, 2009). Health care professionals and the general population should have unencumbered access to information about best practices. Thus, findings from EBP projects require wide dissemination for determining on a much larger scale the full effect that changing practice has on patient/family outcomes (Lavis, Ross, McLeod & Gildiner, 2003). Because implementation science is still relatively new, there is often not enough information about how to change practice effectively (Carney, 2000; Fixsen, Naoom, Blasé, Friedman, & Wallace, 2005). Dissemination about implementation methods for a practice change is just as critical for decreasing the research-to-practice delay, as is communicating the actual results or the effect the intervention had on patients. The purpose of this chapter is to describe dissemination and to identify effective dissemination strategies.

DISSEMINATION MODELS AND THEORIES

In the Iowa model of EBP (Titler & Everett, 2001) dissemination occurs after an organization has piloted a practice change with positive results and then adopted the change as a permanent part of care delivery. Dissemination links back to the beginning of the model because the new information from the practice change serves as knowledge-focused triggers (see Chapter 7) for others in the health care community to continue the EBP process (see Chapter 1, Figure 1-2). Peterson, McMahon, Farkas, and Howland (2005) argued that the scholarship of practice cycle ends when evidence from the EBP process further informs practice through the four strategies of exposure, experience, expertise, and embedding. These strategies differentially target consumers, practitioners, and researchers. Exposure strategies increase knowledge of all recipients of the message, experience strategies increase awareness and positive attitudes of all target groups, expertise strategies are knowledge utilization approaches to develop the competence of clinicians, and embedding strategies through institutionalizing knowledge for the practitioner increase daily use of an innovation.

In many dissemination models, such as the RE-AIM model (Gaglio & Glasgow, 2012; Glasgow, Vogt, & Boles, 1999), there is a connection between dissemination and implementation. Dissemination is from the perspective of the developer of the innovation pushing out the intervention, and implementation is from the perspective of the individual, organization, or community adopting the innovation. The elements of the model, representing each letter in the acronym RE-AIM, include asking how to *reach* the right people, ensure *effectiveness* or impact on health outcomes, promote *adoption* for all who may benefit, *implement* the intervention properly and successfully, and *maintain* long-term change. Those who are disseminating new practices facilitate the implementation process across organizations when making it easy for others to adopt and implement the new approach.

Two concepts consistent with the elements in the RE-AIM model are knowledge transfer and knowledge exchange. Knowledge transfer is imparting knowledge from those who create new knowledge to potential consumers and users (Pentland et al., 2011; Schillinger, 2010, p. 2). Knowledge transfer involves sharing knowledge that is relevant and easily accessible to the potential user. Successful knowledge transfer depends highly on the format and method for the transfer process. Critics of the concept of knowledge transfer identify the seemingly one-way nature of the process and point to an important basic understanding that those in practice determine whether to use an intervention, as well as determine the aspects of a new practice that meet their needs and preferences. Not all EBP interventions work equally well in every setting or are appropriate for widespread dissemination (Kreuter et al., 2012). In addition, during adoption and implementation, clinicians often change or develop an intervention further or morph the practice into something quite different from the original innovation. Some adaptations of the original intervention are positive and improve effectiveness while other changes render the

---

BOX 15-1. DISSEMINATION WORK PLAN—GUIDING QUESTIONS

1. **What is the dissemination strategy?** In terms of products, end users, dissemination partners, communication vehicles

2. **What actions are needed to implement the strategy?** Examples include writing articles, creating posters, presenting at local or national conferences/workshops

3. **What is the timeline for these actions?** Time lines related to publication deadlines, submission of presentation abstracts, meeting schedules

4. **Who will be responsible?** Decisions regarding the team members who will do the work, and the processes for guiding the work in order to meet project deadlines

5. **How will the dissemination strategy be evaluated for effectiveness?** Create an evaluation plan at the start of the dissemination planning process, review original project purpose/goals to ensure the effectiveness of the dissemination activities

6. **How will the team end the project dissemination phase?** Plan ways to celebrate the work and dissemination activities as a means to bring closure to project team members

---

intervention ineffective. A connection between producers and adopters is critical to the dissemination process. Often, researchers develop user networks to keep connected to those implementing the intervention and for identifying effective changes in the innovation.

Knowledge exchange in comparison is an iterative, two-way process between the producer and end user with a focus on collaboration to create a greater understanding of the practice environment and the opportunities for action (Pentland et al., 2011; Schillinger, 2010, p. 2). The concept of knowledge exchange guides the interprofessional team to not only submit the EBP project for publication, but also to use active strategies in facilitating potential end users to implement the change in practice. A primary goal for dissemination is to reduce the time between discovery and routine practice implementation through information, tools, and materials (e.g., intervention manuals, detailing action toolkits, pocket cards, patient teaching sheets, videos, workbooks, and protocols).

DEVELOPING A DISSEMINATION PLAN

The interprofessional EBP team starts to create a dissemination plan at the beginning of the project and continues to develop the plan as the EBP project progresses. Team members with a background in informatics, communication, patient education, organizational learning and staff development, business, social marketing, graphic design, and publishing enhance the work of dissemination. Carpenter, Nieva, Albaghal, and Sorra (2005) created a practical model for the Agency for Healthcare Research and Quality (AHRQ) for dissemination related to patient safety that is helpful in planning dissemination for all types of projects. The first element of the model is deciding what to disseminate, and as part of this decision, the team should consider the following:

- Findings that demonstrate the effectiveness or benefits of a unique and different approach to patient care

- Products the team developed
  - Practice guidelines and interprofessional team-based intervention protocols
  - Interprofessional education modules and toolkits about the new intervention
  - Survey instruments
  - Patient assessment instruments and education materials
  - Changes to the electronic health record that facilitate the new practice

- Interested groups that may want to learn more about the project findings or products

- Project findings or products that will significantly affect the organization or the larger community

- Perspectives of the disciplines involved on the interprofessional team about the most important aspects of the project to disseminate

Deciding exactly what project information to share is often challenging because team members may have differing views as to the most meaningful end-of-project findings and products. Revisiting the original EBP project goals and purpose assists the team in prioritizing the information to share. However, it is essential that the interprofessional team, when planning dissemination, take time to understand the behaviors, values, and beliefs of potential end users and the work context (Carpenter et al., 2005). The interprofessional team should consider whether the practice change saves time, streamlines work processes, and improves patient and family outcomes. Box 15-1 contains questions the team should consider during the initial dissemination planning stage.

An important outcome for the initial dissemination discussion is to identify strategies that create understanding and knowledge across disciplines and that support interprofessional collaboration and team-based practice. Unfortunately, dissemination of EBP interventions has almost exclusively involved single disciplines, which tends to hinder diffusion of innovation overall (Zwarenstein & Reeves, 2006). Dissemination should not only include physicians, nurse practitioners, and physician assistants, but all members of the health care team who may use or support the use of the intervention (e.g., physical, occupational, and respiratory therapists; dieticians; and social workers). Even though an intervention may seem specific to one or only several disciplines, other disciplines may inadvertently decrease the effectiveness of an intervention when using other interventions that interfere or negate the effects of the new practice. In addition, disciplines may need information regarding whom they should refer patients and families so that the discipline with the expertise to use the new intervention or care approach is involved in the case. Physicians and other providers often facilitate access as well as quality of care, and therefore may use an interprofessional protocol as part of their care orders. Thus, including them in the planning and providing these decision makers with evidence generated from the EBP project facilitates dissemination (Grimshaw et al., 2012).

Another factor to consider in the initial planning is the costs of dissemination compared to the available funding. The budget the team created when first developing an interprofessional EBP project should include dissemination expenses. In addition, when submitting for a grant, it is important to include dissemination costs as part of the overall project budget. Many funders are not just interested in the project, but they want to ensure results are widely shared with health care professionals, as well as with stakeholders (Glasgow et al., 2012). The health care and academic organizational partners for the interprofessional EBP program should also assist in providing support for dissemination activities. The program partners may have different resources to assist with dissemination efforts, such as covering costs for posters, travel to a conference, handouts, technology, and media support.

An evaluation strategy is a final element of an initial dissemination plan to determine the effectiveness of the team's dissemination efforts. Evaluation planning *at the start* of the dissemination process ensures continued success throughout the team's dissemination efforts. Dissemination outcomes involve both internal and external evidence that the process is successful. Organizational dissemination outcomes may include the approval of project guidelines as part of the organization's standards, incorporation of assessment processes into the electronic health record, the number of care areas within the organization adopting the new practice, and continued use of educational materials for patients and staff. External evidence for effective dissemination outside of the organization may include the number of presentations and published articles concerning various aspects of the project, requests from potential end users for information and access to project products, requests for consultation, or the number of actual end users adopting the practice change.

IDENTIFYING THE DISSEMINATION AUDIENCE AND END USERS

Once the team has identified the information from the project to disseminate, the next question about end users that the team should address is: Who wants to hear about the project? End users are both internal and external to the EBP project site (Carpenter et al., 2005). Information about potential end users assists with selecting specific audiences in which to communicate about the new practice, which is the second element of the model. The interprofessional team should use the connections each team member has as a way to identify and engage audiences with potential interest in the interprofessional EBP project. Various team members may want to disseminate different aspects of the EBP project; however, the target groups for dissemination primarily depend on the nature of the EBP project, the findings, and the implications (Grimshaw et al., 2012). For example, evidence that a current practice is harmful may require involving policy makers and health care leaders to assist with eliminating the practice, while evidence of an effective intervention may primarily entail an audience of practicing clinicians.

The third element in the AHRQ dissemination model is to identify organizations and networks that may serve as dissemination partners that will connect the interprofessional team to various audiences (Carpenter et al., 2005).

Potential dissemination partners include the following:

- Health care professionals
- Coworkers
- Health care consumer groups
- Research funders
- Care delivery organizations
- Professional organizations and groups
- Policy makers and insurance companies
- Regulatory agencies
- Industry and employers
- Student organizations and groups
- University partners, alumni, faculty, and interested stakeholders

When the team is determining the best potential audiences, they should consider multiple local, regional, national, or international audiences that would assist with the widespread dissemination of the intervention. A variety of audiences are interested in different aspects of EBP projects. One professional group may want specifics about the innovation and methods for implementing the change, whereas a second group may prefer information about the results and recommendations for further research. Education audiences may have an interest in the staff education process, materials, tools, and learning evaluations developed for the project. Additionally, providing information to potential consumers about the project's findings/products may promote widespread interest in the EBP project and possibly enhance adoption of the innovation earlier within and across practice settings. Differentiating several potential audiences allows the team to present multiple aspects of the project findings in various locations and venues, which serves to strengthen and enhance team dissemination efforts.

SELECTING THE RIGHT COMMUNICATION VENUE

Once the team has identified dissemination audiences, the next step is to communicate the message, which is the fourth element in the AHRQ dissemination model (Carpenter et al., 2005). A good question for the team to address is "What communication vehicles will effectively promote dissemination of the project findings and products?" In trying to address this question, the following sub-questions offer additional assistance in the decision-making process:

- What communication vehicles will assist the team in disseminating findings that connect with the needs of the target audience identified in the initial dissemination plan?

- What is the plan for distributing and marketing the new intervention that will reach the largest audience specific to the intervention?

- Are there preliminary findings or unanticipated project results and outcomes that require special communication vehicles and strategies?

- What is the best format in which to deliver the project's findings/products in order to engage the identified end users, project stakeholders, and funders?

- How does audience feedback following initial presentations assist the team in ensuring that future presentations reflect the information about the project the team wants to convey and about what the audience wants to hear?

Communication Venues

To identify communication venues, the interprofessional team should reflect on venues that fit the purpose, goals, and objectives of the project, the aspect of the project that is most important to disseminate, and approaches that align with various team members' expertise and experiences. Table 15-1 includes examples of possible communication venues, ranging from internal and external professional vehicles to social media. For example, one of the goals for the project more than likely includes improving care in a specific practice area within the health care organization. Thus, the dissemination plan would incorporate communicating project findings/products within the health care organization first, using internal communication venues such as newsletters and organizational websites and then eventually expanding dissemination to a broader audience through a variety of venues that include conference presentations and various forms of communication and publishing.

The interprofessional team, when planning dissemination strategies, should also consider how chosen audience(s) prefers to receive information. For example, O'Leary and Mhaolrúnaigh (2012) note that staff nurses prefer to receive information in the form of presentations from other nurses, clinical nurse specialists, practice development coordinators, as well as from other professionals. Staff nurses tend to use guidelines, protocols, the Internet, and books for practice information. Rehabilitation science professionals seem to prefer details on the methodology and results of an EBP project to better implement new findings into their clinical practice settings (Funabashi, Warren, & Kawchuk, 2012). Thus, dissemination to different groups of clinicians may need to take different forms.

The team also considers the funding agency or foundation sponsoring the project when planning dissemination activities (see Chapter 14). Funders are key dissemination partners, and if the team is unable to meet expectations of the funders or communicate the project findings effectively, these groups could withdraw their support, derailing the on-going dissemination efforts. Questions the team should consider when working with financial sponsors include the following:

- Does the sponsor have dissemination vehicles for projects they fund and do they have expectations about using them as part of the funding agreement? They may require publishing project results in their organization's journal, website, or Facebook page.

- If the funders do not require dissemination through their venues, can the team write about the project in the sponsor's newsletters or Web pages? Can the team present the project findings or products at the sponsor's professional conferences, workshops, or meetings?

In addition to using the project sponsor's communication venues, the team should use the informal communication channels within the health care organization and the university to disseminate the project findings or products.

TABLE 15-1	
COMMUNICATION VENUES	
PROFESSIONAL EXTERNAL VENUES	• Professional conferences, workshops, or meetings • Research and EBP journals • Education journals • Clinical practice journals • Quality improvement journals • Professional newsletters
PROFESSIONAL INTERNAL HEALTH CARE ORGANIZATION VENUES	• Organizational newsletters • Organizational face book pages and websites, emails • Online education and simulation platforms for the organization
PROFESSIONAL INTERNAL UNIVERSITY VENUES	• Newsletters and other university media • Web pages • Brown bag lunch presentations • Faculty and staff workshops
SOCIAL MEDIA AND MARKETING VENUES	• Newspapers • Press releases • Popular journals • Television or radio educational segments • Wikis, Twitter • Smartphone Applications • Toolkits

These informal communication networks are often the most effective and expedient ways to immediately disseminate project information. The interprofessional team should consider using the following communication venues in their dissemination efforts:

- Staff meetings, communication books, work emails, unit and organizational newsletters, and department meetings
- Presentations at the organization's committees appropriate for the project, such as clinical practice, quality, or leadership committees
- Student capstone presentations at the university
- Faculty meetings and development workshops
- University library online repositories

The interprofessional team should also consider using mass media to spread information about the project. For example, using a wiki platform (Brown et al., 2013), team member appearances on television or radio educational segments, or writing press releases for local or national media outlets are potentially effective methods to promote a new practice. These types of mass media communication formats can engage the general public, as well as health care professionals. Marketing the team's EBP project, while

a seemingly overwhelming process, is necessary in today's interconnected world. Krueter and Bernhardt (2009) identified that part of the reason for the research–practice gap is the absence of systems and infrastructure for marketing and distributing research and EBP results and products. While business identifies marketing as essential for bringing a new product from development to consumer use, in research and EBP, marketing and distribution functions are generally not assigned, emphasized, or funded appropriately. Lack of marketing support makes it difficult to ensure widespread adoption. Marketing involves transforming the EBP intervention to maximize use and creating polished, professional materials packaged in a manner that the end user expects to receive (Krueter et al., 2012, p. 2124). Marketing an intervention requires the interprofessional team to have clarity around the purpose, use, and individuals who should use the intervention. Some organizations have marketing departments. The interprofessional team should engage these departments in their dissemination activities when possible.

The interprofessional team should also consider using other nontraditional ways to disseminate project findings or products. For example, McGhagie and Webster (2009) suggest simulation scenarios, videos, and Web-based tutorials as additional methods to disseminate scholarly work

(p. 577). Moreover, with the burgeoning use of smartphones in both the private and public sectors, the interprofessional team may want to collaborate with application developers or technology departments to create apps based on the team's EBP project innovation. Additionally, the development and use of a toolkit is often an effective means to market the team's project innovation. An implementation toolkit is the packaging together of materials that when used together or separately facilitates the use of a new program, practice, project, or initiative (http://calswec.berkeley.edu/toolkits/implementation-toolkits). Toolkits often include definitional tools, engagement, and communication tools (e.g., pocket cards for clinicians, announcements, and posters), assessment instruments, planning tools, coaching and learning modules, step-by-step implementation or facilitator guides, evaluation tools, example policy and procedures, and funding or financial processes. The use of a toolkit can promote the EBP project findings/products to a larger audience and enhance a seamless adoption of the project's innovation within and external to the organization.

In addition, part of communication involves determining who the best messengers are for disseminating the results, which will depend on the focus of the communication and the target audience (Scullion, 2002). The source of the communication is often more influential in grabbing the attention of professionals than is the actual message. Professionals are more likely to pay attention to well-known and trusted sources within their discipline, thereby emphasizing the need to use a variety of professional communication mediums and lead authors from the interprofessional team. Messengers might also include a potential end user or consumer, a group, organization, or influential professionals not necessarily part of the interprofessional EBP team, such as a collaborating physician, physician group, health care leader, or researcher (American Geriatric Society, 2015; Grimshaw et al., 2012; Lovelace et al., 2015; Mosser & Begun, 2014; Schuette, 2015).

Publication

Often an initial communication strategy and venue for disseminating an EBP project on a large scale is through publishing (Adams, Farrington, & Cullen, 2012; Milner, 2014). Clinicians and practitioners often do not publish their EBP projects because of lack of experience, skills, and knowledge concerning publishing. In addition, clinicians and practitioners may not recognize the importance of their project and may underestimate the effect it may have on changing practice, improving patient outcomes, and developing other clinicians throughout the country or internationally. Faculty on the interprofessional EBP teams may serve as mentors for publishing and making the process less daunting. To promote dissemination, the interprofessional team should select journals that the majority of clinicians and leaders in the field to whom the intervention pertains will most likely read.

Before beginning the process of publishing, the interprofessional team should review the International Committee of Medical Journal Editors (ICMJE) (2013) standards for publishing, which indicate that all authors on a published EBP paper participated in the work of the project and contributed substantially to writing the article. In addition, according to the standards, authors take accountability for the integrity and content of the article and participate in providing final approval of the manuscript submitted to a journal. The first author has major responsibility for writing and editing the paper and is usually the individual who performed the central role in the project, such as the clinical scholar. However, various team members may take a lead role in publishing different aspects of the project. The lead author is also responsible to ensure that other team members serving as co-authors meet their responsibilities. Acknowledgements within the publication are good ways to recognize contributions of other team members when they do not meet the criteria for authorship. Box 15-2 outlines key considerations for publishing (Adams et al., 2012; ICMJE, 2013; Milner, 2014; Steefel & Saver, 2013).

Many journals now require authors to follow specific guidelines or standards about reported information depending on the type of research or evaluation method used for the EBP project. The need to follow a specific guideline is usually in the author materials that a journal provides. However, following the appropriate guideline when writing about an EBP project's findings regardless of the journal's expectation represents a best practice for transparent and non-biased reporting. Guidelines for "Enhancing the Quality and Transparency of Health Research," are located at www.equator-network.org/. The type of guidelines on that site includes the following:

- CONSORT guidelines for parallel group randomized controlled trials (Moher, Schultz, & Altman, 2001)

- PRISMA guidelines for systematic reviews and meta-analyses (Moher, Liberati, Tetzlaff, & Altman, 2009)

- SQUIRE guidelines for quality improvement in health care (Davidoff, Batalden, Stevens, Ogrinc, & Mooney, 2008; Ogrinc et al., 2008).

- STROBE guidelines for strengthening the reporting of observational studies in epidemiology (von Elm, Altman, Egger, Pocock, Gøtzsche, & Vandenbrouckef, for the STROBE Initiative, 2007).

- COREQ guidelines for qualitative research (Tong, Sainsbury, & Craig, 2007).

MENTOR CHALLENGES

Clinicians new to EBP may not see dissemination as their responsibility, understand the importance of the dissemination phase in EBP, or view dissemination as broadly as needed to ensure adoption of the practice change. As part of

BOX 15-2. PUBLISHING TIPS

- Identify interprofessional team author(s)
  - Include only team members who contributed *directly* to the EBP project.
  - Consider team members who are able to allocate time and effort for writing.
  - Decide if one team member will write the article or if several team members will write different sections of the article.
  - Determine first author, this is the team member who played a major role in the project and is assuming major responsibility for writing.
  - Identify order of co-authors listed after the primary author.
- Select a journal
  - Decide on the most important points and themes of the team's EBP project.
  - Determine the fit of the team project and the readership/audience of the journal.
  - Read/review articles published in selected journals to ensure fit.
- Contact the editor of the chosen journal.
  - Send a query email to the editor to see if the journal is interested in the team's project. Editor contact information is often listed on the journal's website.
  - Include in the query email a concise and engaging summary of the EBP project, why the journal's readers would be interested, significance of the project's findings, and the contributing team member(s) credentials.
- Organize, write, rewrite
  - Review the author guidelines *in detail* before beginning to write; these guidelines are often found in the front of the journal or on the journal's website.
  - Focus your article to fit with the chosen journal's readership and emphasis.
  - Create an outline to streamline and highlight the project information the team wants to convey in the article.
  - Create a process for writing and review, such as team work meetings.
  - Hold team members accountable in meeting writing deadlines.
  - Use plagiarism software to examine manuscript for similarities with other published works.
  - Recruit other professional peers/colleagues to review and edit the first draft, and make revisions to the article based on feedback.
- Submit the article
  - Follow the submission guidelines *exactly* (i.e., formatting guidelines, length requirements). These guidelines are listed in the journal and on the journal's website.
  - Acknowledge others who contributed to the EBP team project at the end of the article.
  - Obtain agreement for the final manuscript with those writing the article and permission from the health care organization to publish.
  - *Note:* it is a breach of publishing ethics to submit the same article, or parts of the same article, to several journals. After selecting a journal, submit to only that journal unless the article is not accepted.
- Review, revise, resubmit
  - After submission, the editor and/or other journal peer reviewers will review and edit the article. Rarely does a journal accept an article for publication with the first review, which is a normal process and should not be looked upon as a rejection
  - Revise the article as requested and resubmit to the journal for final publication.
  - If the article is rejected, review comments and feedback if provided, and revise to submit to another journal.
- Celebrate publishing success with the whole EBP project team!

the dissemination plan, each interprofessional team member should identify his or her desire, willingness, knowledge, and abilities to disseminate aspects of the EBP project internally to the health care organization and the university and externally to the health care community. However, two members essential for disseminating the EBP project internal to the health care organization are the mentor and clinical scholar. These two team members are often able to disseminate the project beyond the original practice area within the health care organization. Other interprofessional team members may end their involvement after completing the original project. Additionally, if the project's innovation becomes part of the new practice culture within the organization, the team must create a plan for ongoing staff education and implementation. The mentor, clinical scholar, staff from clinical practice committees or other organizational groups, and education experts within the health care organization may take the lead for further dissemination. Engaging others within the organization is essential for dissemination. These individuals are often in a position to take responsibility for educating staff and oversee expanding the project.

Team members unable to participate with further dissemination internal to the health care organization may still want to assist with external dissemination of the original work. However, the mentor ensures that team members who are not involved in dissemination still receive formal acknowledgement for their contributions when publishing and presenting the EBP project. A mentor challenge that may occur is preventing remaining team members carrying out the dissemination plan from feeling abandoned when other team members are no longer involved. After leaving the project, many members might continue to assist by providing feedback on manuscripts, abstracts, or professional presentations.

A possible hurdle to overcome in the dissemination process is waning team member motivation. Chapter 14 provides an overview of the issues that affect motivation when a project is wrapping up and includes mentor techniques and supports to enhance team member motivation from the beginning to the end of the project. It is important for the team to use some of these motivational techniques with each other to sustain the team's interest and engagement in the dissemination efforts.

MENTOR TECHNIQUES AND MENTOR SUPPORTS

In the dissemination phase of the EBP project, the mentor is coaching team members to create a feasible dissemination plan that matches the skills and interests of the interprofessional team, but most importantly matches the goals of the EBP project and sponsoring organizations. The mentor is also teaching team members who are

novices in the dissemination tasks how to complete each step. For those new to dissemination, the task of writing and communication about the EBP project could have a high task demand in the form of a large cognitive load. The mentor will need to break down the dissemination activities into manageable, concrete steps, making sure to match team experts with those team members new to the experience. The skill sets needed for developing a presentation and writing a publishable paper might fit better with the academic team members or organizational educators on the team, whereas developing a guideline, protocol, and patient education materials might fit better with practicing clinicians. The insights of student team members, as well as their school or community connections, are extremely helpful in identifying other dissemination audiences and communication venues. Student team members may not necessarily see themselves as capable of doing presentations or writing for publication, but encouraging their participation and involvement in dissemination activities is important for their professional development. Box 15-3 provides recommendations for ensuring the involvement of students in the dissemination of the interprofessional EBP project.

The mentor also assesses team members for their personal access to resources within their own networks that could help the team learn about writing professional publications, submitting content for presentation, and developing materials and products for dissemination. Mentors and program coordinators should connect the team to marketing, distribution, and information/communication specialists within their organizations who might assist with the use of social media and other mechanisms for disseminating information. If the mentor does not have knowledge and experience regarding dissemination strategies and faculty members on the team are unable to assist, the program coordinators will need to seek experts to bring to the team. Often program coordinators are able to provide publishing expertise through helping team members outline a proposed article or presentation, encouraging the team to assign members to each section of the work, and following up with the team regarding missed deadlines. The program coordinators may also want to provide editorial support or bring in others who would assist in making sure an article is well-written and follows the appropriate style of an identified journal (e.g., the university may have access to supports in the student writing center). The program coordinator may also have contacts with journal editors in order to help the team discern whether the EBP project is of interest to the journal or to professional organizations for presentation.

Ultimately, the program coordinators must monitor the output of the dissemination plans because often the success of the interprofessional EBP program is partially measured in terms of how the project affects the goals of the health care organization and the university. The university is interested in the learning outcomes for students (Box 15-4),

BOX 15-3. RECOMMENDATIONS FOR STUDENT INVOLVEMENT IN DISSEMINATION

Student Recommendations

- Do not be afraid to join discussions; students provide valuable input.
- Make time to participate fully on the team. This is an incredible chance to blend the knowledge and experience gained from both the academic and clinical settings.
- Students have insights and connections that other team members may not have and this adds value to the dissemination plan.

Faculty/Education Professionals Recommendations

- Give students an opportunity to discuss their role in the dissemination tasks, particularly those involved at the university or at local conferences involving their disciplines. Assist the student in determining the aspect of the project they would like to disseminate.
- Provide guidance about the possible time demands to help maximize the best match with different aspects of the dissemination.
- Find ways students can assist in smaller components of the dissemination or can work together, such as writing a small section of the article together.
- Look for ways students can use an EBP project dissemination task to achieve other educations goals or requirements.
- Strive to form collegial relationships and work from a position of equality rather than authority when working with students on dissemination activities. They often bring enthusiasm to the presentation, as well as may have creative ideas for ways to present or display information visually.

BOX 15-4. STUDENT PERSPECTIVE

Student Reflection (TD)

As a member of Pi Theta Epsilon, I was asked to join one of the Clinical Scholar programs as it supported the research component of this honor society. The opportunity to be involved in an interprofessional project in a clinical setting appealed because I could apply my newly learned skills in a hospital setting. As a student, I was fascinated, but a little overwhelmed, at the opportunity to implement strategies and pilot a project that I learned about in class. My interest grew as we divided into creation of surveys, training modules, and other project components. Subsequently, my confidence grew as I applied my EBP skills combined with my previous business and implementation proficiencies. I am grateful for the support, knowledge, and opportunities provided by the amazing interprofessional team on this project. Because of this chronic pain project, I plan to specialize in chronic pain when I graduate and I will continue to seek opportunities to support interprofessional research in a clinical practice setting.

Student Reflection (PG)

Sometimes you do what you "gotta" do, so you can do what you "wanna" do. I wanted to do a level II fieldwork experience in home care. Unexpectedly, our fieldwork coordinator contacted me to request my participation in an EBP project studying pain management. I couldn't get up the nerve to say "no," so I heard myself say "yes." I "wanna" do home care so I "gotta" do this evidence-based practice project...or so it seemed. Nevertheless, it proved worthwhile. My role in the project consisted mainly of searching the literature. I searched databases to determine when staff should refer a patient with chronic pain to a Chaplain and gathered information about the need for improved chronic pain management for the IRB application and for the introduction to the study. My other contributions included reading materials and offering input at biweekly meetings with our team. Overall, it was humbling to work with professionals and faculty with much more knowledge and experience than I had. At the same time, it provided me insight into the possibility of integrating EBP into my chosen profession.

the faculty involvement in educational and scholarship activities (Box 15-5), faculty and student involvement in community service, whether team members are interested in advancing their education, and the relationship with the health care organization and the grant funders. The health care organization is primarily interested in the

---

BOX 15-5. FACULTY PERSPECTIVE

Faculty Reflection (JF)

The clinical scholar program has been interesting and rewarding on many levels. We got several students and faculty interested in the program and others have been impressed by the commitment of our department and students in the process. These projects have given the opportunity for people from the other disciplines to get a greater understanding of occupational therapy and how it can contribute to patient care in acute settings. I have gained additional skills and expertise in EBP, knowledge of chronic pain, and research techniques. This experience has also been a great example of cooperation between IRB boards from a university and a health care organization to review the projects when they were ready. This experience gave me more insight into the different types of questions that different IRBs might look at, as well as an understanding of IRB work in acute care settings. Most rewarding has been the interaction with the two students who made significant contributions to the project, their commitment and enjoyment of what they did was evident. We have gone past the traditional student-teacher relationship and have moved into the realm of colleagues. This growth and development is always exciting to an educator and I anticipate productive and interesting careers for both of them.

BOX 15-6. TEAM SUPPORT OF SCHOLAR CASE EXAMPLE

The Clinical Scholar (S.K.) on our interprofessional project team had never written a scholarly paper much less presented at a national conference. She felt very uncomfortable and unprepared to disseminate the results of the team's EBP project. The team was able to guide and teach S. K. on how to create presentations and posters and present them effectively. Support and encouragement were tantamount in helping S. K. overcome her presentations fears. Eventually the team's EBP project was accepted for two poster presentations and a national conference workshop presentation, and S. K. co-presented magnificently!

The team's Clinical Scholar also presented the EBP project to co-workers and Medical Director on her patient care unit. The unit-specific presentation helped to effectively disseminate the EBP project findings and create excitement about the innovation as it was being implemented there.

For several team members, mentoring and partnering with the Clinical Scholar to professionally present our project findings was one of the most gratifying aspects of being involved in this interprofessional EBP project!

---

effect on patient care, reductions in costs of health care, and improvements in the patient care experience; however, they are also interested in the professional development of their clinicians. Clinicians benefit from the mentoring they receive and grow through opportunities to publish and present their work.

An important mentor technique is for the mentor to create opportunities for team members to mentor each other in dissemination activities. For example, team members with prior experience in writing for publication or presenting at conferences should mentor other members who may want to present the project but lack the experience or confidence to do so. Mentoring techniques of the mentor strengthen and enrich the dissemination efforts of the team. The following case example illustrates the importance of team support of the clinical scholar in dissemination of the work of the project (Box 15-6).

When teams do not engage in dissemination activities, the university and the health care organization may determine that the investments in the EBP program were unwarranted, which could affect future offerings. Part of honoring and celebrating the team's accomplishments is for team members to ensure they share the work professionally

and disseminate the project to promote widespread adoption. Box 15-7 provides a summary of the most critical dissemination actions.

SUMMARY

Dissemination of the work of the EBP project using principles of knowledge transfer and exchange is critical. Knowledge exchange is a two-way process between the providers of the new information and potential end users. Dissemination planning includes determining what to disseminate, identifying potential end users of the new practice, cultivating dissemination partners to facilitate the spread of the innovation, selecting the most appropriate communication strategies, and then evaluating the plan. Evaluating the effectiveness of identified actions and modifying the dissemination plan as needed is the best approach for keeping the process realistic, relevant, and successful. The interprofessional team needs to promote a shared attitude that dissemination is crucial to EBP and is something that the team can accomplish.

BOX 15-7. STRATEGIES FOR SUCCESSFUL DISSEMINATION

- Engage in significant project planning for start to finish sustaining the work through the last step of the EBP process, which is dissemination.
- Develop a doable dissemination plan and time line as part of the bigger project plan.
- Evaluate the dissemination plan frequently and modify it as needed.
- Clarify team members' roles and responsibilities in meeting dissemination deadlines.
- Hold each other accountable for completing dissemination tasks.
  - Mitigate team member burnout and disengagement by using motivational strategies to keep interest in the project alive.
  - Use the expertise and experience of each member of the interprofessional team.
  - Provide ongoing support for team members dissemination activities.
- Include communicating to important stakeholders as part of the dissemination plan.
  - Do not forget to disseminate the project findings/products to the organization's leadership team, funders and grant agencies, and those who might be affected by the practice change.
  - Create a plan for ongoing staff education if the innovation becomes part of the new practice culture—be sure to include your organization's education experts, as they are essential for training staff and overseeing expansion of the project's innovation once the original project is completed.
- Use a variety of dissemination venues and communication vehicles based on the goals and objectives of the project.
- Recognize team member's contributions when disseminating the work.
- The most important strategy is to disseminate the results and the products of the project. Not disseminating the work lessens the value of the interprofessional EBP team experience and adds to the research-practice gap.

REFLECTION QUESTIONS

1. How is dissemination different from implementation science?
2. How is the process of dissemination and implementation connected?
3. What are the steps necessary for widespread dissemination of a new practice?
4. What specific communication venues should an interprofessional team use to disseminate the findings and products from an EBP project?

REFERENCES

Adams, S., Farrington, M., & Cullen, L. (2012). Evidence into practice: Publishing an evidence-based practice project. *Journal of PeriAnesthesia Nursing, 27*(3), 193-202. doi: 10.1016/j.jopan.2012.03.004.

American Geriatrics Society (2015). Ten things physicians and patients should question. Choosing Wisely: An initiative of the ABIM Foundation. www.choosingwisely.org.

Balas, E. A., & Boren, S. A. (2000). Managing clinical knowledge for health care improvement. In J. Bemmel and A. McCray (Eds.), *Yearbook of Medical Informatics: Patient centered systems*. Stuttgart, Germany: Schattauer, 65-70.

Brown, T., Findlay, M., von Dincklage, J., Davidson, W., Hill, J., Isenring, E.,...Bauer, J. (2013). Using a wiki platform to promote guidelines internationally and maintain their currency: Evidence-based guidelines for the nutritional management of adult patients with head and neck cancer. *Journal of Human Nutrition and Dietetics, 26*(2), 182-190. doi:10.1111/jhn.12036

Carney, M. (2000). The development of a model to manage change: Reflection on a critical incident in a focus group setting. An innovative approach. *Journal of Nursing Management, 8(15)*, 265-272.

Carpenter, D., Nieva, V., Albaghal, T., & Sorra, J., (2005). Dissemination planning tool: Exhibit A. In K. Henniksen, J. B. Battles, E. S. Marks, & D. I. Lewin (Eds.), *Advances in Patient Safety: From Research to Implementation (Volume 4: Programs, Tools, and Products)*. Rockville, MD: Agency for Health Care Research and Quality (US).

Davidoff, F., Batalden, P., Stevens, D., Ogrinc, G., & Mooney, S. (2008). Publication guidelines for quality improvement in health care: Evolution of the SQUIRE project. *Quality and Safety in Health Care, 17*(Suppl. 1), i3-i9. doi:10.1136/qshc.2008.029066

Dearing, J. W., & Kee, K. F. (2012). Historical roots of dissemination and implementation science. In R. C. Brownson, G. A. Colditz, & E. K. Proctor (Eds.), *Dissemination and Implementation Research in Health*. New York, NY: Oxford University Press. doi:10.1093/acprof:oso/9780199751877.003.0003

Fixsen, D. L., Naoom, S. F., Blasé, K. A., Friedman, R. M. & Wallace, F. (2005). *Implementation research: A synthesis of the literature.* Tampa, Fl., University of South Florida, Louis de la Parte Florida Mental Health Institution, The National Implementation Research Network (FMHI Publication #231).

Funabashi, M., Warren, S., & Kawchuk, G. N. (2012). Knowledge exchange and knowledge translation in physical therapy and manual therapy fields: barriers, facilitators, and issues. *Physical Therapy Reviews, 17*(4), 227-233. doi: 10.1179/1743288x12y.0000000016

Gaglio, B. & Glasgow R. (2012). Evaluation approaches for dissemination and implementation research. In R. C. Brownson, G. A. Colditz, & E. K. Proctor (Eds.), *Dissemination and Implementation Research in Health: Translating Science to Practice.* New York, NY: Oxford University Press, 327-356. doi:10.1093/acprof:oso/9780199751877.003.0016

Glasgow, R. E., Vinson, C., Chambers, D., Khoury, M. J., Kaplan, R. M., & Hunter, C. (2012). National institutes of health approach to dissemination and implementation science: Current and future directions. *American Journal of Public Health, 102*(7), 1274-1281. doi:10.2105/ajph.2012.300755

Glasgow, R. E., Vogt, T. M., & Boles, S. M. (1999). Evaluating the public health impact of health promotion interventions: The RE-AIM framework. *American Journal of Public Health, 89*, 1322-1327.

Green, L. W., Ottoson, J. M., Garcia, C., & Hiatt, R. A. (2009). Diffusion theory and knowledge dissemination, utilization, and integration in public health. *Annual Review of Public Health, 30*, 151-174. doi:10.2105/ajph.89.9.1322

Grimshaw, J. M., Eccles, M. P., Lavis, J. N., Hill, S. J., & Squires, J. E. (2012). Knowledge translation of research findings. *Implementation science, 7*(1), 50. doi:10.1186/1748-5908-7-50.

Grol, R. (2001). Successes and failures in the implementation of evidence-based guidelines for clinical practice. *Medical Care, 39*(8), ll45-ll54.

International Committee of Medical Journal Editors. (2013). Recommendations for the conduct, reporting, editing and publication of scholarly work in medical journals. Retrieved at www.icmje.org/icmje-recommendations.pdf

Kreuter, M. W., & Bernhardt, J. M. (2009). Reframing the dissemination challenge: A marketing and distribution perspective. *American Journal of Public Health, 99*(12), 2123-2127. doi:10.2105/ajph.2008.155218.

Kreuter, M. W., Casey, C. M., & Bernhardt, J. M. (2012). Enhancing dissemination through marketing and distribution systems: A vision for public health. In R. C. Brownson, G. A. Colditz, & E. K. Proctor (Eds.), *Dissemination and Implementation Research in Health: Translation science to practice.* New York, NY: Oxford University Press. doi.10.1093/acprof:oso/9780199751877.001.0001.

Lavis, J., Ross, S., McLeod, C., & Gildiner, A. (2003). Measuring the impact of health research. *Journal of Health Services Research & Policy, 8*(3), 165-170.

Lovelace, K. A., Aronson, R. E., Rulison, K. L., Labban, J. D., Shah, G. H., & Smith, M. (2015). Laying the groundwork for evidence-based public health: Why some local health departments use more evidence-based decision-making practices than others. *American Journal of Public Health, 105*, S189-S197. doi:10.2105/ajph.2014.302306

McGaghie, W. C., & Webster, A. (2009). Scholarship, publications, and career advancement in health professions: AMEE Guide No. 43. *Medical Teacher, 31*, 574-590. doi:10.1080/01421590903050366

McGlynn, E. A., Asch, S. M., Adams, J., Keesey, J., Hicks, J., DeCristofaro, A., & Kerr, E. A. (2003). The quality of health care delivered to adults in the United States. *New England Journal of Medicine, 348*(26), 2635-2645. doi:10.1056/nejmsa022615

Milat, A. J., King, L., Bauman, A., & Redman, S. (2012). The concept of scalability: Increasing the scale and potential adoption of health promotion interventions into policy and practice. *Health Promotion International, 28*(3), 285-298. doi:10.1093/heapro/dar097

Milner, K. A. (2014). 10 steps from EBP project to publication. *Nursing, 44*(11), 53-56.

Moher, D., Liberati, A., Tetzlaff, J., & Altman, D. G. (2009). Preferred reporting items for systematic reviews and meta-analyses: The PRISMA statement. *PLOS Medicine, 6*(7), e1000097. doi:10.1371/journal.pmed.1000097

Moher, D., Schultz, K. F., & Altman, C. G. (2001). The CONSORT statement: Revised recommendations for improving the quality of reports of parallel group randomized trials. *The Lancelot 357*(9263), 1191-1194. doi:10.1016/s0140-6736(00)04337-3

Mosser, G., & Begun, J. W. (2014). *Understanding teamwork in health care.* New York, NY: McGraw-Hill Lange.

O'Leary, D. F., & Mhaolrúnaigh, S. N. (2011). Information seeking behavior of nurses: Where is information sought and what processes are followed? *Journal of Advanced Nursing, 68*(2), 379-390. doi:10.1111/j.1365-2648.2011.05750.x.

Ogrinc, G., Mooney, S. E., Estrada, C., Foster, T., Goldmann, D., Hall, L. W., … Watts, B. (2008). The SQUIRE (Standards for Quality Improvement Reporting Excellence) guidelines for quality improvement reporting: explanation and elaboration. *Quality and Safety in Healthcare, 17*(Suppl): i13-i32. doi:10.1136/qshc.2008.029058.

Pentland, D., Forsyth, K., Maciver, D., Walsh, M., Murray, R., Irvine, L., & Sikora, S. (2011). Key characteristics of knowledge transfer and exchange in healthcare: Integrative literature review. *Journal of Advanced Nursing, 67*(7), 1408-1425. doi:10.1111/j.1365-2648.2011.05631.x

Peterson, E. W., McMahon, E., Farkas, M., & Howland, J. (2005). Completing the cycle of scholarship of practice: A model for dissemination and utilization of evidence-based interventions. *Occupational Therapy in Health Care, 19*(1-2), 31-46. doi:10.1080/j003v19n01_04

Schillinger, D. (2010). An introduction to effectiveness, dissemination and implementation research. In P. Fleischer and E. Goldstein (Eds.), *UCSF Clinical and Translational Science Institute (CTSI) Resource Manuals and Guides to Community-Engaged Research.* Retrieved at https://accelerate.ucsf.edu/files/CE/edi_introguide.pdf.

Schuette, S. (2015). Implementing evidence-based practice throughout a large hospital system. *PT In Motion*, April, 26-32.

Scullion, P. A. (2002). Effective dissemination strategies. *Nurse Researcher, 10*(1), 65-77. doi:10.7748/nr2002.10.10.1.65.c5880

Steefel, L., & Saver, C., (2013). From capstone project to published article. *American Nurse Today, 8*(5), 1-3.

Titler, M. B., & Everett, L. Q. (2001). Translating research into practice: Considerations for critical care investigators. *Critical Care Nursing Clinics of North America, 13*(4), 587-604.

Tong, A., Sainsbury, P., & Craig, J. (2007). Consolidated criteria for reporting qualitative research (COREQ): a 32-item checklist for interviews and focus groups. *International Journal of Qualitative Health Care, 19*(6), 349-357. doi:10.1093/intqhc/mzm042

von Elm, E., Altman, D. G., Egger, M., Pocock, S. J., Gøtzsche, P. C., & Vandenbrouckef, J. P. (2007). The strengthening the reporting of observational studies in epidemiology (STROBE) statement: Guidelines for reporting observational studies. *Epidemiology 18*(6), 800-804. doi:10.1097/ede.0b013e3181577654.

Zwarenstein, M., & Reeves, S. (2006). Knowledge translation and interprofessional collaboration: Where the rubber of evidence-based care hits the road of teamwork. *Journal of Continuing Education in the Health Profession, 26*(1), 46-54. doi:10.1002/chp.50

Supplemental materials for this chapter are available online.
Please refer to the sticker in the front of the book and enter the access code provided.

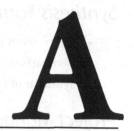

Material on Website

EVIDENCE-BASED PRACTICE EDUCATIONAL SESSIONS

- Chapter 1: Getting Started
- Chapter 2: Partnerships and Organizational Readiness
- Chapter 3: Deliberative and Reflective Mentoring
- Chapter 4: Interprofessional Teams and Clarifying Roles
- Chapter 5: Interprofessional Team Communication
- Chapter 6: Orienting
- Chapter 7: Figuring Out the PICO Question
- Chapter 8: Searching the Literature
- Chapter 9: Appraising the Literature
- Chapter 10: Designing
- Chapter 11: IRB and Grant Funding
- Chapter 12: Implementation Science
- Chapter 13: Evaluating and Analyzing
- Chapter 14: Wrapping Up
- Chapter 15: Disseminating

ONE-MINUTE MENTOR UPDATES

- Effective Problem Solving
- Roles and Responsibilities for Collaborative Practice

- Interprofessional Teams and Teamwork
- Interprofessional Communication
- Values and Ethics for Interprofessional Practice
- Providing Effective Feedback
- Facilitating as Successful Study/Common Challenges
- Time Management in Research/Common Challenges
- Sustaining Motivation & Empowering the Clinical Scholar
- Renewing the Spirit: Yes this is Part of Evidence-Based Practice
- Developing a Dissemination Plan for Your

FORMS FOR EVIDENCE-BASED PRACTICE

Team Forms

- Interprofessional Team Charter
- Field Note Form

Literature Documentation Forms

- Documentation of Database Search
- Documentation of Hand Search
- Documentation of Web Search
- Documentation of Website With Search Engine
- Inclusion/Exclusion Criteria

Moyers, P. A., & Finch-Guthrie, P. L.
*Interprofessional Evidence-Based Practice:
A Workbook for Health Professionals* (pp 243-244).
© 2016 Taylor and Francis Group.

Synthesis Forms

- Intervention Levels & Quality Synthesis
- Comparison of Interventions
- Synthesis of Outcomes

Project Management Forms

- Meeting Agenda
- Milestone Chart
- Gantt Chart

- Project Work Breakdown Structure
- Planning Grid for Project
- Estimating Costs
- Budget Control Chart

Project Implementation Forms

- Learning Planning Tool
- Stakeholder Analysis Tool
- Financial Disclosure

Financial Disclosures

Janet Benz has no financial or proprietary interest in the materials presented herein.

Dr. Mark Blegen has no financial or proprietary interest in the materials presented herein.

Dr. David D. Chapman has no financial or proprietary interest in the materials presented herein.

Therese Whalen Dlugosch has no financial or proprietary interest in the materials presented herein.

Dr. Patricia L. Finch-Guthrie was awarded a $10,000 grant for Mentoring Mentors in an Interprofessional Clinical Scholar Project by The Minnesota Nurses Association Foundation for Chapter 3: Developing Deliberative and Reflective Mentoring, by Penelope A. Moyers, EdD, OT/L, FAOTA, and Patricia L. Finch Guthrie, PhD, RN, St. Catherine University, St. Paul, Minnesota.

Dr. John D. Fleming has no financial or proprietary interest in the materials presented herein.

Susan M. Hageness has no financial or proprietary interest in the materials presented herein.

Dr. Vicky J. Larson has no financial or proprietary interest in the materials presented herein.

Dr. Penelope A. Moyers was awarded a $10,000 grant for Mentoring Mentors in an Interprofessional Clinical Scholar Project by The Minnesota Nurses Association Foundation for Chapter 3: Developing Deliberative and Reflective Mentoring, by Penelope A. Moyers, EdD, OT/L, FAOTA, and Patricia L. Finch Guthrie, PhD, RN, St. Catherine University, St. Paul, Minnesota.

Dr. VaLinda I. Pearson has no financial or proprietary interest in the materials presented herein.

Dr. Sue E. Sendelbach has no financial or proprietary interest in the materials presented herein.

Dr. Mary Fran Tracy has no financial or proprietary interest in the materials presented herein.

Index

Printed in the United States
by Baker & Taylor Publisher Services